CARDIOGENIC SHOCK

CONTEMPORARY CARDIOLOGY

CHRISTOPHER P. CANNON, MD
SERIES EDITOR

CARDIOGENIC SHOCK

Diagnosis and Treatment

Edited by

DAVID HASDAI, MD
Tel Aviv University, Tel Aviv, Israel

PETER B. BERGER, MD
Mayo Clinic, Rochester, MN

ALEXANDER BATTLER, MD
Tel Aviv University, Tel Aviv, Israel

DAVID R. HOLMES, JR., MD
Mayo Clinic, Rochester, MN

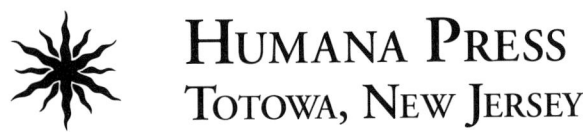

HUMANA PRESS
TOTOWA, NEW JERSEY

© 2002 Humana Press Inc.
999 Riverview Drive, Suite 208
Totowa, New Jersey 07512

humanapress.com

For additional copies, pricing for bulk purchases, and/or information about other Humana titles, contact Humana at the above address or at any of the following numbers: Tel.: 973-256-1699; Fax: 973-256-8341, E-mail: humana@humanapr.com; or visit our Website: http://humanapress.com

Due diligence has been taken by the publishers, editors, and authors of this book to assure the accuracy of the information published and to describe generally accepted practices. The contributors herein have carefully checked to ensure that the drug selections and dosages set forth in this text are accurate and in accord with the standards accepted at the time of publication. Notwithstanding, as new research, changes in government regulations, and knowledge from clinical experience relating to drug therapy and drug reactions constantly occurs, the reader is advised to check the product information provided by the manufacturer of each drug for any change in dosages or for additional warnings and contraindications. This is of utmost importance when the recommended drug herein is a new or infrequently used drug. It is the responsibility of the treating physician to determine dosages and treatment strategies for individual patients. Further it is the responsibility of the health care provider to ascertain the Food and Drug Administration status of each drug or device used in their clinical practice. The publisher, editors, and authors are not responsible for errors or omissions or for any consequences from the application of the information presented in this book and make no warranty, express or implied, with respect to the contents in this publication.

Cover design by Patricia F. Cleary.

This publication is printed on acid-free paper. ∞
ANSI Z39.48-1984 (American National Standards Institute) Permanence of Paper for Printed Library Materials.

Printed in the United States of America.   10 9 8 7 6 5 4 3 2 1

Library of Congress Cataloging-in-Publication Data

Cardiogenic shock : diagnosis and treatment / edited by David Hasdai ... [et al.]
        p;cm.--(Contemporary cardiology)
    Includes bibliographical references and index.
    ISBN 1-58829-025-5 (alk. paper)
    1. Cardiogenic shock. 2. Myocardial infarction--Complications. 3. Heart–Diseases–Complications. I. Hasdai, David. II. Contemporary cardiology (Totowa, N.J.:unnumbered)
    [DNLM: 1. Shock, Cardiogenic. 2. Heart Diseases–complications. WG 300 C26749 2002]
    RC685.C18 C37 2002
    616.1'2–dc21
                                                                    2001039902

PREFACE

Cardiogenic shock, whatever its precipitating cause, is a devastating event. As we have learned from years of clinical research, the mortality rate from shock is alarmingly high, reaching 90% in several series. Indeed, in many cardiac conditions such as myocardial infarction and myocarditis, cardiogenic shock is by far the major reason for death.

Best known as a complication of myocardial infarction, cardiogenic shock also occurs in patients with a wide variety of cardiac disorders, from congenital lesions in both child and adult, to valvular disease, to myocardial or pericardial disease, to mechanical injuries to the heart. The physical findings and imaging modalities used to diagnose these conditions vary, based upon etiology. Transport of the patient with cardiogenic shock to medical centers that deliver unique therapies is often challenging.

Therapies for cardiogenic shock include medical, percutaneous, and surgical procedures, temporary assist devices to allow the injured heart to recover, and artificial hearts to replace those beyond salvage. As newer advances in biotechnology, as well as laboratory work in genomics and proteomics and more traditional basic science, make it to the bedside, there will once again be reason to hope that more patients will survive cardiogenic shock with an acceptable quality of life.

We are honored that so many of the world's leading experts on the causes, consequences, and treatments of cardiogenic shock readily agreed to write chapters for this volume in their particular areas of expertise, and we are impressed by the depth and breadth of the chapters they have written. By bringing together all the various etiologies of cardiogenic shock in this single volume, we present the reader with a comprehensive overview of this dire condition, with emphasis on the unique diagnostic and therapeutic characteristics of each entity.

David Hasdai, MD
Peter B. Berger, MD
Alexander Battler, MD
David R. Holmes, Jr., MD

CONTENTS

Contributors

AHARON AVRAMOVICH, MD • *Department of Anesthesiology, Rabin Medical Center, Petah-Tikva, Israel, and Tel-Aviv University, Tel-Aviv, Israel*

ISRAEL M. BARBASH, MD • *Neufeld Cardiac Research Institute, Sheba Medical Center, Tel-Hashomer, Israel*

ERIC R. BATES, MD • *Division of Cardiology, Department of Internal Medicine, University of Michigan Medical Center, Ann Arbor, MI*

ALEXANDER BATTLER, MD • *Department of Cardiology, Rabin Medical Center, Petah-Tikva, Israel, and Tel-Aviv University, Tel-Aviv, Israel*

PETER B. BERGER, MD • *Internal Medicine and Cardiovascular Diseases, Mayo Clinic, Rochester, MN*

YOCHAI BIRNBAUM, MD • *The Division of Cardiology, University of Texas Medical Branch, Galveston, TX*

ELCHANAN BRUCKHEIMER, MBBS • *Schneider Children's Medical Center Israel, Petah-Tikva, Israel*

HAROLD M. BURKHART, MD • *Division of Cardiovascular Surgery, Mayo Clinic and Mayo Foundation, Rochester, MN*

DAVID G. CABLE • *Division of Cardiovascular Surgery, Mayo Clinic and Mayo Foundation, Rochester, MN*

HOWARD A. COHEN, MD • *Division of Cardiology, University of Pittsburgh Medical Center, Pittsburgh, PA*

JOSEPH A. DEARANI, MD • *Division of Cardiovascular Surgery, Mayo Clinic and Mayo Foundation, Rochester, MN*

DAVID J. DRISCOLL, MD • *Division of Pediatric Cardiology, Mayo Medical School and Foundation, Rochester, MN*

JOHN K. FRENCH, MB, PhD • *Division of Cardiology, Green Lane Hospital, Auckland, New Zealand*

DAVID HASDAI, MD • *Department of Cardiology, Rabin Medical Center, Petah-Tikva, Israel*

RAFAEL HIRSCH, MD • *Department of Cardiology, Rabin Medical Center, Petah-Tikva, Israel, and Tel-Aviv University, Tel-Aviv, Israel*

DAVID R. HOLMES, JR., MD • *Internal Medicine and Cardiovascular Diseases, Mayo Clinic, Rochester, MN*

BERNARD IUNG, MD • *Department of Cardiology, Bichat Hospital, Paris, France*

ROBERT A. KLONER, MD, PhD • *The Heart Institute, Good Samaritan Hospital, Department of Medicine, Keck School of Medicine of the University of Southern California, Los Angeles, CA*

JACOB LAVEE, MD • *Department of Cardiac Surgery, Sheba Medical Center, Tel Hashomer, Israel*

JONATHAN LEOR, MD • *Neufeld Cardiac Research Institute, Tel-Aviv University, Sheba Medical Center, Tel-Hashomer, Israel*

MICHAEL J. LIM, MD • *Division of Cardiology, Department of Internal Medicine, University of Michigan Medical Center, Ann Arbor, MI*

MARK J. LOWELL, MD • *Department of Emergency Medicine, University of Michigan Medical Center, Ann Arbor, MI*

AVIV MAGER, MD • *Department of Cardiology, Rabin Medical Center, Petah-Tikva, Israel, and Tel-Aviv University, Tel-Aviv, Israel*

SURESH R. MULUKUTLA, MD • *Division of Cardiology, University of Pittsburgh Medical Center, Pittsburgh, PA*

OLIVIER NALLET, MD • *Department of Cardiology, Bichat Hospital, Paris, France*

AMIRAM NIR, MD • *Division of Pediatric Cardiology, Hadassah University Hospital, Jerusalem, Israel*

JOHN J. PACELLA, MD • *Division of Cardiology, University of Pittsburgh Medical Center, Pittsburgh, PA*

EHUD RAANANI, MD • *Department of Cardiothoracic Surgery, Rabin Medical Center, Petah-Tikva, Israel, and Tel-Aviv University, Tel-Aviv, Israel*

AZARIA J. J. T. REIN, MD • *Division of Pediatric Cardiology, Hadassah University Hospital, Jerusalem, Israel*

ALEX SAGIE, MD • *Department of Cardiology, Rabin Medical Center, Petah-Tikva, Israel, and Tel-Aviv University, Tel-Aviv, Israel*

YARON SHAPIRA, MD • *Department of Cardiology, Rabin Medical Center, Petah-Tikva, Israel, and Tel-Aviv University, Tel-Aviv, Israel*

ROBERT J. SIEGEL, MD • *The Division of Cardiology, Cedars-Sinai Medical Center, UCLA School of Medicine, Los Angeles, CA*

LIP-BUN TAN, DPHIL, FRCP • *Yorkshire Heart Centre, Leeds General Infirmary, Leeds, UK*

BING HSIEAN TZENG, MD • *Division of Cardiology. Tri-Service General Hospital No. 325, Taipei, Taiwan, Republic of China*

ALEC VAHANIAN, MD • *Department of Cardiology, Bichat Hospital, Paris, France*

MORDEHAY VATURI, MD • *Department of Cardiology, Rabin Medical Center, Petah-Tikva, Israel*

BERNARDO A. VIDNE, MD • *Department of Cardiothoracic Surgery, Rabin Medical Center, Petah-Tikva, Israel, and Tel-Aviv University, Tel-Aviv, Israel*

KEVIN P. WALSH, MD • *Our Lady's Hospital for Sick Children, Dublin, Republic of Ireland*

HARVEY D. WHITE, DSC • *Division of Cardiology, Green Lane Hospital, Auckland, New Zealand*

SIMON G. WILLIAMS, MRCP • *Yorkshire Heart Centre, Leeds General Infirmary, Leeds, UK*

CHEUK-KIT WONG, MD • *Division of Cardiology, Green Lane Hospital, Auckland, New Zealand*

I INTRODUCTION

1

Cardiogenic Shock

Clinical Features

David Hasdai, MD

CONTENTS

Fails my heart, I know not how;
I can go no longer
James Mason Neale (1818–1866)

The gravity of cardiogenic shock may be understood through this simple statement. In this condition, the body can no longer go on functioning because of the failing heart. In contrast to Neale's statement, however, we have made major advances in our understanding about how and why this condition occurs. Moreover, although cardiogenic shock remains an ominous condition, there is a ray of hope that the better diagnostic and therapeutic modalities currently available will result in improved outcomes.

This chapter aims to define and characterize the clinical spectrum of cardiogenic shock.

CATEGORICAL DEFINITION

Cardiac Output

Cardiogenic shock has been defined as a state of tissue hypoxia caused by reduced systemic cardiac output in the presence of adequate intravascular volume *(1)*. This broad definition accounts for the great variability in the diagnosis of shock among different clinicians and investigators. For example, how much does systemic cardiac output need to be reduced to constitute a state of shock? In several series, cardiac index measurements of 2.2 L/min/m^2 or less were considered supportive of the diagnosis *(2–9)*. Others have considered measurements of only 1.8 L/min/m^2 or less to be indicative of cardiogenic shock *(10)*.

In addition to the boundaries of specific index measurements used, there may be variability in measuring methods. Currently, cardiac output is measured primarily

From: *Contemporary Cardiology: Cardiogenic Shock: Diagnosis and Treatment*
Edited by: David Hasdai et al. © Humana Press Inc., Totowa, NJ

using catheters placed in the pulmonary artery. This technique demands some expertise and carries certain, albeit minimal, risks *(11)*. It is, therefore, not universally used in patients with cardiogenic shock *(1)*. In cases where pulmonary artery catheterization is not used, cardiac output can only be estimated.

Tissue Hypoxia

Because there are no widespread bedside assays for tissue hypoxia, surrogate clinical and laboratory indices of tissue function that may reflect tissue hypoxia are sought. However, these indices may not be sensitive enough to identify accurately the gravity of tissue hypoxia, which may range from mild to severe. This problem is underscored among patients with antecedent cardiac disease that has already caused reduced cardiac output and tissue hypoperfusion. In these patients, any additional compromise of cardiac function may result in a disproportionate deterioration of the hemodynamic status resulting in shock, even if the reduction in systemic cardiac output was minimal.

Hypotension

Although systemic hypotension is essential to the diagnosis of the syndrome, the severity of hypotension defining shock varies. Commonly, the cut point for the systolic blood pressure is less than 90 mm Hg *(2–9)* or less than 80 mm Hg *(10,12,13)*. Some also consider the diagnosis of cardiogenic shock in patients with blood pressure measurements greater than 90 mm Hg if they require medications and support devices to maintain normal hemodynamic parameters. A patient may initially have signs associated with the clinical state of cardiogenic shock in the presence of systolic blood pressure measurements greater than 90 mm Hg *(9)*. Therefore, hypotension alone should not be the basis for the diagnosis in the absence of signs of peripheral hypoperfusion, nor should blood pressure measurements within the lower end of the normal range negate the diagnosis of shock in the appropriate clinical scenario.

The method used to measure blood pressure also deserves consideration. Brachial cuff pressure measurements are often inaccurate in states of shock. Arterial blood pressure is more accurately monitored using intra-arterial cannulas.

CLINICAL DEFINITION

The previous section underscored the difficulty of diagnosing cardiogenic shock based on numerical values alone; thus, cardiogenic shock is primarily diagnosed based on clinical findings. This diagnosis can be supported by measured hemodynamic values. Patients with long-standing heart failure frequently fall into the range of values that are used to define shock numerically, although they are clearly not in shock clinically. For cardiogenic shock to be diagnosed, any reduction in cardiac output must be accompanied by signs of hypoperfusion. The systemic signs of hypoperfusion that may be detected in cardiogenic shock include an altered mental state; cold, clammy skin; and oliguria.

As early as 1912, Herrick described the clinical features of cardiogenic shock in patients with severe coronary artery disease: a weak, rapid pulse; feeble cardiac tones; pulmonary rales; dyspnea; and cyanosis *(14)*. These signs are not always present, however. In the full-blown state of shock, some of the characteristic signs of shock are unequivocally evident. In the earlier phases of shock or in less severe circumstances, these signs may be more subtle. For example, a reduction in urine output or slight confusion may represent a state preceding shock. To complicate matters, in certain shock states, these signs are characteristically absent. For example, clear lung fields typically characterize shock resulting from cardiac tamponade or predominantly right ventricular dysfunction. The signs of shock may also be affected by chronic or current medical therapy. For example, a patient taking oral β-blockers on a chronic basis may not be tachycardic during shock, although the heart rate may be much more rapid than in the basal state. Therefore, it is important to evaluate these signs in the context of the specific clinical setting.

Additional systemic features may reflect the severity of shock. For example, prominent jugular venous distention in a patient with shock may indicate severely increased preload. Peripheral cyanosis may reflect reduced cardiac output and severely increased peripheral vascular resistance. These signs, however, are usually not specific to the various etiologies. For example, increased jugular venous distention may occur as a result of severe left ventricular dysfunction as well as right ventricular dysfunction.

FEATURES BASED ON ETIOLOGY

Systemic signs may be detected that shed light on the etiology of cardiogenic shock, but not on the severity of the condition. For example, cutaneous manifestations of infective endocarditis, murmurs of valvular diseases, or murmurs of intracardiac shunts may be readily appreciated during the physical exam. One should not forget, however, that a new cardiac condition could complicate an existing cardiac disease (e.g., myocardial infarction occurring in a patient with long-standing valvular heart disease).

DIFFERENTIAL DIAGNOSIS

The cardiac patient may also have concomitant noncardiac conditions or may be taking medications with the potential of adversely affecting the cardiovascular system. For example, in the elderly patient taking a long list of medications who presents with fever, severe hypotension, and confusion, and is also found to have cardiac dysfunction, it may be difficult to assess accurately the contribution of the cardiac dysfunction to the clinical scenario.

Several noncardiac conditions may cause a state that resembles cardiogenic shock. These conditions should be considered before making the diagnosis of cardiogenic shock. For example, pulmonary embolism can severely reduce cardiac output, with typical clinical features mimicking shock complicating right ventricular infarction such as jugular venous distention. Aortic dissection as a cause of shock often also poses a difficult diagnostic challenge; it can cause excruciating chest or back pain, mimicking the typical anginal pain of acute coronary syndromes. Noncardiac conditions such as aortic dissection can also involve the heart either initially or eventually. Aortic dissection, for example, can propagate retrogradely, causing acute aortic regurgitation or coronary artery dissection.

A thorough physical examination is therefore critical to diagnose cardiogenic shock, to understand the underlying mechanism for shock, and to exclude noncardiac reasons for shock. Moreover, findings easily derived from the physical exam are also of prognostic significance in shock patients *(2,4,6)*. Indeed, these findings may be more important than data derived from invasive and noninvasive imaging techniques.

In the following chapters, the unique clinical features, diagnostic findings, and outcomes for the different etiologies causing cardiogenic shock will be described in depth.

REFERENCES

1. Hasdai D, Topol EJ, Califf RM, Berger PB, Holmes DR Jr. Cardiogenic shock complicating acute coronary syndromes. Lancet 2000;356:749–756.
2. Hasdai D, Califf RM, Thompson TD, et al. Predictors of cardiogenic shock after thrombolytic therapy for acute myocardial infarction. J Am Coll Cardiol 2000;35:136–143.
3. Holmes DR Jr, Califf RM, Van de Werf F, et al. Differences in countries' use of resources and clinical outcome for patients with cardiogenic shock after myocardial infarction: results from the GUSTO trial. Lancet 1997;349:75–78.
4. Hasdai D, Holmes DR Jr, Califf RM, et al. Cardiogenic shock complicating acute myocardial infarction: Predictors of mortality. Am Heart J 1999;138:21–31.
5. Holmes DR Jr, Bates ER, Kleiman NS, et al. Contemporary reperfusion therapy for cardiogenic shock: the GUSTO-I trial experience. J Am Coll Cardiol 1995;26:668–674.
6. Hasdai D, Harrington RA, Hochman JS, et al. Platelet glycoprotein IIb/IIIa blockade and outcome of cardiogenic shock complicating acute coronary syndromes without persistent ST-segment elevation. J Am Coll Cardiol 2000;36:685–692.
7. Hasdai D, Holmes DR Jr, Topol EJ, et al. Frequency and clinical outcome of cardiogenic shock during acute myocardial infarction among patients receiving reteplase or alteplase: results from GUSTO III. Eur Heart J 1999;20:128–135.
8. Holmes DR Jr, Berger PB, Hochman JS, et al. Cardiogenic shock in patients with acute ischemic syndromes with and without ST-segment elevation. Circulation 1999;100:2067–2073.
9. Menon V, Slater JN, White HD, Sleeper LA, Cocke T, Hochman JS. Acute myocardial infarction controlled by systemic hypoperfusion without hypotension: report from the SHOCK trial registry. Am J Med 2000;108:374–380.
10. Antman EM, Braunwald E. Acute myocardial infarction. In: Braunwald E, ed. Heart Disease. A Textbook of Cardiovascular Medicine. 5th ed. WB Saunders, Philadelphia, pp. 1184–1288.
11. Connors AF Jr, Speroff T, Dawson NV, et al. The effectiveness of right heart catheterization in the initial care of critically ill patients. JAMA 1996;276:889–897.
12. Goldberg RJ, Gore JM, Alpert JS, et al. Cardiogenic shock after acute myocardial infarction-incidence and mortality from a community wide perspective 1975–1988. N Engl J Med 1991;325:1117 1122.
13. Goldberg RJ, Samad NA, Yarzebski J, Gurwitz J, Bigelow C, Gore JM. Temporal trends in cardiogenic shock complicating acute myocardial infarction. N Engl J Med 1999;340:1162–1168.
14. Herrick JB. Clinical features of sudden obstruction of the coronary arteries. JAMA 1912;39:2015–2020.

2

Cardiogenic Shock
Physiological and Biochemical Concepts

*Simon G. Williams, MRCP,
Bing Hsiean Tzeng, MD,
and Lip-Bun Tan, DPhil, FRCP, FESC*

INTRODUCTION

Because cardiogenic shock is the culmination of cumulative abnormalities in the heart and because it is associated with the most dire of prognoses, any attempt at its diagnosis and appropriate management demands a clear understanding of the pathophysiological processes involved in the individual patient. For example, treating cardiogenic shock with aggressive diuresis to reduce the central venous pressure when the shock is predominantly secondary to extensive right ventricular infarction may significantly reduce filling of the left ventricle, thereby further exacerbating the cardiogenic shock. Similarly, a misplaced attempt at alleviating the distress of severe dyspnea secondary to acute pulmonary edema by using large doses of morphine or diamorphine may result in marked respiratory depression and precipitate respiratory arrest or alternatively may reduce the arterial pressure so as to compromise the coronary perfusion further, worsening the cardiogenic shock. Erroneous concepts lead to erroneous treatment.

Above all else, it is worth remembering that during cardiogenic shock, the cardiac pump is performing in an unstable state. As a mechanical pump, the heart is unusual in that its performance is somewhat dependent on its own output. When the aortic pressure that it generates falls below the critical pressure for coronary perfusion (usually a mean pressure of about 60 mm Hg), left ventricular myocardium is at risk for

From: *Contemporary Cardiology: Cardiogenic Shock: Diagnosis and Treatment*
Edited by: David Hasdai et al. © Humana Press Inc., Totowa, NJ

ischemia, which can then further impair its pumping performance. Timely treatment should therefore be directed at interrupting the vicious cycle by maintaining the coronary perfusion pressure, thereby ensuring continued cardiac viability. Measures required may include urgent coronary revascularization to salvage threatened viable myocardium, mechanical circulatory support, control of bradyarrhythmia or tachyarrhythmia, removal and counteraction of negative inotropic effects, and correction of metabolic derangement.

PATHOPHYSIOLOGY OF CARDIOGENIC SHOCK

There is more information about the pathophysiology of cardiogenic shock than can be included in this chapter. Therefore, this chapter is necessarily selective and includes only information that is directly relevant to the diagnosis and treatment of cardiogenic shock in clinical practice.

Cardiac and Extracardiac Determinants

When diagnosing cardiogenic shock, it is important to determine whether the presentation of shock is truly cardiogenic. Central cardiac factors need to be distinguished from peripheral and extracardiac factors. The presentation of shock in a coronary care unit does not necessarily preclude the occurrence of shock from other causes than the heart, such as hypovolemic (absolute or relative) shock, septicemic or anaphylactic shock, or shock secondary to a massive pulmonary embolism. It is also possible that more than one type of shock can be present concurrently. Nevertheless, because the heart is not the sole determinant of circulatory collapse, the central contribution of cardiac function and its inadequacy must be considered in relation to the state of the peripheries, including the vasculature, gas exchange, blood constituents, and volume.

Other compounding factors such as intercurrent infection, anemia, hypoxia (secondary to respiratory diseases), hypothermia, hyperpyrexia, dysthyroidism, thiamine deficiency, Addisonian crisis, or other systemic disorders may play a role. Prompt recognition and identification of these compounding factors are necessary before appropriate correction of these defects can be instituted. Drugs with myocardial depressant actions or hypotensive agents (e.g., morphine, diamorphine, β-blockers, arterial vasodilators, streptokinase) may be precipitating or contributory factors toward the onset of shock. Prompt recognition, withdrawal, or counteraction of such harmful effects of drugs may alter the nature and course of shock.

Etiology and Sequence of Events

In true cardiogenic shock, the initiating event occurs in the heart. Most clinicians associate it with myocardial infarction, although the etiology of cardiogenic shock can be the result of any defect in the heart, be it affecting the myocardial function (e.g., ischemia, infarction, stunning, contusion, arrhythmia, heart block, myocarditis), or the integrity of valves (e.g., chordal or papillary muscle rupture, acute regurgitation in endocarditis), or the integrity of cardiac structures (e.g., acute ventricular septal defect [VSD], acute tamponade). Urgent measures should be put in place to deal with these lesions, but while the definitive procedures are being planned and arranged, it is crucial to deal with the hemodynamic and metabolic consequences of the shock.

In addition to a decline in systolic function, there is also a substantial decrease in left ventricular compliance, increasing the filling pressure at a given end-diastolic volume *(1–4)*. The increased left ventricular end-diastolic pressure causes pulmonary congestion, leading to hypoxemia and ischemia, which further reduces coronary perfusion pressure. Myocyte swelling occurs *(5)* as a consequence of an intracellular accumulation of sodium and calcium resulting from anaerobic glycolysis, further decreasing left ventricular compliance *(6)*. The further reduction in compliance and the myocyte swelling lead to an increase in ventricular wall stress, elevating myocardial oxygen requirements. As the myocardium becomes less compliant, the pumping capacity of the heart becomes less efficient, increasing the imbalance between myocardial oxygen requirements and supply.

Soon after the onset of cardiogenic shock, compensatory mechanisms are activated. In mammals, a primary objective of the regulatory system of the circulation is to maintain arterial pressure *(7–10)* to preserve perfusion to the vital organs such as the brain and the heart. This is accomplished by activation of neurohumoral systems, not dissimilar from the responses observed during hemorrhagic shock and exercise. In particular, there are withdrawal of the parasympathetic system and activation of the sympathetic, renin–angiotensin–aldosterone and vasopressin systems, culminating in arterial and venous vasoconstriction, salt and fluid retention, positive chronotropy, and inotropy. Although beneficial in hemorrhagic shock and severe exercise, these compensatory mechanisms may be detrimental in cardiogenic shock. For instance, venoconstriction and salt and fluid retention would increase the preload and arterial vasoconstriction would increase the afterload, thereby overloading the already failing ventricles. Increased heart rate and myocardial contractility would increase the demands in the face of limited supply of oxygenated blood to at-risk myocardial regions (ischemic territories and the subendocardium). The skill of immediate management is therefore to curb the excesses of the compensatory mechanisms without negating some of their potential beneficial effects.

As the shock state persists, hypoperfusion of both the myocardium and peripheral tissues will induce anaerobic metabolism in these tissues and may result in lactic acidosis. An earlier study has shown that the serum lactate level is an important prognostic factor in cardiogenic shock *(11)*. Uncorrected, the accumulation of lactic acid may cause mitochondrial swelling and degeneration, inducing glycogen depletion, which, in turn, impair myocardial function and inhibit glycolysis, leading to irreversible ischemic damage *(12)*. Unfavorable effects on other organ functions follow. The shock state in patients with an acute myocardial infarction leads to a vicious cycle that causes a downward spiral of worsening ischemia: As cardiac output falls, arterial pressure falls and coronary perfusion is lowered, thus exacerbating the low output state. This eventually leads to further ischemia and extension of necrosis in the left ventricle. Several compensatory mechanisms occur during this chain of events that, if left untreated, lead to cardiac pump failure and, ultimately, death.

Compensatory Sympathetic Nervous System Activation

When myocardial function is depressed, several compensatory mechanisms occur. However, the compensatory mechanisms may become maladaptive and actually worsen myocardial ischemia. Initially, as cardiac pump function declines, there is a redistribution of blood flow, in order to ensure adequate perfusion of the heart and brain. Activation of the sympathetic nervous system occurs, resulting in arterial constriction, increased myocardial contractility, and an increase in heart rate.

Systemic vasoconstriction occurs in an attempt to increase blood pressure. This causes the systemic pressure to increase in the aorta during diastole, which initially minimizes the decrease in coronary perfusion. However, this vasoconstriction increases afterload, causing further impairment of cardiac performance and increasing myocardial oxygen demand *(13)*.

α-Mediated adrenergic arteriolar constriction accounts for a reduction in muscular, cutaneous, splanchnic, and renal blood flow, which may induce ischemic injury in these organs *(14)*. This flow mismatch may be further increased by the administration of inotropic or vasodilator agents. α-Adrenergic responses also lead to a postcapillary venular constriction. The combined effect of both arteriolar and venular constriction leads to an increase in capillary hydrostatic pressure causing an egress of fluid from the capillaries, decreasing intravascular volume and causing hemoconcentration. Intravascular volume is also regulated by renal blood flow. As vasoconstriction causes renal blood flow to decrease, the renin–angiotensin–aldosterone system is activated in an attempt to restore intravascular volume to normal and to increase preload.

A reflex increase in heart rate occurs, which further exacerbates myocardial oxygen demand and worsens ischemia. As the sympathetic system is activated further, ventricular extrasystoles become more frequent and cardiac dysrhythmias occur, which decrease cardiac pumping capacity and cardiac output.

CARDIAC DYSFUNCTION IN CARDIOGENIC SHOCK

Hemodynamic Profiling During Cardiogenic Shock

The earliest hemodynamic studies in cardiogenic shock were conducted in the 1950s *(15–17)*. With accumulation of such objective data, concepts of pathophysiology and therapeutic options evolved in the ensuing decades *(13,18–25)*. It is now well established that hemodynamic evaluation is a vital element in the management of patients with cardiogenic shock *(26–28)*.

Gilbert and colleagues were the first to measure cardiac outputs in patients with cardiogenic shock *(15)*. Freis and Smith and their colleagues confirmed decreases in arterial pressure and cardiac output but found systemic vascular resistance rather variable *(16,17)*. Subsequent investigators concentrated on responses to vasoconstrictors as an attempt to raise blood pressure in cardiogenic shock *(13,18–20)*.

Gunnar and colleagues compared post-myocardial-infarction patients with and without shock and found that shock patients had lower mean aortic pressure (mean ± SD: 53 ± 12 mm Hg vs 92 ± 23 mm Hg) and lower cardiac output (measured with indocyanine green dilution method: 2.2 ± 0.9 vs 3.8 ± 1.5 L/min) *(21)*. One of their patients with a cardiac output of 0.61/min died before any treatment could be given. Four patients were unable to increase mean aortic pressure above 80 mm Hg in response to norepineprine infusion, and all of them died within 8 h of the onset of shock. These early hemodynamic data suggested that those with the most compromised cardiac function and least able to respond to inotropic stimulation had the least favorable prognosis.

Smith and colleagues compared the effects of metaraminol (a vasoconstrictor) and isoproterenol on patients in cardiogenic shock who had hypotension, low cardiac output, raised venous pressure, and a systemic vascular resistance index ranging from

1600 to 4500 dyn s cm^5 m^2 *(22)*. They found that metaraminol elevated arterial and venous pressures and systemic vascular resistance at the expense of some reduction in cardiac output. Isoproterenol was found to increase cardiac output and decrease venous pressure and systemic vascular resistance, but in most cases the arterial pressure was also increased (Fig. 1B).

Objectives of Hemodynamic Evaluation

The primary objectives of hemodynamic evaluation in cardiogenic shock are to guide the treatment of this precarious condition *(29)* and to provide prognostic information *(26,27)*. One of the earliest attempts to use hemodynamic evaluation to determine prognosis and to guide therapy was by Ratshin and colleagues *(23)*. All of their cardiogenic shock patients who had left ventricular filling pressure of >15 mm Hg and cardiac index of <2.3 L/min died despite medical therapy. Attempts were also made to assess the reserve function of the failing hearts using dextran infusion, intravenous digoxin, epinephrine, norepinephrine, and isoproterenol, but the results were too varied to draw any useful conclusions.

Swan and colleagues were the first to recognize cardiogenic shock as the extreme manifestation of cardiac power failure *(24)*. Comparing the basal hemodynamics of two cohorts of patients, one with and one without cardiogenic shock post-acute myocardial infarction, the parameter most distinguishing the two cohorts was left ventricular stroke work (26 ± 10 g-m/beat with shock and 81 ± 36 g-m/beat without shock, $p < 0.005$). However, there was significant overlap of the individual basal unstimulated values between survivors and nonsurvivors of shock (Fig. 3). These observations were confirmed by Scheidt and colleagues, who also showed that although various hemodynamic variables are statistically significantly different between the survivors and non-survivors of acute myocardial infarction, individual values showed significant overlaps between the two cohorts *(25)*.

If death is the end point to prevent, identifying individual patients who are most likely to die will require an accurate and reliable predictive hemodynamic indicator. Using a logistic regression modeling technique, the GUSTO-I investigators showed that "cardiac output measurements were of greatest prognostic significance" even when demographic and clinical variables were included in the analysis *(27)*. This is consistent with the concept that in the absence of life-threatening arrhythmia the most important determinant of mortality is cardiac pump function, because it is the inadequacy of this that leads to circulatory collapse and cardiogenic shock.

Which Hemodynamic Variables to Measure?

The heart is a complex organ with many components. Various measurements have been developed in the past to evaluate aspects of cardiac function. Many of the variables are interrelated and concordant, but quite often they are contradictory. For instance, in gross mitral regurgitation, the left ventricular ejection fraction is exaggerated and overestimates cardiac function, whereas in tight aortic stenosis, it provides an underestimate. In cardiogenic shock, being the severest form of cardiac impairment, there is very little room for misinterpretation in the management of patients. Therefore, it is vitally important to conduct the correct measurements and interpret the results appropriately.

The crucial steps involved in evaluating cardiogenic shock are as follows: (1) to establish whether the heart is responsible for the shock (see previous section), (2) to

Table 1
Normal Hemodynamic Values at Rest (for a Healthy Average-Sized Adult Man)[a]

Variables	Values	Comments
Heart rate (min^{-1})	71 (53–89)	May be as low as 30 in elite athletes
Pressures (mm Hg) (1 kPa = 7.5 mm Hg)		
Right atrium	5 (0–9)	Congestive if > 10
Right ventricle, systolic	22 (16–28)	
Right ventricle, end diastolic	5 (0–9)	
Pulmonary artery, S/D	16–28/4–16	PHT if S > 40
Pulmonary artery, mean	15 (6–17)	
Pulmonary artery wedge, mean	8 (2–12)	Congestive if > 15
Left atrium, mean	8 (2–12)	Congestive if > 15
Left ventricle, systolic	100–140	
Left ventricle, end diastolic	8 (2–12)	Congestive if > 15
Aorta, systolic	122 (105–140)	Hypotensive if < 90
Aorta, diastolic	73 (65–90)	
Aorta, mean	93 (80–110)	Hypotensive if < 60
Cardiac flow generation		
Cardiac output (L/min)	6.5 (3.6–9.4)	Cardiogenic shock if < 3.5
Cardiac index (L/min/m^2)	3.6 (2.0–5.2)	Cardiogenic shock if < 2.0
Stroke volume (mL)	93 (53–133)	
LV end-diastolic volume (mL)	75–200	Dependent on method of measurement
LV ejection fraction (%)	55–70	Dependent on method of measurement
Vascular resistances (dyn s/cm^5) (1 mmHg/L min = 80 dyn s/cm^5 = 8 kPa/L^{-1} s)		
Systemic	1070 (660–1480)	Usually > 1500 in cardiogenic shock
Total pulmonary	70 (20–120)	PHT if > 200
Cardiac work		
LV stroke work index (J/m^2)	0.4–0.7	With normal preload
Baseline cardiac power output (W)	0.8–1.3	Very severe cardiogenic shock if < 0.4

Source: Modified from refs. *55* and *113.*

[a] Abbreviations: D, diastolic; dyn, dynes; J, joules; LV, left ventricle; PHT, pulmonary hypertension; S, systolic; SHT, systemic hypertension; W, watts.

assess which component part(s) of the heart is (are) responsible for the circulatory failure, and (3) to measure the extent of the overall organ dysfunction. A readily available imaging technique (usually echocardiography) often fulfills the function of identifying whether the heart is responsible for the shock (step 1) and which components are malfunctioning (step 2). However, it provides only qualitative information about the extent of overall cardiac dysfunction (step 3) and, therefore, invasive hemodynamic measurements and monitoring are required to determine prognosis and provide a quantitative indication of responses to treatment.

Over 100 hemodynamic parameters have been proposed through the ages (Table 1), and each group of investigators advocates its own parameter as the ideal *(30,31)*. When managing critically ill patients in cardiogenic shock, clinicians do not have the luxury of academic uncertainties, but must rely on clarity of thought and prompt actions. With this aim, readers are encouraged to study other chapters in this volume.

Briefly, there are parameters that reflect systolic versus diastolic ventricular function, determinants of cardiac performance such as preload, afterload, chronotropy, and inotropy. Conceptually, for a long time, the holy grail had been the search for an ideal index of myocardial contractility, in the belief that "contractility" is the most accurate representation of how good the heart is, independent of peripheral influences through loading conditions of the ventricle and rate-related phenomena. This concept has been shown to be flawed because indices of contractility obtained from whole ventricular chamber dynamics are at best a summation of the necrotic, ischemic, stunned, hibernating, and normally functioning myocardium, and, at molecular levels, the inotropic aspects of the sliding filaments are inextricably linked to the loading conditions of the myofilaments. Thus, a conceptual paradigm shift away from muscle mechanics toward whole-organ dynamics and functional assessments is more helpful for clinicians in order to select which parameters should be adopted during the management of cardiogenic shock (32,33). To achieve this, it is helpful to return to basics and revisit first principles.

Central Hemodynamics: Concepts and Definitions

By definition, the hallmark of cardiogenic shock is severe primary cardiac pump failure. In true cardiogenic shock, circulatory collapse persists even after optimization of peripheral factors. Understanding the hemodynamic concepts of primary pump failure in cardiogenic shock is vital to correct diagnosis, interpretation of hemodynamic data, and management.

The definition of primary cardiac pump failure hinges on an understanding of the physiological role of the heart in maintaining the circulation. The milestone definition of the function of the heart must be attributed to William Harvey, the discoverer of the circulation, who in 1628 stated "…that the movement of the blood is constantly in a circle, and is brought about by the beat of the heart … for the sake of nourishment…" When the heart stops beating, forces opposing blood flow in the vessels halt the circulation. To restart and maintain the motion, energy is required, which is provided by the cardiac pump.

The primary function of the heart, expressed in modern physiological terms, is to convert biochemical energy into hydraulic energy at rates sufficient to maintain an adequate circulation under normal physiological conditions. In three-dimensional space, the power (work per unit time) of moving a volume of fluid is the product of pressure and flow rate. Thus, the ability of the heart to generate energy and perform external work encompasses not only its ability to generate flow but also its ability to generate pressure. Pressure generation is essential, unless the impedance to flow in the circulation is zero (an impossibility). Adopting the definition of cardiac function as stated here, the definition of primary cardiac pump failure can be simply stated as the failure of the heart, under physiological loading conditions, to produce sufficient hydraulic power output to maintain an adequate circulation at rest and during normal physiological stress.

Components of Pump Failure

It follows that primary cardiac pump failure is the end result of summated effects of the defects in cardiac structures and functions. The defects may include systolic and diastolic dysfunction, dyssynchronous contractile dysfunction, conduction defects and arrhythmias, valvular diseases, and other structural defects, including septal defects.

These may be intrinsic to the heart or extrinsic, such as induced by drugs, malfunctioning devices (e.g., pacemaker-induced tachyarrhythmia), or abnormal neurohumoral
controls. Systolic and diastolic dysfunction includes all causes of cardiomyopathies
(ischemic, dilated, hypertrophic, restrictive), myopericarditis, transplant rejection, constrictive pericarditis, and pericardial effusion. Correct identification of component
defects and their hemodynamic consequences is important to institute appropriate
treatment. For instance, cardiogenic shock in a patient with severe obstructive hypertrophic cardiomyopathy is worsened when treated with standard cardiogenic shock
therapy such as using positive inotropic agents, diuretics, and vasodilators.

Each cardiac lesion may precipitate hemodynamic compromise in a number of
ways. After a massive myocardial infarction, for example, there may be a combination
of component dysfunction such as systolic and diastolic dysfunction, papillary muscle
rupture and mitral regurgitation, acquired ventricular septal defects, conduction defects
(partial bundle branch block or heart blocks), arrhythmias, and pericardial tamponade.

In the Western world, the commonest cause of primary pump failure leading to cardiogenic shock is extensive myocardial infarction *(27,34)*. At autopsy, more than two-
thirds of patients with cardiogenic shock demonstrate stenosis of 75% or more of the
luminal diameter of all three major coronary vessels, usually including the left anterior
descending coronary artery *(35)*. Others have found that patients with cardiogenic
shock had lost at least 40% of the left ventricular myocardium *(36–38)*, although
smaller infarctions or mere ischemia may also precipitate shock *(39)*. Size estimates of
regional infarction need to be adjusted for diffuse cardiomyocyte loss as a result of biological attrition of cardiomyocytes over time *(40)* or as a result of other causes such as
subclinical cardiomyopathies. During ischemia, myocardial metabolism is severely
deranged and cellular energy stores are depleted. It is important to recognize that large
areas of nonfunctional but viable myocardium (stunned and hibernating myocardium)
can contribute to the development of the syndrome. Cardiogenic shock resulting from
or contributed by ongoing ischemic (as opposed to infarcted), stunned, or hibernating
myocardium is likely to have a better prognosis if these factors can be reversed in time.

Baseline Versus Reserve Cardiac Function

It is a truism that how good a heart is, is gaged by how well it maintains the circulation, not at baseline resting states but during the most severe stress. This concept is
even more applicable in cardiogenic shock, because, by definition, the failure of the
cardiac pump to provide an adequate circulation to ensure appropriate tissue perfusion is responsible for the shock state. This implies that the cardiac pump is fully
stimulated by the cardiovascular regulatory system, but this may not be the case in all
circumstances. In cases when the cardiac pump is functioning at its maximum and
circulatory collapse still persists, alternative modes of circulatory support are
required. In other cases, the cardiac pump may underperform for several reasons
(e.g., under the influence of cardiodepressant drugs, marked vagal tone, in the presence of extensive stunned or hibernating myocardium), and the reserve function of
the heart has not been exhausted.

In cardiogenic shock, therefore, a more important feature than the cardiac function
at baseline resting states is the reserve pumping capability of the failing heart (i.e., the
ability to increase pumping capacity during stress). Availability of this mechanistic
information alone would help clinicians to select individual patients who should go

forward for invasive therapy *(28)*. This information may be taken in conjunction with the more probabilistic information contained in the risk factors derived from multivariate analyses of other patient cohorts.

Evaluating the Overall Pump Failure in Shock

The most natural form of stimulating cardiac performance is physiological, through maximal exercise. However, it is impracticable and undesirable to ask patients in cardiogenic shock to perform any form of exercise. An alternative is to use pharmacological means of stressing the heart. In current cardiological practice, the commonest agent used is dobutamine, which can be supplemented with a phosphodiesterase inhibitor (such as milrinone or enoximone), although in intensive care practice, adrenaline is often used instead. Using dobutamine stimulation, Tan and Littler investigated the predictive power of hemodynamic variables measured at baseline and during peak stimulation in consecutive patients admitted to a coronary care unit with cardiogenic shock *(26)*. They found that the presence or absence of reserve function of the failing heart is strongly predictive of prognosis, in contrast to baseline unstimulated states in which there were significant overlaps in all hemodynamic parameters between the survivors and nonsurvivors. When plotted against pulmonary arterial occlusion pressure at baseline unstimulated states, there was a tendency for those with higher cardiac output or left ventricular stroke work and lower left ventricular filling pressure to survive, but there were significant overlaps between the two groups (Fig. 1). When the values during maximal dobutamine stimulation were plotted, the separation between the two groups became more obvious (Fig. 2).

These investigators also tested the hypothesis that the likelihood of prolonged survival is low if patients in cardiogenic shock were unable to exceed the normal resting cardiac power output of 1 W during maximal dobutamine stimulation *(41)*. The results (Fig. 3) showed that at baseline unstimulated states, all patients had cardiac power output values of less than 1 W and there was significant overlap of the values between the survivors and nonsurvivors. Patients with particularly depressed cardiac performance, power output <0.4 W (after optimizing filling pressures), all died. The rest of the cohort showed a diverging response to dobutamine response, with those able to exceed 1 W of power output surviving the 1 yr of follow-up; the nonsurvivors had limited increments in power output *(26)*.

Hemodynamics of Peripheral Factors

VENOUS AND PRELOAD EFFECTS

Hypovolemia, caused by, for example, severe dehydration or hemorrhage, can precipitate shock through underfilling of the ventricles despite normal cardiac function. The threshold for shock is lower if cardiac function is also impaired. In right ventricular infarction leading to predominantly right ventricular failure, the right atrial pressure is elevated relative to the left atrial pressure. To maintain an adequate circulation, the central venous pressure is necessarily elevated to ensure adequate left atrial pressure and left ventricular filling. Maintaining the central venous pressure within the normal range may result in *relative* hypovolemia, manifesting as significant underfilling of the left ventricle, thereby further compromising cardiac function. In the presence of right ventricular infarction and the possibility of relative hypovolemia (shown by raised right atrial pressure and low pulmonary wedge pressure), fluid challenge to

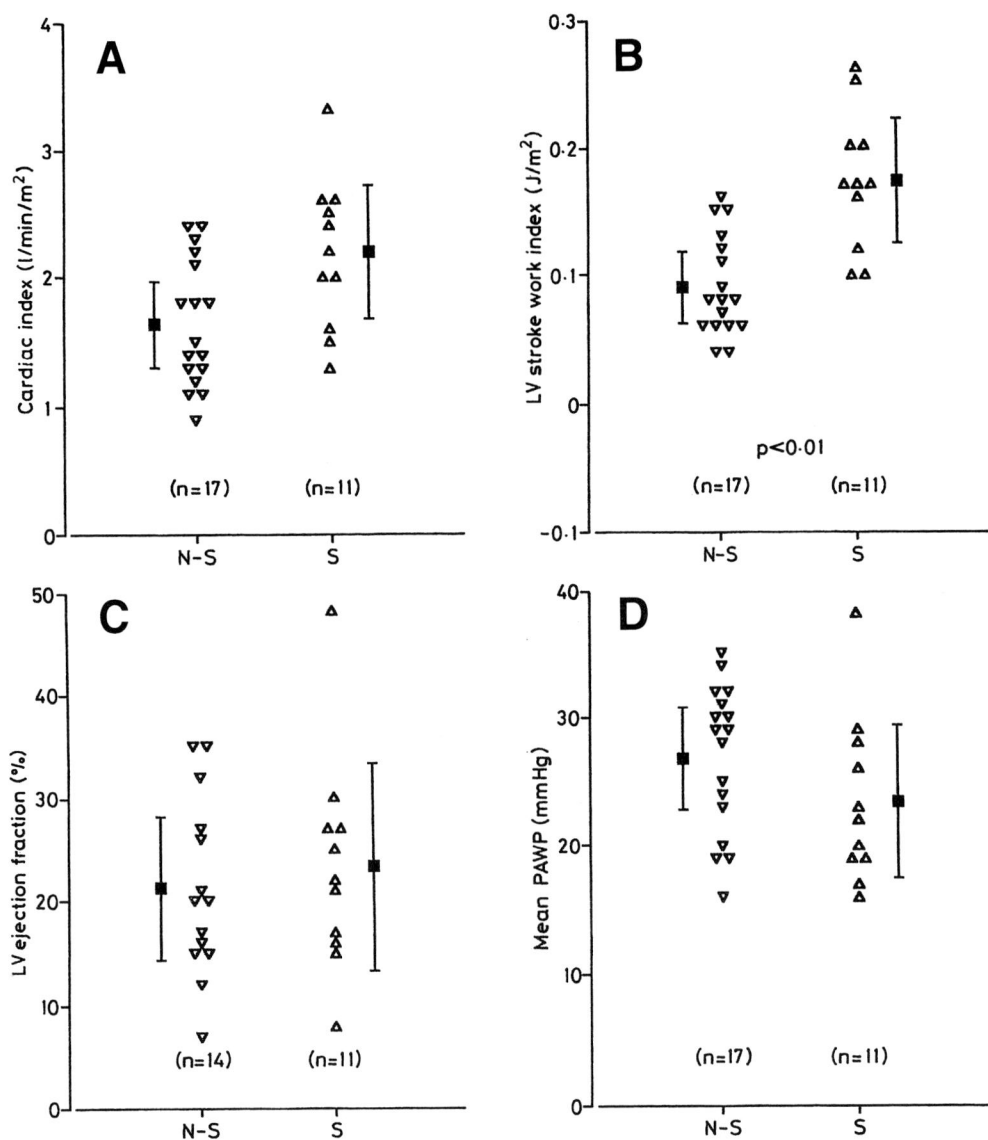

Fig. 1. Baseline resting hemodynamic data of survivors (S) and nonsurvivors (N-S) from consecutive patients admitted to a coronary care unit presenting with cardiogenic shock: **(A)** cardiac index, **(B)** left ventricular stroke work index, **(C)** left ventricular ejection fraction, **(D)** mean pulmonary artery occlusion pressure, **(E)** cardiac index versus pulmonary artery occluded pressure, and **(F)** left ventricular stroke work index versus pulmonary artery occluded pressure. Although the mean values favored the survivors, there were significant overlaps of the individual values between survivors and nonsurvivors. Reprinted with permission from ref. *26.*

raise the pulmonary wedge pressure to >18 mm Hg should be made before diagnosing cardiogenic shock.

On the other hand, overdistension of the left ventricle may precipitate or exacerbate functional mitral regurgitation, effectively resulting in the ventricle functioning in the

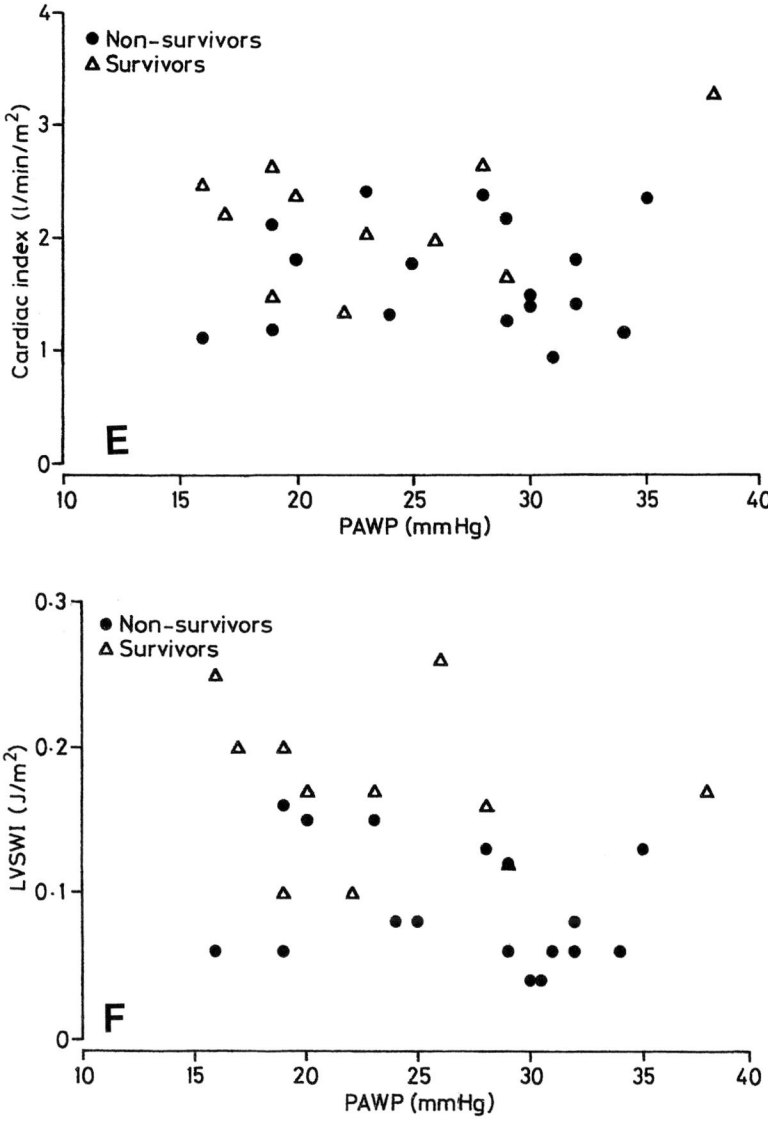

Fig. 1. *(Continued).*

descending limb of Starling's curve. Fluid challenge blindly without hemodynamic monitoring may aggravate this situation. Instead, judicious use of diuretics, venodilation, or even hemofiltration or ultrafiltration may be beneficial.

ARTERIAL AND AFTERLOAD EFFECTS

Any peripheral factors that result in excessive demands on the cardiac pump performance are liable to precipitate or exacerbate cardiogenic shock. In a normal circulation, there is an impedance matching of the cardiac pump and the arterial system such that the hydraulic power output of the heart is maximal *(42)*. Disturbance of this matching would render cardiac function suboptimal. An example is the excessive vasodilatation

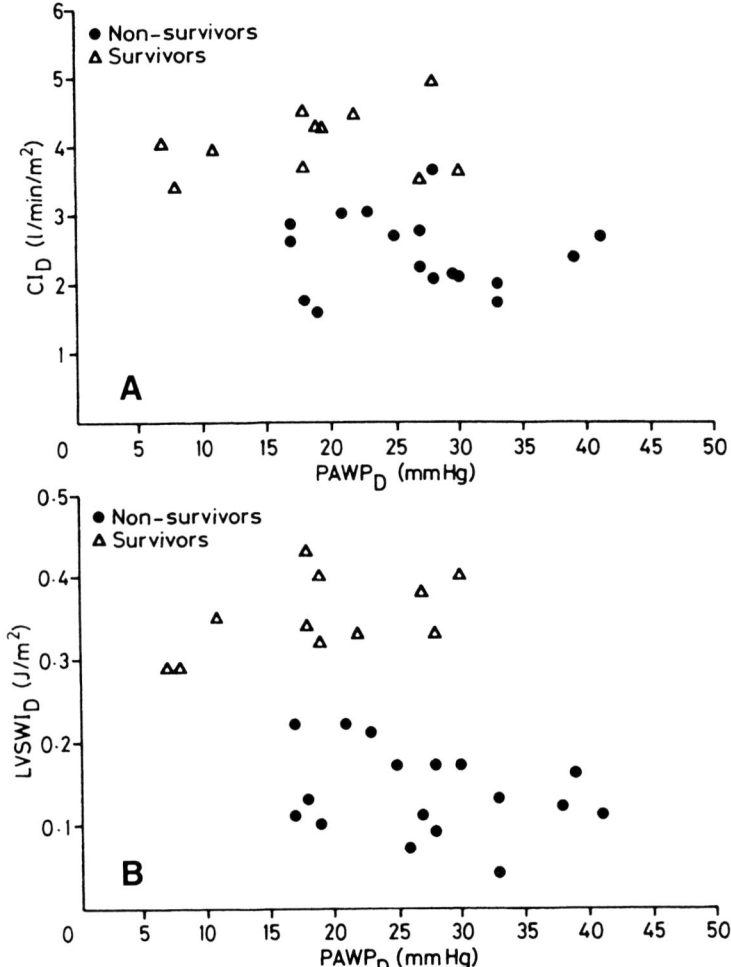

Fig. 2. Hemodynamic data during peak dobutamine stimulation in the same cohort of patients as in Fig. 4, showing clear demarcation of the values of survivors (open triangles) from those of nonsurvivors (filled circles). Reprinted with permission from ref. *26.*

via the nitric oxide pathways, especially of the splanchnic vasculature via the release of endotoxins in septicemic shock *(43–45)*. The threshold for the onset of shock is lower if the cardiac function itself is also impaired (a combination of septicemic and cardiogenic shock). Excessive vasodilatation (through therapeutic use of nitrates or other antianginal agents, morphine or diamorphine) may also exacerbate cardiogenic shock. Similarly, in high-output states (e.g., Paget's disease, arteriovenous malformation, anemia, thyrotoxicosis), shock occurs at lower levels of compromise of cardiac function.

In heart failure, including cardiogenic shock, resulting from activation of the sympathetic and renin–angiotensin–aldosterone systems, there is a tendency for vasoconstriction, which can be excessive for the failing heart and render its function suboptimal *(42)*. Extra elevation of afterload through such mechanisms as treatment with norepinephrine or dopamine (sometimes used in cardiogenic shock), chronic hypertension, aortic steno-

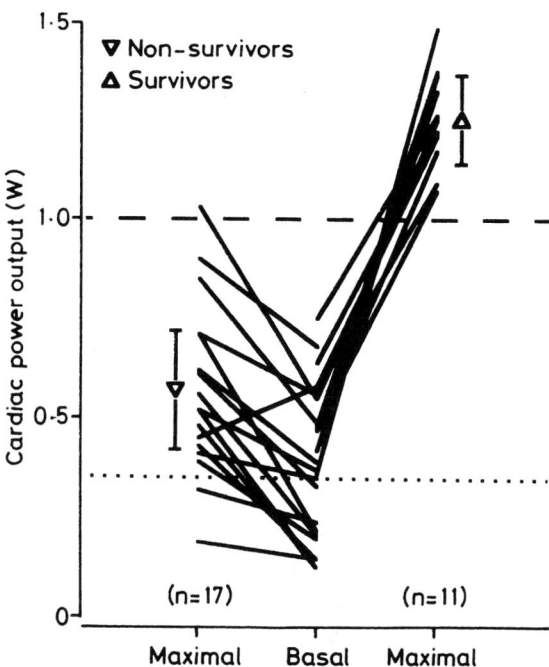

Fig. 3. Cardiac power output at baseline resting states and during peak dobutamine stimulation in the same cohort of patients as in Fig. 4, showing that (1) patients with baseline power output of < 0.4 W all perished, (2) the baseline power outputs of survivors and nonsurvivors were indistinguishable, and (3) patients with peak cardiac power output of > 1 W tended to survive on medical therapy alone. Reprinted with permission from ref. *26*.

sis, or coarctation of the aorta would further exacerbate the mismatch in impedance. In poorly controlled chronic hypertension, there is a further complication in that the autoregulatory levels for blood flow into vital organs are readjusted upward such that higher pressures are required to produce the same blood flow as in normotensives *(46–48)*. In these subjects, the onset of cardiogenic shock (tissue hypoperfusion) can, therefore, occur at higher arterial pressures (e.g., systolic blood pressure >110 mm Hg).

Practical Issues: Monitoring and Interpreting Central Hemodynamics

Because the initiating and primary defect in cardiogenic shock is failure of cardiac function, close monitoring of central hemodynamics is an essential component of managing patients. The objective is to optimize the performance of the heart, to maintain an adequate circulation without stressing the heart unduly. The Schumacker concept of treating septicemic shock by maximizing cardiac output should be avoided in the management of cardiogenic shock *(44)*.

Meticulous management of cardiogenic shock requires invasive measurements via a fluid-filled flotation pulmonary artery catheter and, ideally, invasive monitoring of intra-arterial pressure, in order to assess several important variables that fully reflect cardiac function. Previous concerns about the use of such invasive monitoring are not generally applicable because there were only very few cases of cardiogenic shock included in that study *(49)*. All invasive procedures in seriously ill patients carry some risks and should be conducted by well-trained, experienced personnel.

The parameters that indicate the hemodynamic status of the patient with cardiogenic shock are as follows: (1) cardiac output (determined by heart rate and rhythm and stroke volume), reflecting the blood flow output of the heart; (2) right atrial pressure (RAP) and central venous pressure (CVP), which reflect the right ventricular filling pressure; (3) pulmonary artery wedge pressure (PAWP) and left atrial pressure (LAP), which reflect the left ventricular end-diastolic (filling) pressure; and (4) arterial blood pressure (systolic and diastolic), which reflects the pressure generating capacity of the heart and systemic vasomotor tone. Using these variables, left ventricular stroke work and cardiac power output, which is an indicator of overall cardiac function and incorporates both the pressure- and flow-generating abilities of the heart, can be calculated *(41)*. Cardiac power output is the product of cardiac output × mean arterial pressure × *k*, a conversion factor (2.22×10^{-3}) and is expressed in watts (W). It has been shown to be a powerful prognostic indicator in patients with cardiogenic shock and heart failure *(26,41,50,51)*.

Because nonsurvivors (who had inadequate cardiac reserve at the time of evaluation) and survivors (with adequate reserve) have clear differences between their hemodynamic parameters *(26,27)*, it is possible to triage patients according to their cardiac functional reserve status. Patients with poor reserve are the ones who will not do well with medical therapy alone and need to be considered for aggressive interventions if death is to be avoided. If the peak cardiac power output (CPO) is >1 W, medical therapy—including the use of inotropic agents to maintain adequate pressure and flow—is usually sufficient, unless there is a risk of progression of myocardial damage. If the peak CPO is <1 W (or simple bedside observation of peak attainable systolic blood pressure [BP] of <80 mm Hg despite maximal dobutamine stimulation), then urgent and definitive treatment of primary defects (urgent coronary angioplasty, bypass surgery, other curative operation, or cardiac transplantation) should be sought.

BIOCHEMICAL CONCEPTS

Energetics of the Normal Myocardium

Viewed in terms of energetics, the prime function of the heart is to convert the stored biochemical energy in available substrates and transduce it into mechanical energy, via cardiomyocyte contraction (in a synchronized fashion) to allow the ventricles to deliver hydraulic energy into the systemic and pulmonary vasculature beds *(52)*. Because under normal physiological conditions, cardiac metabolism is oxidative and oxygen is not stored, the most crucial substrate to be supplied for myocardial metabolism is therefore oxygen. The major substrates oxidized in the normal myocardium are fatty acids (67%), glucose (18%), and lactate, although amino acids, ketones, and pyruvate are also used *(53–55)* (Fig. 4). In a normally oxygenated heart, high cellular levels of adenosine triphosphate (ATP) and citrate inhibit glycolysis *(56)*. The energy equivalent of 1 mL of oxygen has been estimated to provide 20.15 J of energy *(57,58)*.

For the entire organ, it is technically quite difficult to measure all of the substrates used, whereas oxygen consumption is relatively easier to measure. Because of this technical limitation, the energy *input* to the heart has traditionally been represented by myocardial oxygen consumption (MVO_2). A more direct measure of energy input into the myocardial contractile elements is the ATP consumption, which can be measured by nuclear magnetic

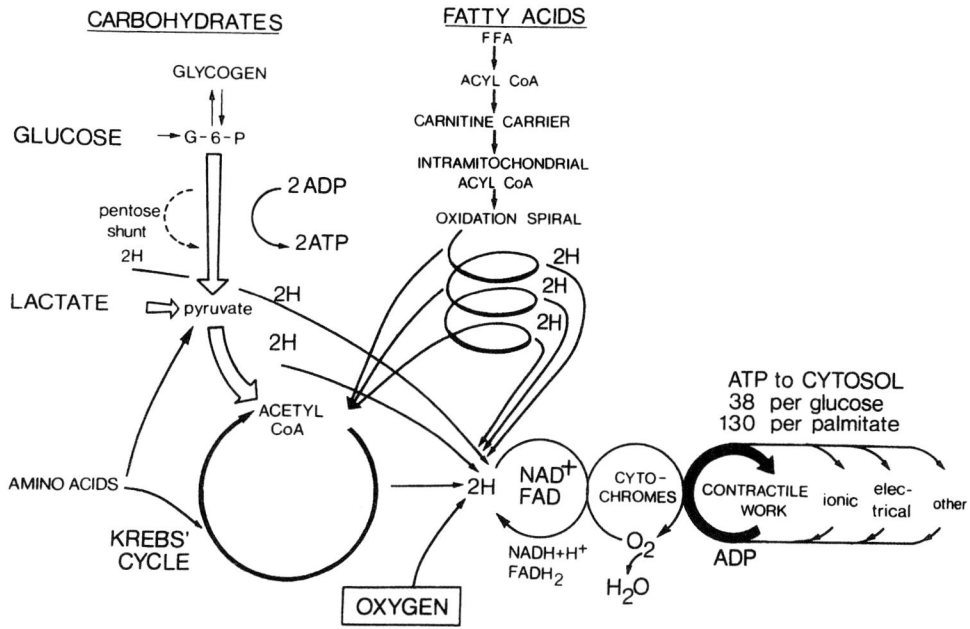

Fig. 4. Free fatty acids, glucose, and lactate are the major substrates of normal myocardium, and their oxidation and final interaction with the cytochrome chain produce the ATP that is the primary fuel for transduction into mechanical energy of myofilament contraction. Reprinted with permission *(109)*.

resonance (NMR) spectroscopy *(59,60)*. Rates of ATP synthesis estimated from magnetization transfer were similar to values calculated from oxygen consumption *(60)*.

The breakdown of ATP to adenosine diphosphate (ADP) (and P_i + free energy) is the direct source of energy for myofilament contraction, the maintenance of ionic gradients, and other vital cellular functions *(61)* (Fig. 5). ADP is reconverted to ATP via oxidative phosphorylation in the mitochondria. In normal myocardium, ATP is maintained relatively constant, despite variations in cardiac performance, through matched changes in the rates of ATP synthesis to its utilization. This is achieved through the buffering mechanism of creatine phosphate (CP) that is present in high concentration in normal myocardium. The transfer of the phosphoryl group from CP to ADP is catalyzed by creatine phosphokinase (CPK or CK) in the following reaction:

$$CP + Mg–ADP = Mg–ATP + creatine$$

which favors the formation of ATP by about 50 times. In vivo, the turnover of the phosphoryl group by CK, measured directly by ^{31}P magnetization transfer, is an order of magnitude faster than net ATP synthesis estimated from oxygen consumption.

The useful energy output of the heart is the hydraulic energy imparted into the circulation. The rest of the energy is dissipated as wasted heat. The ratio of the useful energy output to energy input is the efficiency of the cardiac transduction process. In certain pathological states, such as severe aortic stenosis, the efficiency may be seriously compromised, especially when coupled with modest limitations of oxygen supply (e.g., noncritical coronary artery stenosis), and this may result in an unstable state of cardiogenic shock. How efficiency is affected in cardiac pathophysiological

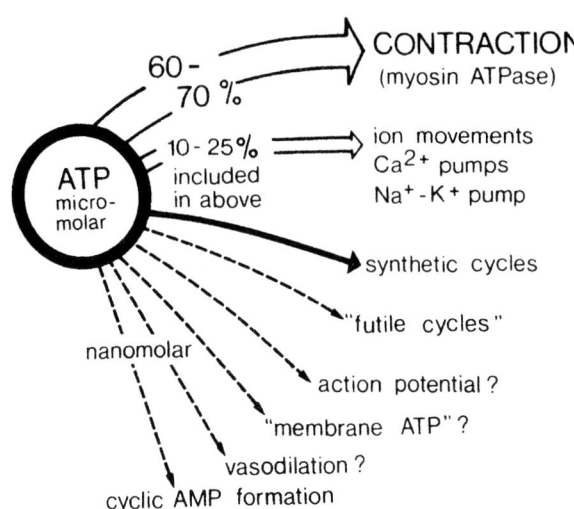

Fig. 5. Cellular functions of ATP in cardiomyocytes. Reprinted with permission *(110)*.

states depends on the relative proportions of the determinants of myocardial oxygen consumption.

The determinants of MVO_2 in terms of the whole organ are as follows: (1) useful external work *(62,63)*, (2) development of wall tension *(64,65)*, (3) noncontractile basal cellular metabolism *(64)*, (4) depolarization and activation *(66)*, (5) heart-rate-related energy expenditure *(67)*, and (6) contractility or inotropy-related energy expenditure *(58,64,68)*. Under different conditions, the three major determinants of myocardial oxygen consumption are systolic wall tension, contractility, and heart rate *(62,63,66,68–72)*, although what proportion of these are wasted as heat and which are converted into useful external work is difficult to ascertain. During normal physiological contractions, probably the highest cost in terms of energy consumption is in the development of left ventricular wall tension *(64,65)*. Wall tension development unaccompanied by forward stroke volume (e.g., during a nonejecting extrasystolic beat) is a wasteful consumption of energy. Similarly, a dilated ventricle requires more energy to develop a much higher wall tension to generate the same intraventricular pressures according to the Law of LaPlace [wall stress = (pressure × radius)/(2 × wall thickness)] *(73)*. MVO_2 is also influenced by the supply of substrates to the heart. The use of free fatty acids increases MVO_2, and catecholamines sensitize the heart to the oxygen-wasting effect of free fatty acids *(63)*. Alteration of myocardial metabolism from mainly free fatty acid to carbohydrate oxidation reduces the extent of myocardial ischemic injury *(74)*.

Energetics and Metabolism of Hypoperfused Myocardium

As a result of circulatory shock and hypoperfusion of the myocardium, aerobic cellular metabolism cannot be maintained. The regeneration of high-energy phosphate compounds, CP and ATP, is impaired and intracellular high-energy reserves therefore decline. When oxygen delivery to the cardiomyocytes is inadequate, oxidative metabolism ceases, cellular citrate and ATP levels fall, and the cell switches to glycolytic anaerobic metabolism to produce a limited amount of ATP. The rate of glucose uptake is accelerated and available glycogen is rapidly depleted *(75,76),* resulting in lactate production instead of lactate uptake by the myocardium *(77–80).* The energy made available from anaerobic glycolysis is only about 6% of that obtainable from oxidative metabolism *(81).* A rough estimate of the efficiencies of glucose metabolism in the production of ATP is as follows *(82):* aerobic oxidation of 1 mol of glucose (free energy of 686 kcal) can produce 36 mol of ATP (7.3 kcal each), giving a conversion efficiency of 38%. Anaerobic metabolism of 1 mol of glucose produces 2 mol of ATP, giving a conversion efficiency of 2.2%. Anaerobic glycolysis is therefore a poor means of compensating for inadequate supply of oxygen *(77),* albeit it may be sufficient to maintain viability of the jeopardized myocytes.

When ischemia is severe, the products of glycolysis accumulate. Anerobic glycolysis yields lactic acid, which results in cellular acidosis that, in turn, inhibits glycolysis and ATP generation ceases. The relative lack of ATP means failure of energy-dependent ion transport pumps, impairing cation transport, with an efflux of potassium and intracellular accumulation of sodium and calcium *(83).* This causes myocyte swelling (see above) and decreasing ventricular compliance. As the ischemia becomes severe, myocardial cell injury becomes irreversible with necrosis; mitochondrial swelling; accumulation of denatured proteins and chromatin in the cytoplasm; lysosomal breakdown; and fracture of the mitochondria, nuclear envelope, and plasma membrane *(83).* Apoptosis may also be responsible for some of the myocyte loss occurring as a result of ischemia; evidence of apoptosis has been found in the border zone of the myocardium during infarction and also sporadically in areas remote from the ischemia *(40,84).* Apoptotic pathways may be activated by inflammatory cascades, oxidative stress, or stretching of myocytes *(84).* The ratio of apoptotic cell death to myocyte necrosis during myocardial ischemia is currently unknown. In these situations, the earliest restoration of oxygenated blood flow is the most rewarding practical solution, provided the jeopardized myocardium is still viable.

In the presence of limited oxygen supply, secondary to coronary artery stenosis or occlusion, considerations about the efficiency of energy transduction also become of paramount importance. In animal experiments following coronary occlusion, interventions that increase myocardial energy expenditure appear to increase the size of the infarction, whereas those that decrease myocardial oxygen consumption reduce the size of the infarction. Reduction of myocardial oxygen demands produced by slowing the heart rate and counteracting the augmentation of sympathetic influences may reduce oxygen demands and thereby the size of the infarction *(68).* However, excessive bradycardia may result in ventricular dilatation that, in turn, will negate or even exceed the energy-saving attempt through reducing the heart rate, resulting in a net increase in myocardial oxygen consumption. The situation becomes very complex in the presence of cardiogenic shock.

Once heart failure is established, recent evidence from NMR spectroscopy studies using myocardium obtained from heart failure patients suggests that the capacity for ATP resynthesis via the CK system is compromised in the failing myocardium *(85,86).* CK activity and ATP, ADP, CP, and free creatine are decreased in failing myocardium. The decrease in the content of the energy reservoir compound, CP, is greater than that for ATP. Phosphoryl transfer via the CK decreases from being 10-fold greater than the rate of ATP synthesis via oxidative phosphorylation in the normal heart to only about threefold greater (assuming no change in the rate of oxidative phosphorylation) in the failing heart. Decreased energy reserve via the CK system for the severely failing heart is likely to reduce the contractile reserve of the heart. It may also contribute to decreased baseline contractile performance *(87)*.

Metabolic Treatment by the Glucose–Insulin–Potassium Infusion

As we have seen previously, several metabolic changes occur during cardiogenic shock, related to the lack of ATP available for cellular energy. ATP is produced from two main sources: glucose and free fatty acids (FFA). When oxygen is abundant during normal perfusion conditions, it is more efficient for the cell to use FFA, as it yields a larger amount of ATP *(88)*. However, during ischemic conditions, the cell switches to glucose metabolism and this causes an accumulation of FFA. Also, sympathetic activation and high catecholamine levels seen during cardiogenic shock lead to increased circulating FFA levels. Myocardial accumulation of FFA leads to depression of myocardial function, membrane instability, and arrhythmias *(89)* and an increase in myocardial oxygen consumption without a parallel increase in myocardial work: the "oxygen-wasting effect of FFA" *(74,90)*.

Although metabolic agents have been routinely used for a number of years as protection against ischemic–reperfusion injury during cardiac surgery *(91,92)*, investigators have only recently adopted a strategy of metabolic alterations as a therapeutic option in the treatment of acute ischemia. There is increasing experimental and clinical evidence of the possible benefit of metabolic treatment of ischemia, which may prevent the development of cardiogenic shock *(93)*. Administration of the polarizing substance, glucose–insulin–potassium (GIK), was first used as a treatment for ischemia in acute myocardial infarction in 1962 by Sodi-Pallares and colleagues *(94)*. GIK is thought to have several possible mechanisms of action in the treatment of ischemia, ranging from its importance in providing a metabolic substrate for an increased energy source, through to its anti-FFA actions *(95)*. All responsible mechanisms may lead to an improvement in contractile performance in ischemic ventricular dysfunction. (See Chapter 5 for a further discussion of GIK.)

Clinical Evidence for GIK Use in Acute Ischemia

A retrospective meta-analysis performed in 1997, involving 1932 patients from nine clinical trials performed during the prethrombolytic era, found GIK to significantly reduce in-hospital mortality versus placebo (16% vs 21%, $p = 0.004$) *(96)*. In a subgroup of four studies using high-dose GIK, in-hospital mortality was reduced by 48%, which is comparable to the mortality reduction seen with reperfusion therapy several years later, suggesting that metabolic protection of the ischemic myocardium may be as important as reperfusion therapy *per se*. However, the results of this meta-analysis must be interpreted with caution, as it suffers from all the drawbacks of the meta-analysis techniques.

Two randomized trials have looked at GIK in the treatment of acute myocardial infarction in the thrombolytic era. The Diabetes Insulin–Glucose in Acute Myocardial Infarction (DIGAMI) trial included 620 diabetic patients with an acute myocardial infarction, all treated with thrombolysis *(97)*. A significant reduction in mortality at 1 yr was seen in the group who received an intensive insulin regimen (insulin–glucose infusion for 24 h, followed by subcutaneous insulin every day for 3 mo or more) versus standard therapy (29% relative reduction [$p = 0.027$]). The results need to be interpreted with caution, however, as the mortality benefit may merely reflect better diabetic control.

The ECLA (Estudios Cardiologicos Latinoamerica) trial involved 407 patients with an acute myocardial infarction, randomized to receive either (1) high-dose GIK (25% glucose, 50 IU insulin, 80 meq potassium/L at 1.5 mL/kg/h), (2) low-dose GIK (10% glucose, 20 IU insulin, 40 meq potassium/L at 1 mL/kg/h), or (3) placebo, in addition to standard therapy (62% of patients were treated with reperfusion therapy [95% thrombolysis, 5% primary percutaneous transluminal coronary angioplasty (PTCA)]) *(98)*. Overall, GIK therapy was associated with a nonsignificant reduction in in-hospital mortality and major and minor in-hospital events. In the subgroup who received reperfusion, the reduction in in-hospital mortality was significant in the GIK-treated group (5.2% vs 15.2%, $p = 0.01$). At 1 yr, there was a trend toward lower mortality in the overall and reperfused groups, although the subgroup of patients who were reperfused and received high-dose GIK had a significant reduction in mortality versus placebo. The results of the ECLA study suggest that high-dose GIK may be more beneficial than either a low-dose regimen or placebo, which is consistent with the findings of the previous meta-analysis *(96)*. This may be due to the fact that the high dose that was used had previously been found to achieve maximal suppression of arterial FFA levels as well as maximal increases in myocardial uptake of glucose in previous experimental studies *(99)*. The finding that there was significant mortality reduction with GIK only in the reperfused group needs to be interpreted with caution, because of the small sample size and conflicting findings from the more statistically robust meta-analysis.

Use of GIK in Cardiogenic Shock

There has been a small amount of work looking at the effects of GIK on patients with severe left ventricular dysfunction immediately following cardiac surgery. This syndrome represents a particular form of cardiogenic shock, and marked metabolic abnormalities such as high concentrations of FFA, hypoxemia, and lactic acidosis are frequently seen. An early small controlled trial consisting of 22 patients saw GIK to significantly decrease plasma FFA levels and increase cardiac index (by up to 40%) after 12 hs of therapy versus a control group treated with standard therapy (inotropic support and intra-aortic balloon pumping, $p < 0.005$) *(100,101)*. Svedjeholm and colleagues showed GIK to enhance the inotropic effect of dobutamine, decrease circulating FFA levels and myocardial FFA uptake, and increase mechanical efficiency *(102)*. Following on from this work, the same group showed GIK to improve hemodynamic function in a group of 16 patients who had signs of cardiac failure after surgery *(102)*. The largest trial performed involved 322 consecutive patients with postoperative heart failure *(103)*. GIK significantly reduced hospital mortality by 35% ($p < 0.02$) and reduced the length of stay in intensive care (compared with a standard control group).

Further randomized trials with larger patient numbers are needed to investigate the effects of GIK further and find out whether adoption of a metabolic strategy prevents the development of, or reverses the changes seen in, cardiogenic shock in the setting of an acute myocardial infarction.

EFFECTS OF SHOCK ON OTHER ORGANS

As the cardiac pump fails, systemic tissue perfusion becomes markedly reduced. This leads to changes and adaptations in several other organs.

Renal Failure

Renal failure is a major complication of circulatory shock, developing within 36–72 h after the onset of the condition. Renal blood flow can be reduced to as low as 10% of normal. α-Adrenergic action and renal nerve sympathetic activity cause vasoconstriction, which diminishes blood flow to the cortical areas leading to renal tubular injury. This progresses to cellular necrosis and tubular obstruction, with accumulation of proteinaceous and cellular debris in the tubular lumen. Back-diffusion and leakage of the glomerular filtrate may cause tubular collapse (104). Initially, there is an increase in sodium and water resorption resulting from the secretion of antidiuretic hormone (ADH) and aldosterone in response to low blood flow—this also enhances back-diffusion. Eventually, the system fails to respond to increases in aldosterone and ADH. Both sodium and urea concentration in the medulla are reduced so that the hypertonic gradient for resorption of water is disabled, leading to loss of the capability of the kidneys to concentrate solute (105).

Pulmonary Function

Early changes include increases in ventilation resulting in an increased ventilation–perfusion mismatch and an increased physiological dead space and alveolar capillary gradient for oxygen. Initially, pulmonary vascular resistance is only mildly elevated, but this increases as hypoxia worsens. Adult respiratory distress syndrome (ARDS) may eventually develop as a result of circulatory collapse and progressive pulmonary injury (106). Primary pulmonary failure is relatively uncommon in patients with cardiogenic shock. Significant lactic acidosis would induce Kussmaul breathing.

Changes in Skeletal Muscle

The resting transmembrane potential declines as a result of decreased blood supply, resulting in impaired membrane transport. The most important muscle affected is the diaphragm, which accounts for decreased efficiency of ventilation and increases oxygen requirements for breathing (107). When oxygen delivery is severely decreased, the increased work requirements may reduce the patient's ability to breathe, resulting in alveolar hypoventilation with hypercarbia and hypoxemia (108), which may require mechanically assisted ventilation. Prolonged hypoperfusion may also result in increasing production of lactate, thus exacerbating respiratory acidosis by metabolic acidosis.

Gastrointestinal System

Massive hepatic necrosis and overt liver failure are uncommon in patients with cardiogenic shock. Nonspecific increases in aspartate aminotransferase (AST), alanine aminotransferase (ALT), and lactate dehydrogenase (LDH) are commonly seen (109). Hepatic congestion renders the liver less able to metabolize lactate, thereby compounding lactic acidosis. Intestinal ischemia leading to submucosal bleeding is relatively uncommon, although it is seen more frequently in elderly patients with preceding atherosclerotic disease of the arteries supplying the intestine. Blood flow to the pancreas is markedly reduced and necrosis is infrequently seen (110).

Blood

With slowing of blood flow, there is intravascular aggregation and clumping of red cells, white cells, and platelets, causing sludging. This process itself may elevate vas-

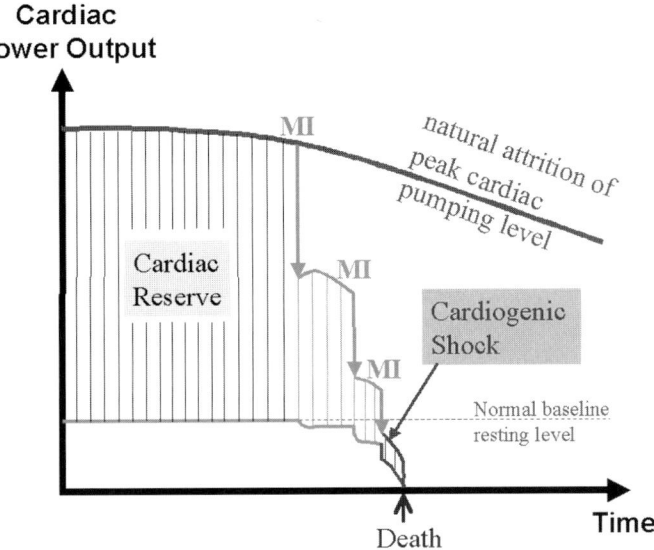

Fig. 6. A conceptual schematic diagram representing progressive deterioration of cardiac pumping capability and reserve with time. Two mechanisms of cardiomyocyte losses are depicted: (1) through natural attrition of myocytes with age and (2) through discrete myocardial infarctions (MI), which cause stepwise reductions in cardiac pumping reserve. After cumulative MIs, when the peak cardiac pumping level falls below the normal baseline resting level, the prognosis is very poor, with a high probability of death unless viable function can be restored without delay through interventions.

cular resistance. Severe shock may result in disseminated intravascular coagulation (DIC). Typical laboratory findings include thrombocytopenia, prolongation of prothrombin time and partial thromboplastin time, decreased levels of factor V and VIII, and an increased concentration of fibrin monomers and fibrin split products.

Brain

Autoregulation maintains constancy of cerebral blood flow protecting the cerebral circulation, but when perfusion pressure falls below the autoregulatory range, the resulting hypoperfusion leads to mental obtundation, drowsiness, and occasional confusional states. It is, however, unusual to see lasting cerebral insult unless there is intrinsic cerebrovascular disease *(111)*.

SUMMARY

The pathophysiological concept of the cumulative effects of myocardial infarctions on cardiac pump function culminating in the onset of cardiogenic shock is depicted in Fig. 6. In the absence of cardiac disease, Olivetti and colleagues *(112)* have shown that the number of cardiac myocytes decreases with age, and compensatory remodeling could not ameliorate the progressive loss of function. When discrete masses of cardiac myocytes are damaged through infarction, stepwise losses of cardiac function occur. When the cardiac reserve function is so compromised that the failing heart becomes barely able to maintain the baseline circulation at rest, cardiogenic shock ensues. Aggressive medical and interventional measures are required to prevent or regain the loss of cardiac functional reserve, through preserving or restoring the viability of cardiomyocyte function.

The pathophysiology of cardiogenic shock involves a vicious downward spiral: myocardial hypoperfusion causing myocardial dysfunction, which, in turn, worsens the hypoperfusion. The key to a good outcome is a prompt recognition of the preshock state in order to initiate therapy early to prevent the onset of cardiogenic shock. Once the state of shock has been reached, therapeutic success depends largely on a systematic approach to diagnosis, clear conceptual understanding of the pathophysiological processes involved, careful hemodynamic monitoring of cardiac performance, and responses to treatment; the immediate goal is sensible priority setting of management plans and adjustment of appropriate therapy. Recent work has suggested that metabolic changes may be just as important as coronary revascularization and this exciting clinical area should be the subject of further research.

REFERENCES

1. Schoen FJ, Bernhard WF, Khuri SF, Koster JK Jr, Van Devanter SJ, Weintraub RM. Pathologic findings in postcardiotomy patients managed with a temporary left ventricular assist pump. Am J Surg 1982;143:508–514.
2. Asou T, Kawachi Y, Imaizumi T, Tokunaga K, Life-saving pericardiectomy in cardiogenic shock due to impairment of diastolic pump function by myocardial swelling. Scand J Thorac Cardiovasc Surg 1995;29:83–85.
3. Risoe C, Hall C, Smiseth OA. Blood volume changes in liver and spleen during cardiogenic shock in dogs. Am J Physiol 1991;261:H1763–H1768.
4. Hollenberg SM, Kavinsky CJ, Parrillo JE. Cardiogenic shock (review). Ann Intern Med 1999;131:47–59
5. Willerson JT, Scales F, Mukherjee A, Platt M, Templeton GH, Fink GS, et al. Abnormal myocardial fluid retention as an early manifestation of ischemic injury. Am J Pathol 1977;87:159–188.
6. Jennings RB. Early phase of myocardial ischemic injury and infarction. Am J Cardiol 1969;24:753–765.
7. Harris P. Evolution and the cardiac patient (review). Cardiovasc Res 1983;17:313–319.
8. Harris P. Evolution and the cardiac patient (review). Cardiovasc Res 1983;17:373–378.
9. Harris P. Evolution and the cardiac patient (review). Cardiovasc Res 1983;17:437–445.
10. Harris P. Congestive cardiac failure: central role of the arterial blood pressure. St Cyres Lecture 1986. Br Heart J 1987;58:190–203.
11. Afifi AA, Chang PC, Liu VY, da Luz PL, Weil MH, Shubin H. Prognostic indexes in acute myocardial infarction complicated by shock. Am J Cardiol 1974;33:826–832.
12. Armiger LC, Herdson PB, Gavin JB. Mitochondrial changes in dog myocardium induced by lowered pH in vitro. Lab Invest 1975;32:223–226.
13. Udhoji VN, Weil MH. Circulatory effects of angiotensin, levarterenol and metaraminol in the treatment of shock. N Engl J Med 1964;270:501–507.
14. Abboud FM, Heistad DD, Mark AL, Schmid PG. Reflex control of the peripheral circulation. Prog Cardiovasc Dis 1976;1:371–403.
15. Gilbert RP, Aldrich SL, Anderson L. Cardiac output in acute myocardial infarction. J Clin Invest 1951;30:640.
16. Freis ED, Schnaper HW, Johnson RL, Schneider GE. Hemodynamic alterations in acute myocardial infarction: I. Cardiac output, mean arterial pressure, total peripheral resistance, "central" and total blood volumes, venous pressure and average circulation time. J Clin Invest 1952;31:131–140.
17. Smith WW, Wickler NS, Fox AC. Hemodynamic studies of patients with myocardial infarction. Circulation 1954;9:352–362.
18. Malmcrona R, Schroder G, Werko L. Hemodynamic effects of metaraminol: II. Patients with acute myocardial infarction. Am J Cardiol 1964;13:15–24.
19. Smulyan H, Cuddy RP, Eich RH. Hemodynamic effects of pressor agents in septic and myocardial infarction shock. JAMA 1964;190:188.

20. Shubin H, Weil MH. Hemodynamic effects of vasopressor agents in shock due to myocardial infarction. Am J Cardiol 1965;15:147.

21. Gunnar RM, Cruz A, Boswell J, Co BS, Pietras RJ, Tobin JR Jr. Myocardial infarction with shock. Hemodynamic studies and results of therapy. Circulation 1966;33:753–762.

22. Smith HJ, Oriol A, Morch J, McGregor M. Hemodynamic studies in cardiogenic shock. Treatment with isoproterenol and metaraminol. Circulation 1967;35:1084–1091.

23. Ratshin RA, Rackley CE, Russell RO. Hemodynamic evaluation of left ventricular function in shock complicating myocardial infarction. Circulation 1972;45:127–139.

24. Swan HJC, Forrester JS, Diamond G, Chatterjee K, Parmley WW. Hemodynamic spectrum of myocardial infarction and cardiogenic shock. A conceptual model. Circulation 1972;45:1097–1110.

25. Scheidt S, Wilner G, Fillmore S, Shapiro M, Killip T. Objective hemodynamic assessment after acute myocardial infarction. Br Heart J 1973;35:908–916.

26. Tan LB, Littler WA. Measurement of cardiac reserve in cardiogenic shock: implications for prognosis and management. Br Heart J 1990;64:121–128.

27. Hasdai D, Holmes DR Jr, Califf RM, Thompson TD, Hochman JS, Pfisterer M, et al. Cardiogenic shock complicating acute myocardial infarction: predictors of death. GUSTO (Global Utilization of Streptokinase and Tissue–Plasminogen Activator for Occluded Coronary Arteries) Investigators. Am Heart J 1999;138:21–31.

28. Williams SG, Wright DJ, Tan LB. Management of cardiogenic shock complicating acute myocardial infarction: towards evidence based medical practice. Heart 2000;83:621–626.

29. Gunnar RM, Loeb HS. Shock in acute myocardial infarction: evolution of physiologic therapy. J Am Coll Cardiol 1983;1:154–163.

30. Waltier DC. Ventricular Function. Williams & Wilkins, Baltimore, 1995.

31. Spodick DH. Assessment of Ventricular Function. Karger, Basel, 1985.

32. Tan LB. Clinical and research implications of new concepts in the assessment of cardiac pumping performance in heart failure. Cardiovasc Res 1987;21:615–622.

33. Tan LB. Evaluation of cardiac dysfuncton, cardiac reserve and inotropic response. Postgrad Med J 1991;67(suppl 1):S10–S20.

34. Hochman JS, Sleeper LA, Godfrey E, et al. Should we emergently revascularize occluded coronaries for cardiogenic shock: an international randomized trial of emergency PTCA/CABG—trial design. Am Heart J 1999;137:313–321.

35. Wackers FJ, Lie KI, Becker AE, et al. Coronary artery disease in patients dying from cardiogenic shock or Congestive heart failure in the setting of acute myocardial infarction. Br Heart J 1976;38:906.

36. Page DL, Caulfield JB, Kastor JA, et al. Myocardial changes associated with cardiogenic shock. N Engl J Med 1972;285:133.

37. Alonso DR, Scheidt S, Post M, et al. Pathophysiology of cardiogenic shock: quantification of myocardial necrosis, clinical, pathologic and electrocardiographic correlation. Circulation 1973;48:588.

38. Goldberg RJ, Samad NA, Yarzebski J, Gurwitz J, Bigelow C, Gore JM. Temporal trends in cardiogenic shock complicating acute myocardial infarction. N Engl J Med 1999;340:1162–1168.

39. Hasdai D, Topol EJ, Califf RM, Berger PB, Holmes DR Jr. Cardiogenic shock complicating acute coronary syndromes. Lancet 2000;356:749–756.

40. Olivetti G, Quaini F, Sala R, et al. Acute myocardial infarction in humans is associated with activation of programmed myocyte cell death in the surviving portion of the heart. J Mol Cell Cardiol 1996;28:2005–2016.

41. Tan LB. Cardiac pumping capability and prognosis in heart failure. Lancet 1986;ii:1360–1363.

42. Williams SG, Cooke GA, Wright DJ, Tan LB. Disparate results of ACE inhibitor dosage on exercise capacity in heart failure: a reappraisal of vasodilator therapy and study design. Int J Cardiol 2001;77:239–245.

43. Wylam ME, Samsel RW, Umans JG, Mitchell RW, Leff AR, Schumacker PT. Endotoxin in vivo impairs endothelium-dependent relaxation of canine arteries in vitro. Am Rev Respir Dis 1990;142:1263–1267.

44. Schumacker PT. Peripheral vascular responses in septic shock. Chest 1991;99:1057–1058.

45. Umans JG, Wylam ME, Samsel RW, Edwards J, Schumacker PT. Effects of endotoxin in vivo on endothelial and smoothe-muscle function in rabbit and rat aorta. Am Rev Res Dis 1993;148:1638–1645.

46. Strandgaard S, Olesen J, Skinhoj E, Lassen NA. Autoregulation of brain circulation in severe arterial hypertension. Br Med J 1973;159:507–510.
47. Marcus ML, Harrison DG, Chilian WM, et al. Alterations in the coronary circulation in hypertrophied ventricles. Circulation 1987;75(suppl I):I-19–I-25.
48. Polese A, De Cesare N, Montorsi P, et al. Upward shift of the lower range of coronary flow autoregulation in hypertensive patients with hypertrophy of the left ventricle. Circulation 1991;83:845–853.
49. SUPPORT Principal Investigators. A controlled trial to improve care for seriously ill hospitalized patients. The Study to Understand Prognoses and Preferences for Outcomes and Risks of Treatments (SUPPORT). JAMA 1995;274:1591–198.
50. Roul G, Moulichon ME, Bareiss P, et al. Prognostic factors of chronic heart failure in NYHA class II or III: value of invasive exercise haemodynamic data. Eur Heart J 1995;16:1387–1398.
51. Williams SG, Cooke GA, Wright DJ, Parsons WJ, Riley RL, Marshall P, et al. Peak exercise cardiac power output: a direct indicator of cardiac function strongly predictive of prognosis in chronic heart failure. Eur Heart J 2001, 22:1496–1503.
52. Tan LB. Cardiac function. In: Glasby MA, Huang CL-H, eds. Applied Physiology for Surgery and Critical Care. Butterworth–Heinemann, Oxford, 1995, pp. 138–150.
53. Bing RJ. Cardiac metabolism. Physiol Rev 1965;45:171.
54. Rushmer RF. Cardiovascular Dynamics. WB Saunders, Philadelphia, 1970.
55. Lentner C, ed. Geigy Scientific Tables. Heart and Circulation. Ciba–Geigy, Basel, 1990.
56. Randle MJ, Morgan HE. Regulation of glucose uptake by muscle. Vitam Horm 1962; 20:199–249.
57. Mirsky I, Ghista DN, Sandler H, eds. Cardiac Mechanics: Physiological, Clinical and Mathematical Considerations. Wiley, New York, 1974.
58. Gibbs CL. Cardiac energetics. In: Langer GA, Brady AJ, eds. The Mammalian Myocardium. Wiley, New York, 1974.
59. Whitman G Jr, Chance B, Bode H, et al. Diagnosis and therapeutic evaluation of a pediatric case of cardiomyopathy using phosphorus-31 magnetic resonance spectroscopy. J Am Coll Cardiol 1985;5:745–749.
60. Bittl JA, Ingwall JS. Reaction rates of creatine kinase and ATP synthesis in the isolated rat heart. A ^{31}P NMR magnetization transfer study. J Biol Chem 1985;260:3512–3527.
61. Opie LH. The Heart: Physiology, Metabolism, Pharmacology and Therapy. Grune & Stratton, London, 1984.
62. Coleman HN, Sonnenblick EH, Braunwald E. Myocardial oxygen consumption associated with external work. The Fenn effect. Am J Physiol 1969;217:291–296.
63. Rooke GA, Feigl ER. Work as a correlate of canine left ventricular oxygen consumption, and the problem of catecholamine oxygen wasting. Circ Res 1982;50:273–286.
64. Gibbs CL, Mommaerts WFHM, Ricchiuti NV. Energetics of cardiac contractions. J Physiol 1967;191:25–46.
65. Rodbard S, Williams CB, Rodbard D, et al. Myocardial tension and oxygen uptake. Circ Res 1964;14:139–149.
66. Klocke FJ, Braunwald E, Ross J Jr. Oxygen cost of electrical activation of the heart. Circ Res 1966;18:357.
67. Boerth RC, Covell JW, Pool PE, Ross J. Increased myocardial oxygen consumption and contractile state associated with increased heart rate in dogs. Circ Res 1969;24:725.
68. Gibbs CL. Cardiac energetics and the Fenn effect. Basic Res Cardiol 1987;82 (suppl 2):61–68.
69. Sonnenblick EH, Ross J Jr, Braunwald E. Oxygen consumption of the heart. Newer concepts of its multifactoral determination. Am J Cardiol 1968;22:328–360.
70. Braunwald E, Sarnoff SJ, Case RB, Stainsby WN, Welch GH. Hemodynamic determinants of coronary flow: effect of changes in aortic pressure and cardiac output on the relationship between myocardial oxygen consumption and coronary flow. Am J Physiol 1958;192:157–163.
71. Braunwald E. Control of myocardial oxygen consumption: physiologic and clinical considerations. Am J Cardiol 1971;27:416–432.
72. Braunwald E. Myocardial oxygen consumption: the quest for its determinants and some clinical fall-out. JACC 1999;34:1365–1368.
73. Li JK-L. Comparative cardiac mechanics: LaPlace's Law. J Theor Biol 1986;118:339–343.
74. Vik-Mo H, Mjos OD. Influence of free fatty acids on myocardial oxygen consumption and ischemic injury. Am J Cardiol 1981;48:361–365.

75. Brachfeld N, Scheuer J. Metabolism of glucose by the ischemic dog heart. Am J Physiol 1967;212:603–606.
76. Danforth WH, Naegle S, Bing RJ. Effects of ischemia and reoxygenation on glycolytic reactions and adenosine triphosphate in heart muscle. Circ Res 1960;8:965–971.
77. Shea TM, Watson RM, Protrowski SF, Dermksian G, Case RB. Anaerobic myocardial metabolism. Am J Physiol 1962;203:463–469.
78. Huckabee WE. Relationship of pyruvate and lactate during anaerobic metabolism. V. Coronary adequacy. Am J Physiol 1961;200:1169–1176.
79. Parker JO, Chiong MA, West RO, Case RB. Sequential alterations in myocardial lactate metbolism, ST segments and left ventricular function during angina induced by atrial pacing. Circulation 1969;40:113–131.
80. Kubler W. Glycolytic pathway in the myocardium. In: Muir JR, ed. Prospects in the Management of Ischaemic Heart Disease. CIBA Lab, Horsham, UK, 1972.
81. Green DE, Goldberger RF. Pathways of metabolism in heart muscle. Am J Med 1961;30:666–678.
82. Lehninger AL. Bioenergetics. Benjamin, New York, 1971.
83. Hollenberg SM, Parrillo JE. Shock. In: Fauci AS, Braunwald E, Wilson JD, et al., eds. Harrison's Principles of Internal Medicine. 14th ed. McGraw-Hill, New York, 1998, pp. 214–222.
84. Bartling B, Holtz J, Darmer D. Contribution of myocyte apoptosis to myocardial infarction. Basic Res Cardiol 1998;93:71–84.
85. Nascimben L, Pauletto P, Pessina AC, Reis I, Ingwall JS. Decreased energy reserve may cause pump failure in human dilated cardiomyopathy. Circulation 1991;84(suppl II):II-563.
86. Massie BM, Conway M, Yonge R, et al. P(31) nuclear magnetic resonance evidence of abnormal skeletal muscle metabolism in patients with congestive heart failure. Am J Cardiol 1987;60:309–315.
87. Nascimben L, Friedrich J, Liao R, Pauleto P, Pessina AC, Ingwall JS. Enalapril treatment increases cardiac performance and energy reserve via the creatine kinase reaction in myocardium of Syrian myopathic hamsters with advanced heart failure. Circulation 1995;91:1824–1833.
88. Neely JR, Morgan HE. Relationship between carbohydrate and lipid metabolism and the energy balance of heart muscle. Annu Rev Physiol 1974;36:413–459.
89. Oliver MF, Opie LH. Effects of glucose and fatty acids on myocardial ischemia and arrhythmias. Lancet 1994;343:155–158.
90. Liedtke AJ. Lipid burden in ischemic myocardium. J Moll Cell Cardiol 1988;20(suppl II):65–74.
91. Svedjeholm R, Hakanson E, Vanhanen I. Rationale for metabolic support with amino acids and glucose–insulin–potassium (GIK) in cardiac surgery. Ann Thorac Surg 1995;59(2 suppl):S15–S22.
92. Svedjeholm R, Huljebrant R, Hakanson E, Vanhanen I. Glutamate and high-dose glucose–insulin–potassium (GIK) in the treatment of severe cardiac failure after cardiac operations. Ann Thorac Surg 1995;59:S23–S30.
93. Apstein CS. Increased glycolytic substrate protection improves ischemic cardiac dysfunction and reduces injury. Am Heart J 2000;139(suppl2):S107–S114.
94. Sodi-Pallares D, Testelli M, Fishleder F. Effects of an intravenous infusion of a potassium–insulin–glucose solution on the electrocardiographic signs of myocardial infarction. Am J Cardiol 1962;9:166–181.
95. Apstein CS. Glucose–insulin–potassium for acute myocardial infarction: remarkable results from a new prospective, randomized trial. Circulation 1998;98:2223–2226.
96. Fath-Ordoubadi F, Beatt KJ. Glucose–insulin–potassium therapy for treatment of acute myocardial infarction: an overview of randomized placebo-controlled trials. Circulation 1997;96:1152–1156.
97. Malmberg K, Ryden L, Hamsten A, Herlitz J, Waldenstrom A, Wedel H. Effects on insulin treatment on cause specific one-year mortality and morbidity in diabetic patients with acute myocardial infarction: DIGAMI study group: diabetes insulin–glucose in acute myocardial infarction. Eur Heart J 1996;17:1337–1344.
98. Diaz R, Paolasso EA, Piegas LS, et al. Metabolic modulation of acute myocardial infarction. The ECLA (Estudios Cardiologicos Latinoamerica) Collaborative Group. Circulation 1998;98:2227–2234.
99. Stanley AW, Moraski RE, Russell RO, et al. Effects of glucose–insulin–potassium on myocardial substrate availability and utilization in stable coronary artery disease: studies on myocardial carbohydrates, lipid and oxygen arterial-coronary sinus differences in patients with coronary artery disease. Am J Cardiol 1975;36:929–937.
100. Coleman GM, Gradinac S, Taegtmeyer H, Sweeney M, Frazier OH. Efficacy of metabolic support with glucose–insulin–potassium for left ventricular pump failure after aortocoronary bypass surgery. Circulation 1989;80(suppl I):I91–I96.

101. Gradinac S, Coleman GM, Taegtmeyer H, Sweeney MS, Frazier OH. Improved cardiac function with glucose-insulin-potassium after aortocoronary bypass grafting. Ann Thorac Surg 1989;48:484–489.

102. Svedjeholm R, Hallhagen S, Ekroth R, Joachimsson PO, Ronquist G. Dopamine and high-dose insulin infusion (glucose–insulin–potassium) after a cardiac operation: effects on myocardial metabolism. Ann Thorac Surg 1991;51:262–270.

103. Taegtmeyer H, Goodwin GW, Doenst T, Frazier OH. Substrate metabolism as a determinant for postischemic functional recovery of the heart. Am J Cardiol 1997;80:3A–10A.

104. Donohoe JF, Venkatachalam MA, Bernard DB, Levinsky NG. Tubular leakage and obstruction after renal ischemia: structural–functional correlations. Kidney Int 1978;13:208–222.

105. Brown R, Babcock R, Talbert J, Gruenberg J, Czurak C, Campbell M. Renal function in critically ill postoperative patients: sequential assessment of creatinine osmolar and free water clearance. Crit Care Med 1980;8:68–72.

106. Rinaldo JE, Rogers RM. Adult respiratory-distress syndrome: changing concepts of lung injury and repair. N Engl J Med 1982;306:900–909.

107. Johnson G III, Henderson D, Bond RF. Morphological differences in cutaneous and skeletal muscle vasculature during compensatory and decompensatory hemorrhagic hypotension. Circ Shock 1985;15:111–121.

108. Henning RJ, Shubin H, Weil MH. The measurement of the work of breathing for the clinical assessment of ventilator dependence. Crit Care Med 1977;5:264–268.

109. Shubin H, Weil MH. Acute elevation of serum transaminase and lactate dehydrogenase during circulatory shock. Am J Cardiol 1963;11:327–332.

110. Herlihy BL, Lefer AM. Alterations in pancreatic acinar cell organelles during circulatory shock. Circ Shock 1975;2:143–146.

111. Johansson B, Standgaard S, Lassen NA. On the pathogenesis of hypertensive encephalopathy. The hypertensive breakthrough of autoregulation of cerebral blood flow with forced vasodilatation, flow increase, and blood brain-barrier damage. Circ Res 1974;35:167–177.

112. Olivetti G, Melissari M, Capasso JM, Anversa P. Cardiomyopathy of the aging human heart. Myocyte loss and reactive cellular hypertrophy. Circ Res 1991;68:1560–1568.

113. Milnor WR. Cardiovascular Physiology. Oxford University Press, New York, 1990.

II CARDIOGENIC SHOCK COMPLICATING ACUTE CORONARY SYNDROMES

3

Cardiogenic Shock Complicating Non–ST-Segment Elevation Acute Coronary Syndrome

*David R. Holmes, Jr., MD,
and David Hasdai, MD*

CONTENTS

A man aged 55 in good health was seized with severe pain in the lower precordial region. When I saw him twelve hours from the attack, there was moderate cyanosis and mild dyspnea. The chest was full of fine and coarse moist rales; there was a running feeble pulse of 140. Urine was scanty.

Herrick, Dec. 7, 1912

Classically, cardiogenic shock has been considered a sequela of ST-segment elevation myocardial infarction, most commonly caused by left ventricular dysfunction resulting from ongoing ischemia and cell necrosis. In keeping with this scenario, most of the current literature on cardiogenic shock confines itself to ST-segment elevation. It must be remembered, however, that Herrick's classic description of cardiogenic shock in 1912 predated the discovery and application of electrocardiography, emphasizing the important fact that in the setting of acute myocardial infarction, shock may occur irrespective of the direction of the electrocardiographic abnormalities.

In the setting of non–ST-segment elevation, there are limited data on the incidence, timing, risk factors, and outcome of shock compared with the abundant information available regarding ST-segment elevation. This has important implications, as the incidence of non–ST-segment elevation infarction appears to be increasing. Furman et al., in a population-based study, found that although the incidence of Q-wave

From: *Contemporary Cardiology: Cardiogenic Shock: Diagnosis and Treatment*
Edited by: David Hasdai et al. © Humana Press Inc., Totowa, NJ

Table 1
Baseline Patient Characteristics in ST-Elevation Versus Non–ST-Segment
Elevation Shock Patients

	GUSTO IIb			SHOCK Registry		
	ST elevation	No ST elevation	p	ST elevation (n = 729)	No ST elevation (n = 152)	p
Age (yr)	70	73	0.015	67.9	71.4	<0.001
Prior MI (%)	24	44	<0.001	36.7	55.7	<0.001
Prior CABG (%)	4	18	<0.001	8.4	18.5	<0.001
CHF (%)	4	12	0.001	16.5	35.2	<0.001
Hx CRI (%)	—	—	—	8.4	20.7	<0.001
DM (%)	21	34	0.002	33.2	31.3	0.703
PVD (%)	—	—	—	16.4	28.4	0.007

Abbreviations: MI = myocardial infarction, CABG = coronary artery bypass graft surgery, CHF = congestive heart failure, CRI = chronic renal insufficiency, DM = diabetes mellitus, PVD = peripheral vascular disease.

infarction declined from 1975 to 1997, the incidence of non–Q-wave infarction increased significantly *(1)*.

INCIDENCE

The incidence of cardiogenic shock irrespective of electrocardiographic abnormalities has been studied in large population-based analyses as well as in subset analyses of randomized clinical trials. One of the largest populations studied to date involved the Global Use of Strategies to Open Occluded Coronary Arteries (GUSTO IIb) trial *(2)*. In this trial, shock was a predefined subset, and it occurred in 2.6% of patients with non–ST-segment elevation; this was approx 50% less than its incidence in patients with ST-segment elevation (odds ratio [OR] 0.50, 95% confidence interval [CI] 0.413, 0.612, $p < 0.001$) *(3)*. In the multicenter SHOCK (SHould we emergently revascularize Occluded coronaries for Cardiogenic shocK) Registry, there were 881 patients with cardiogenic shock secondary to predominant left ventricular (LV) failure *(4)*. Of this relatively pure patient group, 152 patients were classified as having non–ST-segment elevation infarction. The incidence of shock has also been analyzed in the PURSUIT (Platelet glycoprotein IIb/IIIa in Unstable angina: Receptor Suppression Using Integrilin Therapy) trial of patients with acute coronary syndromes but without persistent ST-segment elevation *(5)*. Of the 9449 patients enrolled, 2.5% (237) developed shock after enrollment.

CLINICAL SETTING (TABLE 1)

Cardiogenic shock with non–ST-segment elevation infarction also occurs in patients with different clinical characteristics than those with ST-segment elevation. A prototypical scenario of shock with ST-segment elevation is a large anterior infarction with no collaterals and a massive amount of jeopardized or necrotic myocardium. In the GUSTO IIb trial, in contrast to ST-segment elevation, shock in the setting of non–ST-segment elevation occurred in higher-risk patients—older age *(73* yr vs 70 yr, $p < 0.034$), higher frequency of prior myocardial infarction (44% vs 24%, $p < 0.001$), prior coronary bypass

Table 2
Angiographic Findings

	GUSTO IIb			SHOCK Registry		
	ST↑	No ST↑	p	ST↑	No ST↑	p
Patients	90	91		351	52	
Diseased vessels			<0.001			<0.001
0/1	32.9	8.9		24.8	6.9	
2	36.8	26.6		21.7	16.4	
3	30.0	64.6		53.5	76.7	
Infarct-related artery			<0.001			0.001
LAD	46.1	24.2		50.1	36.5	
Circ	4.5	17.6		13.4	34.6	
RCA	43.8	16.5		30.2	17.3	
Other						
TIMI grade			0.012			0.513
0	57.0	28.8		66.9[a]	66.7[a]	
1	8.9	11.5				
2	11.4	17.3		18.8	26.7	
3	22.8	42.3		14.4	6.7	

Abbreviations: LAD = left anterior descending coronary artery; Circ = circumflex coronary artery; RCA = right coronary artery.

[a] These are the percentages of patients in combined TIMI grades 0/1.

graft surgery (18% vs 4%, $p < 0.001$), and diabetes mellitus (34% vs 21%, $p = 0.005$). In the SHOCK Registry, non–ST-segment-elevation patients were also at higher risk from the standpoint of adverse baseline characteristics, including older age, more prior myocardial infarction, congestive heart failure, renal insufficiency, and prior coronary artery bypass graft surgery (all $p < 0.001$) (6). Each of these characteristics has been associated with a higher risk of mortality in association with infarction.

There were other striking similarities between the GUSTO IIb and SHOCK Registry datasets:

1. Shock occurred later after symptom onset in non–ST-segment elevation patients than in those with ST-segment elevation. In GUSTO IIb, patients with non–ST-segment elevation developed shock a median of 76.2 h after the onset of infarction in contrast to ST-segment-elevation patients in whom the median time interval from onset of infarction to shock was 9.6 h. In the SHOCK Registry, the time from myocardial infarction onset to shock onset was also different: 8.9 h for non–ST-segment-elevation infarction versus 5.9 h for ST-segment-elevation infarction.

2. There was more recurrent ischemia or reinfarction in the non–ST-segment-elevation group. In GUSTO IIb, recurrent ischemia occurred more than twice as frequently in non–ST-segment elevation (54.8% vs 29.5%, $p < 0.001$), and reinfarction occurred almost three times as frequently (32.0% vs 12.4%, $p < 0.001$). In the SHOCK Registry, there was a trend toward more recurrent ischemia in non–ST-segment elevation (25.7% vs 17.4%, $p = 0.058$), although the proportion of patients with reinfarction was similar.

3. Patients with non–ST-segment elevation had more three-vessel disease than did patients with ST-segment-elevation (Table 2). In the GUSTO IIb experience, 64.6% of non–ST-

Table 3
Predictors of Shock Developing Among Patients in PURSUIT Who Had Acute
Coronary Syndromes But Did Not Have Persistent ST-Segment Elevation

Variable	Chi square	p-Value	Odds ratio	95% CI
Age (yr)	40.31	0.0001	1.05	1.03–1.06
ST ↓ (>0.5 mm)	15.90	0.0001	1.77	1.34–2.34
Sys BP (mmHg)	10.53	0.001	0.99	0.98–0.996
Angina	8.39	0.004	1.92	1.24–2.98
Pulse (beats/min)	7.84	0.005	1.01	1.004–1.022
Height (cm)	6.57	0.009	0.98	0.97–0.995
Enrolling MI	4.48	0.03	1.35	1.02–1.78
Rales [a] ≤1/3 (vs none)	5.34	0.02	1.56	1.07–2.27
Rales >1/3 (vs none)	3.92	0.048	2.18	1.008–4.70

Source: Reprinted with permission from ref. *5.*

Abbreviations: ST↓ = ST-segment depression; Sys BP = systolic blood pressure at the time of enrollment; Enrolling MI = myocardial infarction at the time of enrollment.

[a] The presence of rales was categorized as restricted to the lower third of the lungs or above and both situations were compared with the absence of rales.

segment-elevation patients had three-vessel disease compared with 30.3% for ST-segment elevation; correspondingly, in the SHOCK Registry, 76.7% of patients with non–ST-segment elevation had three-vessel disease versus 53.5% for ST-segment elevation ($p = 0.001$).

4. A final point of similarity was the fact that in both datasets, the infarction size as assessed by creatine kinase elevation was significantly lower in the non–ST-segment-elevation group.

In the PURSUIT trial, from which patients with persistent ST-segment elevation were excluded, the 2.5% of patients who developed shock were also at higher risk in terms of baseline characteristics, including older age, more frequent hypertension, prior coronary artery disease, and heart failure. In addition, patients who developed shock more commonly had ST-segment depression at baseline. As was true in the GUSTO IIb and SHOCK Registry experiences, shock typically developed after admission; in PURSUIT, it most commonly developed more than 48 h after enrollment (median 94.0 h).

In summary, the clinical setting of cardiogenic shock with non–ST-segment elevation is characterized by more adverse baseline characteristics, more advanced coronary artery disease, but somewhat smaller infarctions. Shock in this population is more often the result of recurrent ischemia, reinfarction or, perhaps, diffuse subendocardial ischemia leading to the vicious cycle of hemodynamic deterioration and exacerbation of the ischemia.

PREDICTION OF SHOCK

The ability to predict the development of shock would be important in helping to identify new strategies that might improve outcome. Given the fact that with non–ST-segment elevation, shock usually occurs with some delay after the onset of infarction, a prediction algorithm might be able to be developed and tested. Evaluating this in the PURSUIT study, Hasdai et al. *(7)* identified factors associated with development of shock (Table 3) — most important, older age and ST depression greater than 0.5 mm. Using these factors, they developed a scoring algorithm (Table 4). As can be seen, the point score uses easily available clinical data and ranges from 95 to 266. Over this range, the probability of developing shock ranges from 0.1% to 35%. The concordance index of the original logistic model was 0.710 and of the validated model was 0.670. Hasdai et al. then tested the validity of this model from the PURSUIT database in the GUSTO IIb patients and found a concordance index of 0.682, again indicating reliability of the model in predicting shock.

OUTCOME

Once cardiogenic shock has occurred, the rate of mortality is dismal and not different irrespective of the status of ST-segment deviation. In the GUSTO IIb trial, 72.5% of non–ST-segment-elevation patients with shock died versus 63.0% of ST-segment-elevation patients. In the SHOCK Registry, the mortality was also high and comparable: 62.5% for non–ST-segment elevation and 60.4% for ST-segment elevation ($p = 0.649$). In the PURSUIT trial, 65.8% of shock patients died within 30 d. In a subset analysis among shock patients, those who had presented with infarction had a higher incidence of mortality at 30 d (77.2% compared with 52.7%, $p = 0.001$).

Of interest, in the PURSUIT trial, which tested the efficacy of the glycoprotein IIb/IIIa receptor inhibitor, eptifibatide, patients who developed shock and had been given the drug had a lower incidence of 30-d death (58.5% mortality vs 73.5% for placebo). The odds ratio of death within 30 d in patients treated with eptifibatide was 0.51 (95% CI 0.28–0.94, $p = 0.03$). Whether this effect was the result of chance remains unclear. Angioplasty was performed in only approx 29% of the PURSUIT patients, so it is unlikely that the reduction in mortality was related to improved outcome from percutaneous intervention. Platelet glycoprotein IIb/IIIa receptor inhibitors may have beneficial effects on the microvasculature (see Chapter 5 for further discussion of glycoprotein IIb/IIIa inhibitors). In these shock patients, there may be severe abnormalities of microvascular tone, which further increase subendocardial ischemia. Improvement of these abnormalities with a IIb/IIIa receptor antagonist may improve outcome in this manner.

The effect of revascularization strategies in patients with cardiogenic shock has been controversial because of selection bias. In patients with ST-segment elevation, large registry studies and a smaller randomized trial have documented improved outcome if revascularization could be achieved, either by percutaneous coronary intervention (PCI) or coronary artery bypass graft surgery *(7,8)*. There is very limited data on revascularization for non–ST-segment-elevation shock. In the SHOCK Registry, angioplasty was performed postshock less often in patients with non–ST-segment elevation than ST-segment elevation (17.8% vs 34%, $p = 0.001$). The authors used multivariate adjustment for patient age and treatment selected, including intra-aortic balloon pump, lytic therapy, angiography, and bypass surgery. They found a nonsignificant survival benefit for patients with non–ST-segment elevation.

CONCLUSION

Cardiogenic shock is not confined to the stereotypical setting of first infarction, large anterior wall involvement, and ST-segment elevation. Although shock occurs more frequently in the setting of ST-segment elevation, it also occurs without ST-segment

Table 4
Scoring Algorithm Predicting the Development of Shock

Step 1: Find points for each characteristic

Age		SBP		Pulse		Height		Miscellaneous risk factors	
Years	*Pts.[a]*	*mm/Hg*	*Pts.*	*bpm*	*pts.*	*cm*	*Pts.*	*Factor*	*Pts.*
30–39	12	40–59	77	40–59	7	130–139	49	Enrollment MI	8
40–49	25	60–79	71	60–79	14	140–149	43	Angina	18
50–59	38	80–99	65	80–99	21	150–159	38	ST depression	16
60–69	50	100–119	59	100–119	27	160–169	32	Rales ≤ 1/3 of lungs	12
70–79	62	120–139	53	120–139	34	170–179	27	Rales > 1/3 of lungs	21
80–89	75	140–159	48	140–159	41	180–189	22		
90–99	88	160–179	42	160–179	48	190–199	16		
≥100	100	180–199	36	180–200	55	200–209	11		
		200–219	30						
		220–239	24						
		240–259	18						
		260–279	12						
		≥280	6						

Step 2: Sum points		*Step 3: Look up risk corresponding to points*	
Factor	*Points*	*Total points*	*Probability of shock*
Age		95	0.1%
SBP		158	1%
Pulse		203	5%
Height		223	10%
MI		236	15%
Angina		245	20%
ST↓		253	25%
Rales		260	30%
Total		266	3%

Abbreviations: MI = myocardial infarction. SBP = systolic blood pressure. ST↓ = ST-segment depression.

Note: To predict the occurrence of cardiogenic shock, determine the points for each characteristic. The probability of shock development corresponds to the total number of points.

[a] Pts, = points.

Source: Reprinted with permission from ref. 5.

elevation, albeit less commonly. Patients with non–ST-segment elevation shock have more adverse baseline clinical and angiographic characteristics; they present later after the onset of infarction and more often as a result of recurrent ischemia or recurrent infarction.

Algorithms are now available to predict the development of shock. The ability to predict patients at highest risk for shock taken together with the longer time before shock develops offers the chance to design and test strategies to prevent this problem, which, when it develops, is associated with strikingly increased mortality.

REFERENCES

1. Furman MI, Dauerman HL, Goldberg RJ, Yarzbeski J, Lessard D, Gore JM. Twenty-two year (1975 to 1997) trends in the incidence, in-hospital and long-term case fatality rates from initial Q-wave and non-Q-wave myocardial infarction: a multi-hospital community-wide perspective. J Am Coll Cardiol 2001;37:1571–1580.
2. The GUSTO IIb Investigators. A comparison of recombinant hirudin with heparin for the treatment of acute coronary syndromes. N Engl J Med 1996;335:775–782.
3. Holmes DR Jr, Berger PB, Hochman JS, et al. Cardiogenic shock in patients with acute ischemic syndromes with and without ST-segment elevation. Circulation 1999;100:2067–2073.
4. Jacobs AK, French JK, Col J, et al. Cardiogenic shock with non-ST-segment elevation myocardial infarction: a report from the SHOCK Trial Registry. J Am Coll Cardiol 2000;36(3 suppl A):1091–1096.
5. Hasdai D, Harrington RA, Hochman JS, et al. Platelet glycoprotein IIb/IIIa blockade and outcome of cardiogenic shock complicating acute coronary syndromes without persistent ST-segment elevation. J Am Coll Cardiol 2000;36:685–692.
6. Hochman JS, Boland J, Sleeper LA, et al. Current spectrum of cardiogenic shock and effect of early revascularization on mortality. Results of an International Registry. Circulation 1995;91:873–881.
7. Hasdai D, Califf RM, Thompson TD, et al. Predictors of cardiogenic shock after thrombolytic therapy for acute myocardial infarction. J Am Coll Cardiol 2000;35:136–143.
8. Berger PB, Holmes DR Jr, Stebbins A, Bates ER, Califf RM, Topol EJ. Impact of an aggressive invasive catheterization and revascularization strategy on mortality in patients with cardiogenic shock in the Global Utilization of Streptokinase and Tissue Plasminogen Activator for Occluded Coronary Arteries (GUSTO I) trial. Circulation 1997;96:122–127.

4

Cardiogenic Shock Complicating ST-Segment Elevation Acute Coronary Syndrome

Peter B. Berger, MD, and David Hasdai, MD

Contents

EPIDEMIOLOGY OF SHOCK

Severe left ventricular dysfunction sufficient to cause cardiogenic shock can result from each of the acute coronary syndromes, including ST-elevation myocardial infarction, non–ST-elevation myocardial infarction, and unstable angina without infarction *(1)*. This chapter will focus on shock resulting from ST-elevation myocardial infarction. In part, because the definition of cardiogenic shock and the study population with acute coronary syndromes have varied in different series, the reported incidence of cardiogenic shock complicating acute coronary syndromes has also varied. In two large, international series of patients receiving thrombolytic therapy for acute myocardial infarction, the reported incidence of shock differed between countries, being greatest in the United States; whether this was the result of differing adherence of the diagnosis, different vigilance for identifying diagnostic criteria, the result of different therapies used in the countries, or true geographic variability, is unknown *(2,3)*.

The most common cause and most studied etiology of cardiogenic shock is acute ST-segment-elevation myocardial infarction (Table 1). In three large, international series of patients with ST-segment-elevation myocardial infarction receiving thrombolytic therapy for acute myocardial infarction, the incidence of cardiogenic shock ranged from 4.2% to 7.2% *(2–4)*. In earlier placebo-controlled studies, thrombolytic therapy was shown to reduce the frequency of cardiogenic shock by 25–45% *(5,6)*. However, the reported incidence of cardiogenic shock among ST-segment-elevation myocardial infarction receiving thrombolytic therapy suffers from selection bias, in

From: *Contemporary Cardiology: Cardiogenic Shock: Diagnosis and Treatment*
Edited by: David Hasdai et al. © Humana Press Inc., Totowa, NJ

Table 1
Baseline Characteristics and Outcomes of Patients with Cardiogenic Shock
With and Without ST-Segment Elevation

	ST↑	No ST↑
Incidence (%)	4.2	2.5
Median time from randomization to shock (h)	9.6	76.2
Baseline characteristics		
Median age (yr)	70	73
Diabetes mellitus (%)	21	34
Hyperlipidemia (%)	28	42
Hypertension (%)	40	59
Prior myocardial infarction (%)	24	44
Prior coronary bypass surgery (%)	4	18
Prior heart failure (%)	4	12
Prior angina (%)	52	85
3-Vessel coronary artery disease (%)	30	65
30-d Mortality (%)	63	73

that patients with cardiogenic shock are often not enrolled in multicenter random-ized trials. In population-based studies, the proportion of patients with acute myocardial infarction presenting with shock is much greater. Evidence of selection bias in the enrollment of patients with cardiogenic shock is provided by the observa-tion that in randomized trials, approx 90% of patients with shock developed it after enrollment and only approximately 10% had shock on arrival. However, in a popu-lation-based study of unselected patients enrolled with acute myocardial infarction, 56% of shock patients had shock upon arrival *(7)*. The lower enrollment of patients in randomized trials with cardiogenic shock at the time of enrollment is probably multifactorial, relating, in part, to difficulty in obtaining informed consent in high-risk populations, reluctance to enroll patients in such trials given the additional time requirements to obtain informed consent, and the widespread belief that direct angioplasty is superior to thrombolytic therapy for patients with cardiogenic shock. Among patients who have been enrolled in trials of thrombolytic therapy, the median time to the development of shock is 10 or 11 h, and nearly all patients who develop shock do so within 48 h of admission *(1,2,4)*.

PREDICTORS OF SHOCK

Because of the high mortality from cardiogenic shock, it is important to identify patients at high risk for developing shock so that preventive measures can be instituted, and if shock occurs nonetheless, treatment can be rapidly initiated. Algorithms have been devised to predict the occurrence of in-hospital cardiogenic shock among patients with acute coronary syndromes. An algorithm for patients with persistent ST-segment-elevation myocardial infarction was devised for patients randomized to thrombolytic therapy in the GUSTO-I trial (Table 2) that was subsequently validated in the Global Use of Strategies to Open occluded coronary arteries (GUSTO-III) trial with relatively high concordance *(8)*.

Table 2
Algorithm Predicting the Development of Cardiogenic Shock for Patients
with ST-Segment-Elevation Myocardial Infarction

Step 1. *Find points for each predictive factor*

Age		Heart rate		Systolic BP		Diastolic BP	
Yr	*Points*	*Beats/min*	*Points*	*mm Hg*	*Points*	*mm Hg*	*Points*
20	6	40	3	80	59	40	4
30	12	60	0	100	49	60	5
40	19	80	8	120	39	80	7
50	25	100	14	140	32	100	9
60	31	120	17	160	27	120	11
70	37	140	19	180	23	140	13
80	43	160	22	200	18	160	15
90	49	180	24	220	14	180	16
		200	27	240	9	200	18
		220	29	260	5		
		240	32	280	0		
		260	34				

Weight		Treatment		Killip class	
Kg	*Points*	*Tx*	*Points*	*Killip class*	*Points*
40	19	tPA	0	1	0
60	17	SK-IV	5	2	9
80	15	tPA + SK	3	3	17
100	12	SK-SQ	6		
120	10				
140	8				
160	6				
180	4				
200	2				
220	0				

MI Location		Miscellaneous Risk Factors	
Location	*Points*	*Factor*	*Points*
Anterior	8	Previous MI	5
Inferior	1	Previous CABG	6
Other	0	No previous PTCA	6
		Female	3
		Hypertension	2
		US	5

Step 2. Add points for all predictive factors: Age + Heart rate + Systolic blood pressure + Diastolic blood pressure + Weight + Treatment + MI location + Killip class + Miscellaneous risk factors = Total points

Table 2
(Continued)

Step 3. *Determine risk corresponding to total points*

Points	Probability of in-hospital cardiogenic shock (%)
92	1
103	2
110	3
114	4
118	5
130	10
137	15
142	20
146	25
149	30
152	35
155	40
158	45
160	50

Note: In step 1, find the value most closely matching the patient's risk factor and circle the points.

In step 2, add the total points for all predictive factors.

In step 3, determine the predicted occurrence of cardiogenic shock corresponding to the total number of points.

Abbreviations: BP = blood pressure; tPA = tissue-plasminogen activator, SK = streptokinase, IV = intravenous, SQ = subcutaneous, MI = myocardial infarction, CABG = coronary artery bypass grafting, PTCA = percutaneous transluminal coronary angioplasty, US = United States.

Source: Reprinted from Hasdai D, Topol EJ, Califf RM, Berger PB, Holmes DR Jr: Cardiogenic shock complicating acute coronary syndromes. Lancet 2000;356:749–756 with permission of The Lancet Ltd.

Among patients with ST-segment elevation, older age was the variable most strongly associated with shock; for every 10-yr increase in age, the risk of shock increased by 47%. Other predictors derived from the physical examination, such as systolic blood pressure, heart rate, and Killip class, were also strong predictors of subsequent development of shock. These parameters provided more than 85% of the information needed to predict shock in this model.

These algorithms underscore the importance of the history and physical examination. These physical examination variables were of much greater significance for predicting shock than variables such as prior myocardial infarction or infarct location *(8)*.

A limitation of these algorithms is that their ability to predict who will develop shock is only moderate. For example, in the GUSTO-I model of patients with ST-segment-elevation myocardial infarction, a patient with all of the characteristics associated with increased risk of developing shock had only a 50% chance of developing shock. However, patients without high-risk variables are very unlikely to develop shock during the hospitalization, and so this model has a better negative predictive value than positive predictive value and is better able to identify a low-risk group, which may still be of clinical benefit.

THERAPY AND PROGNOSIS

Pharmacologic Therapy

The initial treatment of cardiogenic shock resulting from left ventricular dysfunction requires the intravenous administration of dopamine or other vasopressors, or perhaps dobutamine if the systemic vascular resistance is high. Volume status should be optimized, and either diuretics or fluids should be administered if the left ventricular filling pressure is determined (or estimated) to be high or low, respectively. Oxygen should be administered; if hypoxemia persists or if there is an abnormal mental status despite supplemental oxygen, mechanical ventilation may be necessary. Nitrates should be avoided because they may worsen hypotension.

Patients with causes of shock other than left ventricular dysfunction should be rapidly identified, as their treatment often differs significantly from that given above.

Whether right-heart catheterization is necessary to titrate therapy is controversial. Although much information can be gleaned from right-heart catheterization, no guidelines or algorithms have been established for the management of shock patients based on the measurements derived from right-heart catheterization. Although studies have shown that patients have better outcomes when they received more invasive treatments, including right-heart catheterization, right-heart catheterization has not always been an independent predictor of improved outcome *(9),* and other studies have reported a higher mortality in patients with cardiogenic shock undergoing right-heart catheterization *(10).* The role of right-heart catheterization in patients with cardiogenic shock remains controversial, but is likely to be most beneficial when noninvasive assessment of a patient's hemodynamic status is inconclusive or provides contradictory information.

Thrombolytic Therapy

Thrombolytic therapy clearly reduces the frequency with which shock develops in patients with ST-segment-elevation myocardial infarction without shock at the time of treatment *(5,6).* Tissue plasminogen activator is more effective than streptokinase at preventing the development of shock. However, whether any thrombolytic agent reduces the mortality when administered to patients who already have shock is controversial.

Because the outcome of cardiogenic shock is closely linked to the patency of the culprit coronary arteries, it might be expected that thrombolytic therapy would reduce mortality among patients with shock at the time of treatment *(11).* However, the results of randomized trials administering thrombolytic therapy for patients who have already developed shock has been disappointing. The Gruppo Italiano per lo Studio della Streptochinasi nell' Infarto Miocardico (GISSI-I) study *(12),* a controlled trial comparing streptokinase with control therapy for patients with ST-segment-elevation infarction, included 280 patients with cardiogenic shock at study entry. The mortality at 21 d was 69.9% among the 146 patients who received streptokinase and 70.1% among the 134 patients in the group who received control, nonthrombolytic therapy. Registry data such as those from the Should We Emergently Revascularize Occluded Coronaries for Cardiogenic Shock (SHOCK) Registry, indicating that administration of thrombolytic therapy is associated with a lower mortality, are biased in that patients who did not get thrombolytic therapy were at increased risk of dying independent of treatment received (13). In the randomized portion of the SHOCK Trial (see below), thrombolytic therapy was an independent correlate of 12-mo survival on univariate analysis, but not after adjustment for confounding factors (14). The lack of apparent benefit of thrombolytic agents in treating cardiogenic shock may be the result of reduced lysis of coronary thrombi in patients with low perfusion pressures (15,16). The use of intra-aortic balloon counterpulsation may increase the efficacy of thrombolytic therapy in patients with hypotension by increasing the perfusion pressure.

An argument for administering thrombolytic therapy to shock patients is contained in Chapter 5. The final answer about whether and to what extent thrombolytic therapy reduces mortality once shock has developed remains controversial.

Intra-aortic Balloon Counterpulsation

Intra-aortic balloon counterpulsation (IABP) can stabilize patients with cardiogenic shock. Intra-aortic balloon counterpulsation reduces systemic afterload without increasing myocardial oxygen demand, and increases diastolic coronary arterial perfusion, although not beyond a severe coronary stenosis (17). Although many studies suggest that balloon counterpulsation reduces mortality in patients with cardiogenic shock, most patients in these studies who received balloon counterpulsation also underwent a coronary revascularization procedure; few data support the ability of intra-aortic balloon counterpulsation to improve the survival of patients with shock independent of revascularization. In the SHOCK Registry, although patients who received both thrombolytic therapy and an IABP had the lowest mortality rate, patients who did not receive these interventions had more adverse baseline clinical characteristics associated with mortality (18). Berger et al. reported that although intra-aortic balloon counterpulsation was associated with a reduced mortality at 30 d in the GUSTO-I trial, most patients who received intra-aortic balloon counterpulsation also underwent coronary revascularization (19). Balloon counterpulsation was not associated with a mortality reduction independent of coronary revascularization. Intra-aortic balloon counterpulsation is clearly effective at stabilizing patients with shock for a sufficient time that revascularization may be performed, such as during transfer from the community hospital to a facility where percutaneous or surgical revascularization can be performed (20). Balloon counterpulsation also appears to increase the safety of a coronary revascularization procedure among patients in shock at the time of the procedure. Drawbacks to balloon counterpulsation include that expertise is required for safe placement and not all physicians are comfortable placing them, particularly physicians that practice at hospitals without a catheterization laboratory. Most physicians, particularly those less experienced at placing balloon pumps, prefer to insert balloon pumps in a catheterization laboratory under fluoroscopic guidance, which is not available at all hospitals, particularly at hospitals where balloon counterpulsation might be useful to stabilize a patient during transfer to a tertiary-care facility. Intra-aortic balloon pumps have been associated with an increased risk of bleeding, particularly if thrombolytic therapy is administered. Furthermore, time is required to place an intra-aortic balloon pump, and if not done quickly, it may significantly delay the time to revascularization, a more definitive therapy for the treatment of cardiogenic shock that must be performed rapidly if it is to be of maximal benefit. There are important contraindications to balloon counterpulsation, including significant peripheral or aortic vascular disease and aortic insufficiency. However, despite the scant randomized data supporting its use, many believe that intra-aortic balloon counterpulsation is underutilized in the management of patients with cardiogenic shock *(2,3,21)*. Despite a lack of strong or direct evidence supporting the use of an IABP in shock patients not undergoing revascularization, the data supporting such a practice are outlined in Chapter 5, where it is argued that an IABP should be placed in all shock patients.

Revascularization

Early studies of coronary revascularization for cardiogenic shock focused on surgical revascularization, and several small surgical series reported relatively good outcomes have also been reported in surgical series patients with cardiogenic shock *(22–25)*. Berger et al. reported that revascularization among shock patients was associated with improved 30-d and 1-yr survival in the GUSTO-I trial, even after adjustment for differences in characteristics among patients who did and did not undergo revascularization *(19,26)*. At 1 yr, the survival curves for patients who did and did not undergo revascularization were continuing to diverge *(26)*.

Retrospective analyses of patients who did and did not undergo revascularization for shock must be viewed with caution, as there is selection bias in clinical practice regarding the use of mechanical revascularization *(9,19,26,27)*. The clinical and angiographic profile of patients undergoing angioplasty or surgery is almost always more favorable than that of patients treated with medical therapy without revascularization, which is unfortunate because most data indicate that the highest-risk, most ill patients are most likely to derive benefit from revascularization procedures.

RANDOMIZED TRIALS OF REVASCULARIZATION

There have been two prospective randomized trials evaluating the role of revascularization among patients with cardiogenic shock. In the SMASH Trial (Swiss Multicenter Trial of Angioplasty for Shock), 55 patients with myocardial infarction complicated by cardiogenic shock were randomized to undergo revascularization (surgical or percutaneous) versus treatment with medical therapy alone *(28)*. Unfortunately, SMASH was stopped prematurely because of low enrollment, in part resulting from the perception of physicians that revascularization was beneficial based on retrospective analyses of registries. However, in this small, undersized cohort, a 9% absolute reduction in 30-d mortality was seen among patients treated with revascularization (69% vs 78%, $p = 0.68$ log rank test) that did not achieve statistical significance.

In the second randomized study, the SHOCK trial, patients who developed cardiogenic shock within the first 36 h of acute myocardial infarction (either ST-segment elevation or new left bundle-branch block) were eligible for enrollment; patients with mechanical causes for shock or predominantly right ventricular infarction were excluded. In SHOCK, an aggressive, invasive approach (angioplasty or coronary artery bypass surgery, generally with intra-aortic balloon pumping) was compared with medical treatment, often including thrombolytic therapy and intra-aortic balloon pumping; in the medical therapy arm, revascularization was permitted 54 h after study entry *(29)*. Randomization was required within 12 h of shock onset. Most patients randomized to the invasive approach ($n = 152$) underwent coronary angiography (97%), and 87%

underwent revascularization (surgical or percutaneous). Thirty-day mortality (the primary end point of the study) was 46.7% in the invasive therapy arm versus 56.0% in the conservative arm ($p = 0.11$). Although this large difference did not reach statistical significance, mortality at 6 mo was significantly lower in the revascularization group (50.3% vs 63.1%, $p = 0.027$), and the difference in survival widened, slightly, at 12 mo of follow-up *(30)*. The predefined primary end point of the trial, 30-d mortality, was not significantly reduced by revascularization because the assumptions on which the trial was sized (that there would be a 20% reduction in 30-d mortality for patients with shock treated with early revascularization) were not achieved. There was a lower than anticipated mortality among patients treated medically and a lower than anticipated reduction in mortality associated with early revascularization. In a prespecified subgroup analysis, the benefit of early revascularization was seen only in patients younger than 75 yr of age, in whom the 30-d mortality was 56.8% for the medical therapy arm versus 41.4% for the revascularization arm, relative risk 0.73 (95% confidence interval of 0.56–0.95). However, 30-d survival among medically treated patients older than 75 yr tended to be better than that of older patients in the early revascularization arm (53.1% vs 75.0%, relative risk 1.41 [95% confidence interval of 0.95–2.11], $p = \text{NS}$).

The Kaplan–Meier survival curves for the revascularization arm of the trial revealed an increase in mortality among the first 5 d after randomization. However, after the first 5 d, there was a clear survival benefit in favor of revascularization. The 13% absolute reduction in mortality at 6 mo associated with the aggressive revascularization strategy (50.3% vs 63.1%, $p = 0.027$) was both statistically and clinically significant, and most clinicians (and the investigators of the SHOCK trial) believe that the trial confirmed the benefits of early revascularization for cardiogenic shock after acute myocardial infarction. Indeed, on the basis of the SHOCK trial, the ACC/AHA guidelines for the treatment of patients with acute myocardial infarction have classified early revascularization for shock as a "class one indication," meaning that there is clear and convincing evidence of benefit of early revascularization of shock patients, and that it should be performed, particularly for those under 75 yr of age.

During the performance of the SHOCK trial, a registry of patients at all participating sites with cardiogenic shock not enrolled in the randomized trial was maintained. Nonrandomized patients (including patients who were eligible to be enrolled in the study) were older and sicker, and the in-hospital mortality of such patients was significantly higher than those enrolled in the study. This was only partly the result of the fact that only patients suitable for revascularization were randomized. Of 1492 patients screened for enrollment in the trial, only 302 were enrolled, compared with 1190 patients screened for enrollment who were not randomized. Significant changes in technology and adjunctive medical therapy occurred during the performance of this trial. During the initial performance of the SHOCK trial, stents were infrequently used; the use of stents was estimated to be 0% in 1993–1994 and 19% in 1995–1996, rising to 74% in 1997–1998. Platelet glycoprotein IIb/IIIa inhibitors were used in no patients in 1993–1994, in 27% in 1995–1996, and in 59% of patients in 1997–1998. Both stents and platelet glycoprotein IIb/IIIa inhibitors improve the outcome of percutaneous revascularization in many clinical and anatomic subgroups and are likely to improve outcome in shock patients as well *(31)*.

Several caveats must be considered when applying the results of these randomized trials to the individual patient with shock. There is often a natural selection process favoring patients who survived the initial phase of shock to be enrolled in a randomized trial; the results of revascularization in clinical practice may not be as good as those achieved in such trials *(29)*. The results achieved with revascularization in the trials are generally derived from hospitals experienced in the rapid performance of revascularization in critically ill patients. For example, in the SHOCK trial, the median time from randomization to revascularization was 0.9 h for patients undergoing angioplasty and 2.7 h for patients undergoing surgery *(30)*. Such prompt institution of revascularization treatment may not be able to be duplicated at many hospitals. Also, the success of angioplasty performed by less experienced operators may be significantly lower than that of the randomized trials, resulting in worse outcomes.

Nonetheless, the data are convincing that rapid revascularization reduces mortality in patients with acute myocardial infarction complicated by cardiogenic shock.

Future Trends

The outcome of cardiogenic shock complicating acute coronary syndromes may be improving. Goldberg et al. *(32)* demonstrated that the outcome of patients with cardiogenic shock complicating acute myocardial infarction (Q-wave and non-Q-wave) improved during a 23-yr period, with the greatest improvement in the last decade (1990s): There was greater than a 70% in-hospital mortality among patients with cardiogenic shock from 1975 through 1990, declining to 61% between 1993 and 1995 and to 59% in 1997. This trend was evident despite the fact that patients with shock were older and sicker in recent years. Similarly, the outcome of patients with myocardial infarction and shock has improved over time in Israel, with 30-d mortality rates of 87% in 1992, 84% in 1994, and 73% in 1996 ($p = 0.02$ for trend) (Jonathan Leor, written communication, 1999). Although such observations can be influenced by changing different diagnostic criteria or surveillance for patients with shock, these reports, along with the increasingly frequent performance of revascularization and results of randomized trials, suggest that current therapeutic approaches to shock are more effective than prior approaches.

Algorithms of Outcome

Clinicians must frequently make difficult decisions concerning aggressiveness of care of patients with cardiogenic shock complicating acute coronary syndromes. These decisions are often made in the face of substantial uncertainty regarding the prognosis of the individual patient. Because mortality in these patients is high and large amounts of resources can be expended in a potentially futile effort, clinicians may consider not offering aggressive measures to high-risk patients or withdrawal of aggressive measures in others. Recent results of trials, however, suggest that aggressive and highly expensive care is often worthwhile. In order to help identify patients who might derive particular benefit from such therapies, an algorithm was derived from the GUSTO-I database *(33)* that allows clinicians to make more accurate estimates of the probability of survival for patients with shock complicating ST-segment-elevation myocardial infarction (Table 3). Similar to algorithms predicting the occurrence of cardiogenic shock, this algorithm reveals that the likelihood of survival is heavily influenced by the patient's age and physical findings at the time of diagnosis. These data may help clinicians understand the likelihood of survival if aggressive measures are instituted to patients with shock.

Table 3
Algorithm Predicting 30-d Mortality Rates of Patients with Cardiogenic Shock and ST-Segment-Elevation Myocardial Infarction Based on Demographic, Clinical, and Hemodynamic Variables

Step 1. *Find points for each predictive factor*

Age		Height		Baseline heart rate		Baseline systolic BP		Time to thrombolytic treatment	
Years	Points	cm	Points	Beats/min	Points	mm Hg	Points	Hours	Points
20	0	140	66	40	8	20	36	0	10
30	3	150	46	60	12	40	28	2	4
40	5	160	30	80	17	60	20	4	10
50	8	170	37	100	21	80	12	6	16
60	12	180	30	120	25	100	5	8	15
70	21	190	23	140	29	160	1	10	13
80	40	200	15	160	33	180	2	12	11
90	60	210	8	180	37	200	3	14	9
100	80			200	42	220	5		
						240	6		

Miscellaneous Risk Factors

	Points		Points
Prior infarction	13	Smoking status	
Prior angina	8	Current	0
Infarction location		Former	1
Anterior	13	Never	8
Inferior	0	No extramyocardial factors corrected	8
Other	10	Altered sensorium	18
Killip class		Cold, clammy skin	18
1	0	Oliguria	29
2	11	Ventricular-septal defect	34
3	20	Ventricular rupture	74
4	1	Arrhythmia	10
Diabetes	13		

Step 2. *Add points for all predictive factors: Age + Height + Baseline heart rate + Baseline systolic blood pressure + Time to thrombolytic treatment + Miscellaneous risk factors = Total points*

Step 3. *Determine risk corresponding to total points*

Points	Probability of 30-d mortality
103	10%
126	20%
141	30%
154	40%
165	50%
176	60%
189	70%
204	80%
227	90%

Source: Reprinted from Hasdai D, Topol EJ, Califf RM, Berger PB, Holmes DR Jr: Cardiogenic shock complicating acute coronary syndromes. Lancet 2000;356:749–756 with permission of The Lancet Ltd.

Clinical and Economic Implications

The treatment of patients with cardiogenic shock imposes a large economic burden on health care systems; the 5–10% of patients with shock consume more resources than the care of all other patients with acute myocardial infarction who do not develop shock. Nonetheless, the utilization of such intensive resources appears appropriate, given that when patients with shock survive the initial hospitalization, the outcome is good; 85% of shock patients who survive 30 d will be alive at 1 yr *(26)*. Given the high early mortality of even those patients with shock who receive early revascularization, the best approach would be to develop therapies that prevent shock from occurring in the first place. Unfortunately, other than administering early reperfusion therapy to patients with acute myocardial infarction, such therapy has not yet been discovered. If such therapy is developed, it remains difficult to identify patients who would benefit from it the most. Even the previously described algorithms to identify patients with acute coronary syndromes (with or without ST-segment elevation) at highest risk of developing shock are limited because more than half of even such high-risk patients will not develop shock, even when only standard, currently available therapies are administered.

Right Ventricular Infarction

Because of the important differences among the etiology, diagnosis, and prognosis of patients with cardiogenic shock resulting from the right versus left ventricular dysfunction, we will address the entity of right ventricular infarction separately. Right ventricular infarction, as detected by right precordial ST-segment elevation or by echocardiography, occurs in approximately one of every three patients with acute inferior ST-segment-elevation infarction; however, it is hemodynamically significant in only half of the patients *(34–39)*. Prompt diagnosis is important, because cardiogenic shock resulting from right ventricular infarction is generally reversible. However, therapies that are often administered to patients with shock resulting from left ventricular dysfunction must be avoided, such as nitrates and diuretics, and others often avoided in patients with left ventricular dysfunction should be administered, such as normal saline, large amounts (several liters) of which may be required.

Thrombolytic Therapy for Right Ventricular Infarction

As with cardiogenic shock resulting from left ventricular infarction, thrombolytic therapy is able to reduce the development of shock in inferior ST-segment-elevation infarction due to right ventricular dysfunction *(40,44)*.

Patients with right ventricular infarction have larger infarction, greater impairment of left ventricular function, and more complications, including cardiac arrest and heart block, than patients without right ventricular infarction and cardiogenic shock *(42)*. Therefore, the prompt recognition of right ventricular involvement during inferior infarction identifies a subset of patients with a worse prognosis who are particularly good candidates for interventions aimed at myocardial salvage.

Prognosis of Right Ventricular Infarction Complicated by Shock

If patients with right ventricular infarction survive the initial hospitalization, most (although not all) studies suggest that they do not have a significantly higher mortality in the year following discharge *(44,43,44)*. In fact, the majority of right ventricular wall motion abnormalities resolve and are not detectable on echocardiography or radionuclide ventriculography weeks to months following the infarction *(41)*. Therefore, it is possible that the term "right ventricular infarction" may be a misnomer. The majority of such patients may, in fact, have severe ischemia and stunning of the right ventricle without substantial necrosis. The reasons why the right ventricle appears to be more resistant to infarction than the left ventricle are unclear but probably include lower oxygen requirements of the right ventricle as a result of its smaller muscle mass and lesser work load, a greater total amount of available blood flow to the right than left ventricle resulting from greater coronary blood flow during systole, more extensive collateralization of the right ventricle from the left coronary system, and, perhaps, even diffusion of oxygen from intracavitary blood flow directly through the thin wall of the right ventricle.

CONCLUSIONS

Based on the results of the SHOCK trial *(29)*, the SMASH trial *(28)*, and the many registries of shock patients, early angiography (and revascularization, when appropriate) should be performed in patients with cardiogenic shock resulting from left ventricular dysfunction from acute myocardial infarction whenever possible, as rapidly as possible and by experienced operators. Rapid reperfusion should also be administered to patients with cardiogenic shock because of right ventricular dysfunction. When such patients develop shock at a hospital in which urgent revascularization cannot be performed, clinicians should consider whether the patient can be transported safely to an institution where angiography and revascularization can be performed. The more widespread use of intracoronary stents and antiplatelet agents in patients with cardiogenic shock may attenuate the early hazards associated with percutaneous revascularization procedures in such critically ill patients and further improve the outcomes of patients with shock above those achieved in the randomized trials and registries to date.

REFERENCES

1. The Global Use of Strategies to Open Occluded Coronary Arteries (GUSTO) IIb Investigators. A comparison of recombinant hirudin with heparin for the treatment of acute coronary syndromes. N Engl J Med 1996;335:775–782.
2. Holmes DR Jr, Bates ER, Kleiman NS, et al. Contemporary reperfusion therapy for cardiogenic shock: the GUSTO-I trial experience. J Am Coll Cardiol 1995;26:668–674.
3. Hasdai D, Holmes DR Jr, Topol EJ, et al. Frequency and clinical outcome of cardiogenic shock during acute myocardial infarction among patients receiving reteplase or alteplase: results from GUSTO III. Eur Heart J 1999;20:128–135.
4. Holmes DR Jr, Berger PB, Hochman JS, et al. Cardiogenic shock in patients with acute ischemic syndromes with and without ST-segment elevation. Circulation 1999;100:2067–2073.
5. AIMS Trial Study Group. Effect of intravenous APSAC on mortality after acute myocardial infarction: preliminary report of a placebo-controlled clinical trial. Lancet 1988;1:545–549.
6. Wilcox RG, von der Lippe G, Olsson CG, Jensen G, Skene AM, Hampton JR. Trial of tissue plasminogen activator for mortality reduction in acute myocardial infarction: Anglo-Scandinavian Study of Early Thrombolysis (ASSET). Lancet 1988;1:525–530.
7. Barbash IM, Hasdai D, Behar S, et al. Usefulness of pre- versus postadmission cardiogenic shock during acute myocardial infarction in predicting survival. Am J Cardiol 2001;87:1200–1203.
8. Hasdai D, Califf RM, Thompson TD, et al. Predictors of cardiogenic shock after thrombolytic therapy for acute myocardial infarction. J Am Coll Cardiol 2000;35:136–143.
9. Holmes DR Jr, Califf RM, Van de Werf F, et al. Differences in countries' use of resources and clinical outcome for patients with cardiogenic shock after myocardial infarction: results from the GUSTO trial. Lancet 1997;349:75–78.

10. Connors AF Jr, Speroff T, Dawson NV, et al. The effectiveness of right heart catheterization in the initial care of critically ill patients. SUPPORT Investigators. JAMA 1996;276:889–897.

11. Bengtson JR, Kaplan AJ, Pieper KS et al. Prognosis in cardiogenic shock after acute myocardial infarction in the interventional era. J Am Coll Cardiol 1992;20:1482–1489.

12. Gruppo Italiano per lo Studio della Streptochinasi nell' Infarto Miocardico. Effectiveness of intravenous thrombolytic therapy in acute myocardial infarction. Lancet 1986;1:397–401.

13. Jacobs AK, French JK, Col J, et al. Cardiogenic shock with non-ST-segment elevation myocardial infarction: a report from the SHOCK Trial Registry. J Am Coll Cardiol 2000;36:1091–1096.

14. Hochman JS, Sleeper LA, White HD, et al. One-year survival following early revascularization for cardiogenic shock. JAMA 2001;285:190–192.

15. Prewitt RM, Gu S, Garber PJ, Ducas J. Marked systemic hypotension depresses coronary thrombolysis induced by intracoronary administration of recombinant tissue-type plasminogen activator. J Am Coll Cardiol 1992;20:1626–1633.

16. Prewitt RM, Gu S, Schick U, Ducas J. Intraaortic balloon counterpulsation enhances coronary thrombolysis induced by intravenous administration of a thrombolytic agent. J Am Coll Cardiol 1994;23:794–798.

17. Kern MJ, Aguirre F, Bach R, Donohue T, Siegel R, Segal J. Augmentation of coronary blood flow by intra-aortic balloon pumping in patients after coronary angioplasty. Circulation 1993;87:500–511.

18. Sanborn TA, Sleeper LA, Bates ER, et al. Impact of thrombolysis, intra-aortic balloon pump counterpulsation, and their combination in cardiogenic shock complicating acute myocardial infarction: a report from the SHOCK Trial Registry. J Am Coll Cardiol 2000;36:1123–1129.

19. Berger PB, Holmes DR Jr, Stebbins AL, Bates ER, Califf RM, Topol EJ. Impact of an aggressive invasive catheterization and revascularization strategy on mortality in patients with cardiogenic shock in the Global Utilization of Streptokinase and Tissue Plasminogen Activator for Occluded Coronary Arteries (GUSTO-I) Trial: an observational study. Circulation 1997;96:122–127.

20. Stomel RJ, Rasak M, Bates ER. Treatment strategies for acute myocardial infarction complicated by cardiogenic shock in a community hospital. Chest 1994;105:997–1002.

21. Anderson RD, Ohman EM, Holmes DR Jr., et al. Use of intra-aortic balloon counterpulsation in patients presenting with cardiogenic shock: observations from the GUSTO-I Study. J Am Coll Cardiol 1997;30:708–715.

22. Dunkman WB, Leinbach RC, Buckley MJ, et al. Clinical and hemodynamic results of intraaortic balloon pumping and surgery for cardiogenic shock. Circulation 1972;46:465–477.

23. Bardet J, Masquet C, Khan JC, et al. Clinical and hemodynamic results of intra-aortic balloon counterpulsation and surgery for cardiogenic shock. Am Heart J 1977;93:280–288.

24. DeWood MA, Notske RN, Hensley GR, et al. Intraaortic balloon counterpulsation with and without reperfusion of myocardial infarction shock. Circulation 1980;61:1105–1112.

25. Subramanian VA, Roberts AJ, Zema MJ, et al. Cardiogenic shock following acute myocardial infarction: late functional results after emergency cardiac surgery. NY State J Med 1980;80:947–952.

26. Berger PB, Tuttle RH, Holmes DR Jr, et al. One-year survival among patients with acute myocardial infarction complicated by cardiogenic shock, and its relation to early revascularization: Results from the GUSTO-I trial. Circulation 1999;99:873–878.

27. Hochman JS, Boland J, Sleeper LA, et al. Current spectrum of cardiogenic shock and effect of early revascularization on mortality. Circulation 1995;91:873–881.

28. Urban P, Stauffer JC, Bleed D, et al. A randomized evaluation of early revascularization to treat shock complicating acute myocardial infarction: the (Swiss) Multicenter trial of Angioplasty for SHock — (S)MASH. Eur Heart J 1999;96:1030–1038.

29. Hochman JS, Sleeper LA, Webb JG, et al. Early revascularization in acute myocardial infarction complicated by cardiogenic shock. N Engl J Med 1999;341:625–634.

30. Hochman JS, Sleeper LA, Webb JG, et al. Effects of early revascularization for cardiogenic shock on 1 year mortality: The SHOCK trial results. Circulation 1999;100(suppl I):I-369.

31. Hasdai D, Harrington RA, Hochman JS, et al. Platelet glycoprotein IIb/IIIa blockade and outcome of cardiogenic shock complicating acute coronary syndromes without persistent ST-segment elevation. J Am Coll Cardiol 2000;36:685–692.

32. Goldberg RJ, Samad NA, Yarzebski J, Gurwitz J, Bigelow C, Gore JM. Temporal trends in cardiogenic shock complicating acute myocardial infarction. N Engl J Med 1999;340:1162–1168.

33. Hasdai D, Holmes DR Jr, Califf RM, et al. Cardiogenic shock complicating acute myocardial infarction: predictors of mortality. Am Heart J 1999;138:21–31.

34. Starling MR, Dell'Italia LJ, Chandhuri TK, Boros BL, O'Rourke RA. First transit and equilibrium radionuclide angiography in patients with inferior transmural myocardial infarction: criteria for the diagnosis of associated hemodynamically significant right ventricular infarction. J Am Coll Cardiol 1984;4:923–930.

35. Sharpe ND, Botvinick EH, Shames DM, et al. The noninvasive diagnosis of right ventricular infarction. Circulation 1978;57:483–490.

36. Shah PK, Maddahi J, Berman DS, Pichler M, Swan HJC: Scintigraphically detected predominant right ventricular dysfunction in acute myocardial infarction: clinical and hemodynamic correlates and implications for therapy and prognosis. J Am Coll Cardiol 1985;6:1264–1272.

37. Dell'Italia LJ, Starling MR, O'Rourke RA: Physical examination for exclusion of hemodynamically important right ventricular infarction. Ann Intern Med 1983;99:608–611.

38. Erhardt LR, Sjogren A, Wahlberg I. Simple right-sided precordial lead in the diagnosis of right ventricular involvement in inferior myocardial infarction. Am Heart J 1976;91:571–576.

39. Croft CH, Nicod P, Corbett JR, et al. Detection of acute right ventricular infarction by right precordial electrocardiography. Am J Cardiol 1982;50:421–427.

40. Kalan JM, Gertz SD, Kragel A, Berger PB, Roberts WC, Ryan TJ. Effects of tissue plasminogen activator therapy on right ventricular infarction studied at necropsy as part of the Thrombolysis in Myocardial Infarction (TIMI) study. Int J Cardiol 1993;38:151–158.

41. Berger PB, Ruocco NA, Ryan TJ, et al. Frequency and significance of right ventricular dysfunction during inferior wall left ventricular myocardial infarction treated with thrombolytic therapy (results from the Thrombolysis in Myocardial Infarction (TIMI II) Trial). Am J Cardiol 1993;71:1148–1152.

42. Berger PB, Ryan TJ. Inferior infarction: high risk-subgroups. Circulation 1990;81:401–411.

43. Pfisterer M, Emmenegger H, Soler M, Burkhart F. Prognostic significance of right ventricular ejection fraction for persistent complex ventricular arrhythmias and/or sudden cardiac death after first myocardial infarction: relation to infarct location, size, and left ventricular function. Eur Heart J 1986;7:289–298.

44. Gadsboll N, Hoilund-Carlsen PF, Madsen EB, et al. Right and left ventricular ejection fractions: relation to one-year prognosis in acute myocardial infarction. Eur Heart J 1987;8:1201–1209.

III   Contemporary Treatment of the Patient with Cardiogenic Shock Complicating Acute Coronary Syndromes

5

Medical Treatment for Cardiogenic Shock

John K. French, MB, PhD,
Cheuk-Kit Wong, MD,
and Harvey D. White, DSc

CONTENTS

INTRODUCTION
THROMBOLYTIC THERAPY
INTRA-AORTIC BALLOON PUMP COUNTERPULSATION
RIGHT-HEART CATHERIZATION
GLYCOPROTEIN IIB/IIA RECEPTOR ANTAGONISTS
INOTROPES AND VASOPRESSORS
N-MONOMETHYL-L-ARGININE
METABOLIC SUPPORT AGENTS
SODIUM/HYDROGEN-EXCHANGE INHIBITORS
ANTIOXIDANTS
GLUCOSE – INSULIN – POTASSIUM INFUSION
CONCLUSIONS
REFERENCES

INTRODUCTION

Cardiogenic shock occurs in 7–10% of patients with acute myocardial infarction and is usually associated with extensive infarction of the left ventricle. It has remained the leading cause of death among patients hospitalized for acute myocardial infarction in the reperfusion era *(1,2)*, although changes in treatment in recent years have reduced the mortality rate. For instance, the long-term Worcester Heart Attack Study of patients from all hospitals in Worcester, Massachusetts reported that the mortality rate from cardiogenic shock (defined throughout as a systolic blood pressure of <80 mm Hg and evidence of end-organ hypoperfusion in the absence of hypovolemia) fell from an average of 77% prior to 1993 to approx 60% in 1993–1997, whereas the use of revascularization procedures increased from 10% to 42%, intra-aortic balloon pump counterpulsation (IABP) from 16% to 42%, and thrombolytic therapy from 8% (in 1986–1988) to 25% (Fig. 1) *(3)*. The report did

From: *Contemporary Cardiology: Cardiogenic Shock: Diagnosis and Treatment*
Edited by: David Hasdai et al. © Humana Press Inc., Totowa, NJ

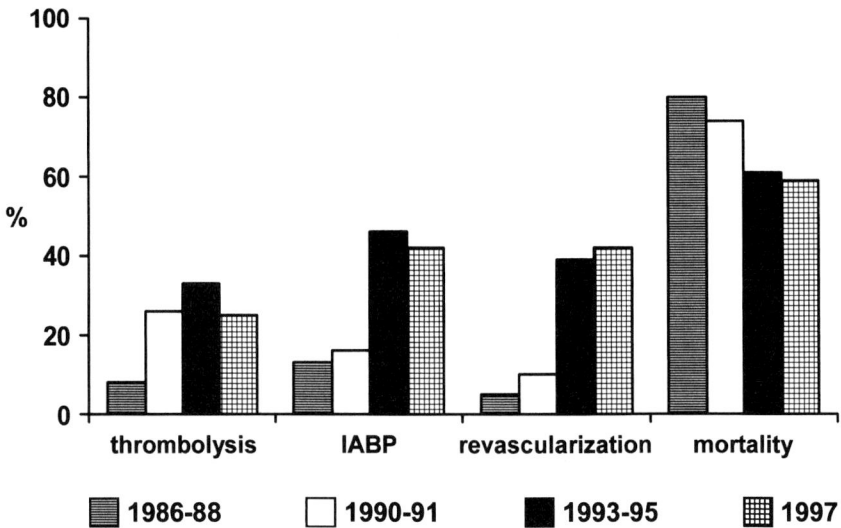

Fig. 1. Changes between 1986 and 1997 in the usage of thrombolytic therapy, IABP, and revascularization (individually reported percutaneous and surgical revascularization rates combined), and mortality over the same period among patients with cardiogenic shock in the Worcester Heart Attack Study *(3)*.

not, however, elaborate on what changes may have occurred since 1975 in the timing of therapies relative to the onset of shock.

This chapter discusses the changing roles of supportive medical therapies (including new pharmacological agents) in the management of cardiogenic shock complicating acute myocardial infarction. For example, in the Should We Emergently Revascularize Occluded Coronaries for Cardiogenic Shock (SHOCK) Trial, 86% of all patients were treated with IABP, 83% with ventilators, 94% with pulmonary artery catheterization, and 55% with thrombolytic therapy. Although the primary purpose of the trial was to compare the treatment strategies of emergency revascularization and initial medical stabilization, the high usage rates of the aforementioned therapies may well have contributed to the comparatively low overall mortality rate of 51% at 30 d *(4)*.

THROMBOLYTIC THERAPY

Most large randomized controlled trials comparing thrombolytic therapy with placebo or control treatment have excluded patients with cardiogenic shock, so there is little randomized evidence regarding the use of thrombolytic therapy in this subgroup of patients. The GISSI-1 Study enrolled 435 patients with Killip class III and 279 patients with Killip class IV symptoms. Although the 30-day mortality rate was lower with streptokinase (33.0% vs 39.0% with control therapy in class III patients and 69.9% vs 70.1% in class IV patients), the difference was not significant *(5)*. In the Fibrinolytic Therapy Trialists' Collaborative Overview, thrombolytic therapy (versus placebo or control treatment) was found to save 7 lives per 100 treated in patients with a systolic blood pressure of <100 mm Hg and a heart rate of >100 beats/min *(6)*.

In the SHOCK Trial Registry, patients with ST-elevation myocardial infarction treated with thrombolytic therapy had a lower 30-d mortality rate than those not treated with thrombolytic therapy (54% vs 64%, $p = 0.005$) *(7)*. It should be noted, however, that those not given thrombolytic therapy had higher baseline risk factors, as they were more likely to be older and female, and had higher rates of diabetes mellitus, hypertension, congestive heart failure, and prior myocardial infarction *(8)*.

The SHOCK Trial enrolled patients who met the electrocardiographic criteria for thrombolysis *(9)*. Thrombolytic therapy was given to 63% of patients and was associated with lower 12-mo mortality rates in those randomized to undergo initial medical stabilization (with or without IABP), but not in those randomized to undergo emergency revascularization (49% of patients). Patients in the initial medical stabilization group who received thrombolytic therapy alone had a 12-mo mortality rate of 44%. Thrombolytic therapy use was a predictor of 12-mo mortality on univariate analysis (relative risk 0.5; $p = 0.008$), but not after adjustment for covariates (relative risk 0.72; $p = 0.15$) *(10)*.

We believe that it is beneficial to achieve epicardial artery (and myocyte) reperfusion as soon as possible after the onset of acute myocardial infarction *(11,12)*, and, indeed, the nonrandomized data suggest that thrombolytic therapy improves the prognosis of patients with cardiogenic shock complicating acute myocardial infarction. We therefore recommend that thrombolytic therapy be given to all patients without absolute contraindications who meet the electrocardiographic and time criteria for thrombolysis *(9)* and who are unlikely to have reperfusion achieved by percutaneous coronary intervention within 60 min.

INTRA-AORTIC BALLOON PUMP COUNTERPULSATION

Intra-aortic balloon pump counterpulsation (IABP) has been used in patients with cardiogenic shock complicating acute myocardial infarction since the 1970s *(13)*. Studies in animal models have provided support for its use in conjunction with thrombolytic therapy to enhance diastolic coronary blood flow and improve thrombolytic efficacy. In a canine hypertensive model, IABP facilitated the dissolution of thrombus by tissue-plasminogen activator, reducing the reperfusion time from 39 to 13 min ($p = 0.02$) *(14)*.

Small retrospective studies in the early 1990s found that the combination of IABP and thrombolytic therapy was associated with lower in-hospital mortality rates than thrombolytic therapy alone *(15–18)*, and this was subsequently supported by the large National Registry of Myocardial Infarction-2, which reported that adjunctive use of IABP with thrombolytic therapy was associated with a lower mortality rate of 49% vs 67% *(19)*.

In the Global Utilization of Streptokinase and tPA for Occluded Coronary Arteries (GUSTO)-I Trial, which administered thrombolytic therapy to all patients, the 30-d mortality rate in the 2972 patients who developed shock prior to or after randomization was 56% *(1)* and there was a trend toward lower mortality in those who received early IABP *(20)*. However, these data should be interpreted cautiously, as they exclude patients who died before reaching the catheterization laboratory, and angiographic data were unavailable for many patients. Patients in the United States tended to be treated more aggressively than those in other countries with regard to the use of IABP (35% vs 7%), angioplasty (26% vs 8%), and coronary artery bypass surgery (16% vs 4%), which may have contributed to the lower mortality rate in the United States (50% vs 66%; $p < 0.001$ for all comparisons) *(20)*.

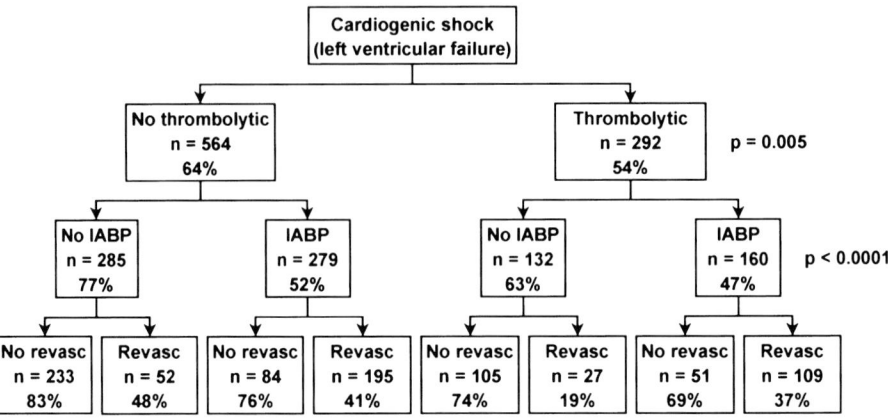

Fig. 2. In-hospital mortality rates of SHOCK Trial Registry patients with predominant left ventricular failure. Patients given thrombolytic therapy had significantly lower mortality rates than those not given thrombolytic therapy in the overall cohort (*p*=0.005), and this benefit was independent of the usage of IABP (interaction *p* = 0.126). There were differences in in-hospital mortality among the four subsets of patients treated with thrombolysis with IABP, thrombolysis without IABP, IABP alone, or neither. Treatments were selected by local physicians. In each of these subsets, patients who underwent revascularization (revasc) had lower mortality rates than those who were not revascularized. Redrawn with permission from: Sanborn TA, Sleeper LA, Bates ER, et al. Impact of thrombolysis, intra-aortic balloon pump counterpulsation, and their combination in cardiogenic shock complicating acute myocardial infarction: a report from the SHOCK Trial Registry. J Am Coll Cardiol 2000;36:1123–1129.

In the SHOCK Trial Registry, patients treated with IABP in combination with thrombolytic therapy had the lowest in-hospital mortality rate (47%) of the four initial treatment strategies (Fig. 2). Patients with ST-elevation myocardial infarction who did not receive IABP and/or thrombolytic therapy had the worst baseline risk status *(7)*.

A combined analysis of the GUSTO-I and GUSTO-III thrombolytic trials showed that patients treated with IABP had an odds ratio of 0.73 for mortality at 30 d. The in-hospital mortality rate was nonsignificantly higher in patients who received IABP within 6 h than in those who received it after 6 h (53% vs 41%, *p* = 0.17), but this may have been because those receiving it earlier were more severely ill and were thought to be at greater risk of dying *(21)*.

The only trial to examine the role of IABP in conjunction with thrombolytic therapy was the Thrombolysis and Counterpulsation to Improve Cardiogenic Shock Survival (TACTICS) Trial, which enrolled patients with a systolic blood pressure of <100 mm Hg unresponsive to fluids within 3 h of the commencement of thrombolytic therapy. Recruitment was terminated after 57 patients had been randomized. The mortality rates at 30 d were 33% in the 30 patients randomized to receive IABP (which included three patients who did not receive the assigned treatment) versus 43% in the patients randomized to thrombolysis alone (*p* = NS), of whom 30% crossed over to receive IABP *(22)*.

IABP was recommended in the SHOCK Trial protocol and used in 87% of patients for a median duration of approx 3 d. The small group of 40 patients (13%) who did not receive IABP were likely to have been highly selected. In some, death occurred before IABP could be initiated, whereas others may have achieved successful reperfusion and been considered sufficiently low risk not to warrant IABP. The use of IABP was also less common in patients with peripheral vascular disease ($p = 0.03$). Overall, IABP usage was not an independent predictor of mortality at 12 mo. However, in patients with systemic hypoperfusion whose hemodynamics and end-organ perfusion were improved by IABP, the mortality rates were lower at 12 mo in both the initial medical stabilization and the emergency revascularization treatment groups (both $p < 0.01$). The combination of IABP and thrombolytic therapy did not significantly increase the incidence of bleeding requiring transfusion, although patients who also underwent revascularization were at higher risk of bleeding *(23)*.

Based on these data, all patients with cardiogenic shock should receive IABP for at least 3 d or longer if clinically indicated for recovery from myocardial stunning. The issue of whether heparin needs to be continued once IABP is instituted has not been systematically studied, but it is our practice to maintain an activated partial thrombo-plastin time (aPTT) of 50–70 s *(24)*, as anticoagulation helps to reduce the risk of venous thrombosis in patients with cardiogenic shock *(25)* and may also enhance the likelihood of achieving infarct artery patency and reduce the risk of left ventricular thrombus formation.

RIGHT-HEART CATHETERIZATION

In patients with cardiogenic shock complicating acute myocardial infarction, man-agement of hemodynamic perturbations in the pulmonary and systemic circulation may require different approaches. Thus, clinicians have often considered it helpful to directly measure the pulmonary artery pressure using pulmonary artery (Swan–Ganz) catheters, which also have particular utility in cases of right ventricular infarction because of the need for high right heart filling pressures to maintain cardiac output and renal perfusion.

A randomized trial evaluating right-heart catheterization in critically ill patients, some of whom had cardiogenic shock, was terminated early because of poor enroll-ment, as many physicians at the enrolling centers in Ontario believed that randomiza-tion was unethical *(26)*. A more recent retrospective study found that there was a mortality hazard associated with right-heart catheterization in critically ill patients, although this hazard did not persist after adjustment for confounding factors (relative hazard 1.02, 95% confidence interval [CI] 0.55–1.89, $p = 0.94$) *(27)*.

An analysis of right-heart catheterization data from 949 patients in the GUSTO-I Trial found that the mortality rate was lower in patients who underwent right-heart catheterization than in those who did not (45.2% vs 63.4%). The lowest 30-d mortality rate was observed in patients with a cardiac output of 5.1 L/mm/m^2 and a pulmonary capillary wedge pressure of 20 mm Hg. Patients with a higher cardiac output had a slightly higher mortality rate, perhaps reflecting the influence of both mechanical causes of cardiogenic shock and decreased peripheral resistance *(28)*.

The SHOCK Trial Registry reported no increase in in-hospital mortality among patients undergoing right-heart catheterization *(29)*. In the SHOCK Trial, there was a very high rate of right-heart catheterization (94%) because measurement of pulmonary capillary wedge pressure was an inclusion criterion for most patients (except for those who had anterior myocardial infarction with radiological pulmonary edema); thus, it is not possible to assess its impact on 12-mo mortality rates *(4)*.

Although no randomized studies have evaluated the benefits of accurate hemodynamic assessment, we recommend the use of pulmonary artery catheters in patients without major bleeding contraindications.

GLYCOPROTEIN IIb/IIIa RECEPTOR ANTAGONISTS

There is considerable evidence that outcomes are improved by the use of glycoprotein IIb/IIIa receptor antagonists prior to *(30)* and at the time of percutaneous coronary intervention *(31)*. (See a further discussion of glycoprotein IIb/IIIa receptor inhibitors in Chapter 3.) In the setting of acute myocardial infarction and cardiogenic shock, microvascular flow *(32–35)* may be enhanced *(36,37)*. Recently, several small nonrandomized studies have reported improved outcomes with abciximab in patients undergoing percutaneous intervention for cardiogenic shock complicating acute myocardial infarction *(38,39)*.

When the SHOCK Trial commenced in 1993, the use of IIb/IIIa antagonists (predominantly abciximab) was rare, but by the final year of the trial in 1998, 61% of patients undergoing percutaneous intervention were treated with a IIb/IIIa antagonist *(4)*. However, this treatment was not randomized, so it is not possible to evaluate its contribution to the better outcomes achieved by emergency revascularization.

In the PURSUIT Trial of 9449 patients with acute coronary syndromes without persistent ST elevation, eptifibatide had no effect on the incidence of cardiogenic shock (1.2% vs 1.3% with placebo, odds ratio-0.95, 95% CI-0.72–1.25, $p = 0.71$), but it did reduce the mortality rate at 30 d (odds ratio-0.51, 95% CI-0.28–0.94, $p = 0.03$) *(40)*.

The available data favor administration of a IIb/IIIa antagonist, particularly abciximab, in patients with cardiogenic shock who are undergoing percutaneous intervention, unless the risk of bleeding is considered to be too great. It has not yet been defined just how soon IIb/IIIa antagonists can be safely administered after full-dose thrombolytic theraphy.

INOTROPES AND VESOPRESSORS

In patients with cardiogenic shock, a mean arterial pressure of 60 mm Hg is generally necessary for tissue perfusion. Studies in patients with septic shock have shown that further elevation of the mean blood pressure by norepinephrine did not improve systemic perfusion but did increase myocardial oxygen demands *(41)*.

Dopamine and dobutamine are the most commonly used inotropic agents. They have different effects on the hemodynamics, cardiac output, and systemic vascular resistance (Table 1).

Low-dose dopamine (0.5–2 µg/kg/min) acts on the dopaminergic receptors, causing vasodilatation and theoretically preserving renal blood flow and natriuresis, an observation based mainly on data from human volunteers *(42)*. However, a recent Australasian placebo-controlled trial in intensive care patients reported no nephro-protective benefit from low-dose dopamine *(43)*. Dopamine's myocardial inotropic and chronotropic effects are mediated through several myocardial β-1-adrenergic receptors and are most evident with doses above 5 µg/kg/min. As the infusion rate rises, peripheral α-adrenergic vasoconstriction activity increases, raising the blood pressure. Because dopamine

Table 1
Inotropes and Vasopressors

	Heart rate	Blood pressure	Cardiac output	Systemic vascular resistance
Dopamine	↑	→↑	↑	↓→↑
Dobutamine	↑	→↑	↑	↑
Norepinephrine	↑	↑	→↑	↑
Milrinone	↑	↓→	↑	↓→

selectively affects multiple receptors in a dose-dependent manner, the variable plasma-dopamine clearance in very sick patients can lead to unpredictable serum concentrations and, consequently, variable clinical benefits *(44)*.

Dobutamine is a synthetic racemic mixture of dextro- and levo-isomers and possesses both α- and β-adrenergic agonistic activity. Its major effect is to increase myocardial contractility through the β-adrenergic receptors, whereas the peripheral α and β effects tend to balance out, with only a small peripheral vasodilatory effect overall. The drug is usually initiated at 2 μg/kg/min and titrated upward according to the patient's response, usually to a maximum of 20 μg/kg/min. Dobutamine is often used together with low-dose dopamine for the inotropic effect of the former and the putative renal vasodilator effect of the latter *(42)*.

Norepinephrine is a potent α-adrenergic agonist with less marked β-1-adrenergic agonistic properties and a short half-life of 2–4 min. Through dose-related vasoconstriction, the drug infusion can be titrated upward from an initial low dose of 0.02–0.04 μg/kg/min to a dose that maintains adequate systemic blood pressure, often in conjunction with dopamine and dobutamine. However, the cardiac effects of these agents include worsening ischemia and serious arrhythmia, and the vasoconstriction induced by norepinephrine can lead to end-organ ischemia; thus, prolonged treatment is best avoided.

Milrinone, a bipyridine analog of amrinone, is a second-generation phosphodiesterase inhibitor that prevents the breakdown (thereby raising cellular levels) of cyclic adenosine monophosphate (cAMP), the final common pathway for raising intracellular calcium and increasing inotropy. This mechanism of action differs from that of catecholamines, which raise cAMP levels by increasing its production in cardiac myocytes; thus, the two types of drug can be used synergistically to enhance myocardial contractility *(45)*. In patients who have previously received β-blockers, a β-adrenergic agonist such as dobutamine may have to be administered at very high doses (e.g., >10 μg/kg/min), whereas milrinone maintains its efficacy even when there is full β blockade *(46)*. Even though milrinone can be expected to increase myocardial oxygen demands resulting from its direct positive inotropic effect, its substantial vasodilatory properties usually offset any detrimental increase in oxygen demands *(47)*. However, this vasodilatory effect also makes milrinone difficult to use as monotherapy in patients with cardiogenic shock. Milrinone has a relatively long plasma half-life, and in order to rapidly achieve a therapeutic plasma level, a 50-μg/kg bolus should be given over a 10-min period, followed by a constant infusion of 0.375–0.75 μg/kg/min. Patients should be watched very closely, as further hypotension can occur.

There have been no large-scale controlled studies comparing different combinations of inotropes in patients with cardiogenic shock. Their efficacy can be influenced by the underlying etiology of the cardiogenic shock and the extent of residual myocardial perfusion, contractility, and vasoconstriction. It is more difficult for the drug to reach the myocardium in a patient with diffuse coronary disease or an occluded infarct-related artery than in a patient who has undergone successful revascularization. In the SHOCK Trial Registry, a period of nonhypotensive peripheral hypoperfusion often preceded the full-shock syndrome, as maximal systemic vasoconstriction had prevented hypotension occurring but had worsened hypoperfusion (48). These patients had a high 30-d mortality rate of 43%. Judicious use of vasodilators may help to improve cardiac output and outcomes, but this hypothesis has not yet been tested in randomized trails.

N-MONOMETHYL-L-ARGININE

In animal models of septic or endotoxin shock, there is evidence that upregulation of cytokine-inducible nitric oxide synthase may play a role in reducing microvascular catecholamine responsiveness in the peripheral vasculature (49) and depressing the contractile function of the heart (50). N-Monomethyl-L-arginine (L-NMMA), a nitric oxide synthase inhibitor, has been tested in 11 patients with refractory cardiogenic shock who were judged to be in a poor state after maximal treatment with high-dose catecholamines, IABP, mechanical ventilation, and judicious percutaneous revascularization. Within 5–10 min of administering L-NMMA (a 1-mg/kg bolus followed by a 1-mg/kg/h infusion for 5 h), the mean arterial pressure rose from 75 ± 9 to 106 ± 19 mm Hg and urine output increased from 68 ± 30 to 158 ± 67 mL/h. The cardiac index initially dropped by 15% from 2.0 ± 0.6 to 1.7 ± 0.5 L/min, but gradually returned to the pretreatment value. No adverse effects were noted, and 10 of the 11 patients were successfully weaned from mechanical ventilation and IABP, with seven surviving at 1-mo follow-up (51). In a randomized controlled trial of 26 patients by the same investigators, the 1-mo mortality rates were 33% in patients given L-NMMA and 77% in those given a placebo ($p = 0.04$) (52).

METABOLIC SUPPORT AGENTS

Reperfusion injury may occur following thrombolysis or percutaneous coronary intervention (PCI). The possible benefits of metabolic modulation depend not only on restoration of cellular perfusion in the infarct zone, thus minimizing reperfusion injury, but also on countering metabolic derangement in the noninfarct zone, which may also suffer ischemia to some extent. The mechanism of reperfusion injury is complex and includes production of oxygen free radicals, activation of neutrophils, changes in intracellular calcium levels, activation of the complement cascade, and tissue edema. Many attempts have been made to prevent reperfusion damage in animal models, and some drugs have been tested in humans.

Adenosine, an endogenous purine nucleoside, antagonizes many of the biochemical and physiological mechanisms implicated in reperfusion injury. In a study of 54 patients undergoing primary angioplasty for acute myocardial infarction, 4 mg of adenosine or control saline was injected through the catheter lumen while the balloon was inflated over the infarct-related lesion, resulting in less no-reflow phenomenon and better ventricular function at 7 d in the patients who received adenosine *(53)*.

In a multicenter randomized placebo-controlled trial of 236 patients, 70 µg/kg/min of adenosine infused over 3 h as an adjunct to thrombolytic therapy reduced the infarct size by 33% as assessed by scintigraphy on d 6 *(54)*. The exact mechanism of adenosine's cardioprotective effect is not fully understood. Proposed mechanisms include inhibition of neutrophil activation, prevention of endothelial damage, improved glucose metabolism with decreased cellular acidosis and calcium overload, and reduced levels of tumor necrosis factor, which has negative inotropic effects and induces myocyte apoptosis.

SODIUM/HYDROGEN-EXCHANGE INHIBITORS

Intracellular sodium/hydrogen exchange plays an important role during ischemia. In the early phase, the high-energy phosphate stores are depleted and the cell switches to anaerobic metabolism, raising intracellular pH and reducing the activity of the ATP-dependent sodium/potassium exchanger. The falling pH activates cellular sodium/hydrogen exchange, leading initially to intracellular sodium accumulation. Subsequently, the sodium/calcium-exchange mechanism causes intracellular calcium accumulation, ultimately precipitating cell death *(55,56)*.

The cellular sodium/hydrogen exchange continues as long as there is an abnormal pH gradient with the extracellular environment. Upon reperfusion, the acidic extracellular fluid in the microcirculation is washed out, increasing the pH gradient, and the ion-exchange process continues, culminating in cell necrosis.

Cariporide is the first agent in a new class of sodium/hydrogen-exchange inhibitors to be tested in clinical trials. Cariporide potently and selectively reduces calcium flux into the ischemic myocyte after reperfusion. In a randomized placebo-controlled trial of 100 patients, administration of cariporide prior to primary angioplasty reduced enzyme leakage and preserved ventricular function *(57)*. In the Guard During Ischemia Against Necrosis (GUARDIAN) Trial, 11,590 patients with unstable angina or non-ST-elevation myocardial infarction or undergoing high-risk percutaneous or surgical revascularization were randomized to receive either a placebo or one of three doses of cariporide. Overall, there was no significant benefit from cariporide. However, in patients undergoing high-risk bypass surgery with a high risk of reperfusion injury, high-dose cariporide (120 mg every 8 h) reduced the incidence of perioperative myocardial infarction *(58)*. In the recent ESCAMI Trial, 959 patients undergoing reperfusion therapy for acute myocardial infarction (of whom about 35% underwent primary PCI) were randomized to receive one of two doses (100 mg or 150 mg) of eniporide or a placebo. There was no difference in enzymatic infarct size, and clinical outcomes were similar. Cardiogenic shock occurred in 1.9% vs 2.8% vs 3.2% respectively ($p = $ NS) *(59)*.

ANTIOXIDANTS

There have been no trials of antioxidants and free-radical scavengers in patients with cardiogenic shock. In a placebo-controlled study of 120 patients undergoing primary angioplasty for acute myocardial infarction, recombinant human superoxide dismutase (a free-radical scavenger) was given intravenously prior to angioplasty. There was no improvement in ventricular function *(60)*.

In a placebo-controlled trial of 47 patients with acute myocardial infarction, *N*-acetylcysteine was used adjunctively with reperfusion therapy, resulting in smaller infarct sizes as determined by the electrocardiographic QRS score and better echocardiographic left ventricular function at d 7 *(61)*. Larger trials are ongoing.

GLUCOSE – INSULIN – POTASSIUM INFUSION

In patients with acute myocardial infarction, infusion of glucose, insulin, and potassium (GIK) reduces blood levels—and, consequently, myocardial uptake—of free fatty acids, which cause membrane damage, arrhythmogenesis, and impaired contractility *(62)*. (See further discussion of GIK in Chapter 2.) In addition to increasing glycolytic flux in myocardial cells, GIK helps to minimize cellular changes resulting from ongoing ischemia *(63)*.

A meta-analysis of studies performed in the prethrombolytic era, totaling 1932 patients, showed that GIK infusions reduced in-hospital mortality by 28% *(64)*. A recent prospective study, in which patients received either a high- or low-dose GIK infusion, found that GIK was beneficial, particularly in the subgroup receiving reperfusion therapy (relative risk of in-hospital mortality 0.34, $p = 0.008$) and the frequency of cardiogenic shock was 4.6% in those who received GIK compared with 7.6% in those who did not (relative risk 0.60, 95% CI 0.21-1.69, $p = $ NS) *(65)*. There have been no published studies of GIK use in patients with cardiogenic shock.

CONCLUSIONS

Since the late 1980s, the mortality rates from cardiogenic shock complicating acute myocardial infarction have fallen from 70–80% to 50–60% *(1,3,20,48)*. The reasons for this include the use of thrombolytic therapy to achieve expeditious reperfusion, support measures such as intra-aortic balloon counterpulsation, right-heart catheterization-guided therapies, and urgent revascularization. New myocardial protection agents currently in development have the potential to reduce reperfusion injury and improve metabolic and cellular conditions. To date, most studies of these agents have excluded patients with cardiogenic shock, and trials are needed to specifically evaluate their use in this subgroup of patients.

REFERENCES

1. Berger PB, Holmes DR Jr, Stebbins AL, et al. Impact of an aggressive invasive catheterization and revascularization strategy on mortality in patients with cardiogenic shock in the Global Utilization of Streptokinase and Tissue Plasminogen Activator for Occluded Coronary Arteries (GUSTO-I) Trial: an observational study. Circulation 1997;96:122–127.
2. White HD. Cardiogenic shock: a more aggressive approach is now warranted [editorial]. Eur Heart J 2000;21:1897–1901.
3. Goldberg RJ, Samad NA, Yarzebski J, et al. Temporal trends in cardiogenic shock complicating acute myocardial infarction. N Engl J Med 1999;340:1162–1168.
4. Hochman JS, Sleeper LA, Webb JG, et al. Early revascularization in acute myocardial infarction complicated by cardiogenic shock. N Engl J Med 1999;341:625–634.
5. Gruppo Italiano per lo Studio della Streptochinasi nell'Infarto Miocardico (GISSI). Effectiveness of intravenous thrombolytic treatment in acute myocardial infarction. Lancet 1986;i:397–402.
6. Fibrinolytic Therapy Trialists' (FTT) Collaborative Group. Indications for fibrinolytic therapy in suspected acute myocardial infarction: collaborative overview of early mortality and major morbidity results from all randomised trials of more than 1000 patients. Lancet 1994;343:311–322.

7. Sanborn TA, Sleeper LA, Bates ER, et al. Impact of thrombolysis, intra-aortic balloon pump counterpulsation, and their combination in cardiogenic shock complicating acute myocardial infarction: a report from the SHOCK Trial Registry. J Am Coll Cardiol 2000;36:1123–129.

8. Jacobs AK, French JK, Col J, et al. Cardiogenic shock with non-ST-segment elevation myocardial infarction: a report from the SHOCK Trial Registry. J Am Coll Cardiol 2000;36:1091–1096.

9. French JK, Williams BF, Hart HH, et al. Prospective evaluation of eligibility for thrombolytic therapy in acute myocardial infarction. Br Med J 1996;312:1637–1641.

10. Hochman JS, Sleeper LA, White HD, et al. One-year survival following early revascularization for cardiogenic shock. JAMA 2001;285:190–192.

11. White HD. Future of reperfusion therapy for acute myocardial infarction [editorial]. Lancet 1999;354:695–697.

12. Andrews J, Straznicky IT, French JK, et al. ST-segment recovery adds to the assessment of TIMI 2 and 3 flow in predicting infarct wall motion after thrombolytic therapy. Circulation 2000;101:2138–2143.

13. Scheidt S, Wilner G, Mueller H, et al. Intra-aortic balloon counterpulsation in cardiogenic shock. N Engl J Med 1973;288:979–984.

14. Gurbel PA, Anderson RD, MacCord CS, et al. Arterial diastolic pressure augmentation by intra-aortic balloon counterpulsation enhances the onset of coronary artery reperfusion by thrombolytic therapy. Circulation 1994;89:361–365.

15. Silverman AJ, Williams AM, Wetmore RW, et al. Complications of intraaortic balloon counterpulsation insertion in patients receiving thrombolytic therapy for acute myocardial infarction. J Interven Cardiol 1991;4:49–52.

16. Waksman R, Weiss AT, Gotsman MS, et al. Intra-aortic balloon counterpulsation improves survival in cardiogenic shock complicating acute myocardial infarction. Eur Heart J 1993;14:71–74.

17. Stomel RJ, Rasak M, Bates ER. Treatment strategies for acute myocardial infarction complicated by cardiogenic shock in a community hospital. Chest 1994;105:997–1002.

18. Kovack PJ, Rasak MA, Bates ER, et al. Thrombolysis plus aortic counterpulsation: improved survival in patients who present to community hospitals in cardiogenic shock. J Am Coll Cardiol 1997;29:1454–1458.

19. Barron HV, Every NR, Parsons LS, et al. The use of intra-aortic balloon counterpulsation in patients with cardiogenic shock complicating acute myocardial infarction: data from the National Registry of Myocardial Infarction 2. Am Heart J 2001;141:933–939.

20. Holmes DR Jr, Califf RM, Van de Werf F, et al. Difference in countries' use of resources and clinical outcome for patients with cardiogenic shock after myocardial infarction: results from the GUSTO Trial. Lancet 1997;349:75–78.

21. Hudson MP, Granger CB, Stebbins AL, et al. Cardiogenic shock survival and use of intraaortic balloon counterpulsation: results from the GUSTO I and III Trials [abstract]. Circulation 1999;100 (Suppl I):I-370.

22. Ohman EM, Nanas J, Stomel R, et al. A prospective randomized trial of thrombolysis and counterpulsation to improve cardiogenic shock survival: preliminary results of the TACTICS Trial [abstract]. Eur Heart J 2000;21(Abstract Suppl):15.

23. French JK, Miller D, Palmieri S, et al. Cardiogenic shock treated with thrombolytic therapy and intra-aortic balloon counter pulsation: a report from the SHOCK Trial [abstract]. Circulation 1999;100(Suppl I):I-370.

24. Granger CB, Hirsh J, Califf RM, et al. Activated partial thromboplastin time and outcome after thrombolytic therapy for acute myocardial infarction: results from the GUSTO-I Trial. Circulation 1996;93:870–878.

25. Samama MM, Cohen AT, Darmon J-Y, et al. A comparison of enoxaparin with placebo for the prevention of venous thromboembolism in acutely ill medical patients. N Engl J Med 1999;341:793–800.

26. Guyatt G. A randomized control trial of right-heart catheterization in critically ill patients: Ontario Intensive Care Study Group. J Intensive Care Med 1991;6:91–95.

27. Connors AFJ, Speroff T, Dawson NV, et al. The effectiveness of right heart catheterization in the initial care of critically ill patients. SUPPORT Investigators. JAMA 1996;276:889–897.

28. Hasdai D, Holmes DR Jr, Califf RM, et al. Cardiogenic shock complicating acute myocardial infarction: predictors of death. Am Heart J 1999;138:21–31.

29. Menon V, Sleeper LA, Fincke R, et al. Outcomes with pulmonary artery catheterization in cardiogenic shock [abstract]. J Am Coll Cardiol 1998;31(Suppl A):397A.

30. The CAPTURE Investigators. Randomised placebo-controlled trial of abciximab before and during coronary intervention in refractory unstable angina: the CAPTURE Study. Lancet 1997;349:1429–1435.

31. Topol EJ, Califf RM, Weisman HF, et al. Randomised trial of coronary intervention with antibody against platelet IIb/IIIa integrin for reduction of clinical restenosis: results at six months. Lancet 1994;343:881–886.

32. The EPILOG Investigators. Platelet glycoprotein IIb/IIIa receptor blockade and low-dose heparin during percutaneous coronary revascularization. N Engl J Med 1997;336:1689–1696.

33. Topol EJ, Mark DB, Lincoff AM, et al. Outcomes at 1 year and economic implications of platelet glycoprotein IIb/IIIa blockade in patients undergoing coronary stenting: results from a multicentre randomised trial. Lancet 1999;354:2019–2024.

34. The ESPRIT Investigators. Novel dosing regimen of eptifibatide in planned coronary stent implantation (ESPRIT): a randomised, placebo-controlled trial. Lancet 2000;356:2037–2044.

35. The EPISTENT Investigators. Randomised placebo-controlled and balloon-angioplasty-controlled trial to assess safety of coronary stenting with use of platelet glycoprotein-IIb/IIIa blockade. Lancet 1998;352:87–92.

36. Antman EM, Giugliano RP, Gibson CM, et al. Abciximab facilitates the rate and extent of thrombolysis: results of the Thrombolysis in Myocardial Infarction (TIMI) 14 Trial. Circulation 1999;99:2720–2732.

37. Topol EJ, Yadav JS. Recognition of the importance of embolization in atherosclerotic vascular disease. Circulation 2000;101:570–580.

38. Schultz RD, Heuser RR, Hatler C, et al. Use of c7E3 Fab in conjunction with primary coronary stenting for acute myocardial infarctions complicated by cardiogenic shock. Cathet Cardiovasc Diagn 1996;39:143–148.

39. Giri S, Mitchel JF, Hirst JA, et al. Synergy between intracoronary stenting and abciximab in improving angiographic and clinical outcomes of primary angioplasty in acute myocardial infarction. Am J Cardiol 2000;86:269–274.

40. Hasdai D, Kitt MM, Harrington RA, et al. Impact of platelet glycoprotein IIb/IIIa blockade on outcome of cardiogenic shock among patients with acute coronary syndromes without persistent ST-segment elevation [abstract]. Circulation 1999;100(Suppl I):I-433.

41. LeDoux D, Astiz ME, Carpati CM, et al. Effects of perfusion pressure on tissue perfusion in septic shock. Crit Care Med 2000;28:2792–2732.

42. Denton MD, Chertow GM, Brady HR. "Renal-dose" dopamine for the treatment of acute renal failure: scientific rationale, experimental studies and clinical trials. Kidney Int 1996;50:4–14.

43. Australian and New Zealand Intensive Care Society (ANZICS) Clinical Trials Group. Low-dose dopamine in patients with early renal dysfunction: a placebo-controlled randomised trial. Lancet 2000;356:2139–2143.

44. Juste RN, Moran L, Hooper J, et al. Dopamine clearance in critically ill patients. Intensive Care Med 1998;24:1217–1220.

45. Colucci WS, Denniss AR, Leatherman GF, et al. Intracoronary infusion of dobutamine to patients with and without severe congestive heart failure: dose-response relationships, correlation with circulating catecholamines, and effect of phosphodiesterase inhibition. J Clin Invest 1988;81:1103–1110.

46. Lowes BD, Simon MA, Tsvetkova TO, et al. Inotropes in the beta-blocker era. Clin Cardiol 2000;23(Suppl III):III-11–III-16.

47. Grose R, Strain J, Greenberg M, et al. Systemic and coronary effects of intravenous milrinone and dobutamine in congestive heart failure. J Am Coll Cardiol 1986;7:1107–1113.

48. Menon V, Slater JN, White HD, et al. Acute myocardial infarction complicated by systemic hypoperfusion without hypotension: report of the SHOCK Trial Registry. Am J Med 2000;108:374–380.

49. Hollenburg SM, Broussard M, Osman J, et al. Microvascular reactivity, blood pressure, and survival are improved in septic iNOS-deficient knockout mice [abstract]. J Am Coll Cardiol 2000;35(Suppl A):312A.

50. Greenberg SS, Ouyang J, Zhao X. Inducible nitric oxide synthase mRNA and protein in ventricular myocyte mitochondria in endotoxic shock [abstract]. Circulation 1998;98(Suppl I):I-132.

51. Cotter G, Kaluski E, Blatt A, et al. L-NMMA (a nitric oxide synthase inhibitor) is effective in the treatment of cardiogenic shock [abstract]. Circulation 1999;100(Suppl I):I-371.

52. Cotter G, Kaluski E, Milovanov O, et al. LINCS: L-NMMA in cardiogenic shock: preliminary results from a prospective randomized study. Presented at the American Heart Association Scientific Sessions 2001; Anaheim, California, USA; November 11–14, 2001.

53. Marzilli M, Orsini E, Marracini P, et al. Beneficial effects of intracoronary adenosine as an adjunct to primary angioplasty in acute myocardial infarction. Circulation 2000;101:2154–2159.

54. Mahaffey KW, Puma JA, Barbagelata A, et al. Adenosine as an adjunct to thrombolytic therapy for acute myocardial infarction: results of a multicenter, randomized, placebo-controlled trial: the Acute Myocardial Infarction Study of Adenosine (AMISTAD) Trial. J Am Coll Cardiol 1999;34:1711–1720.
55. Scholz W, Albus U. Na+/H+ exchange and its inhibition in cardiac ischemia and reperfusion. Basic Res Cardiol 1993;88:443–455.
56. Scholz W, Albus U. Potential of selective sodium-hydrogen exchange inhibitors in cardiovascular therapy. Cardiovasc Res 1995;29:184–188.
57. Rupprecht H-J, vom Dahl J, Terres W, et al. Cardioprotective effects of the Na+/H+ exchange inhibitor cariporide in patients with acute anterior myocardial infarction undergoing direct PTCA. Circulation 2000;101:2902–2908.
58. Théroux P, Chaitman BR, Danchin N, et al. Inhibition of the sodium–hydrogen exchanger with cariporide to prevent myocardial infarction in high-risk ischemic situations: main results of the GUARDIAN Trial. Circulation 2000;102:3032–3038.
59. Zeymer U. The ESCAMI Study. Presented at the Hot Line I session, European Society of Cardiology XXIII Congress; Stockholm, Sweden; September 2, 2001.
60. Flaherty JT, Pitt B, Gruber JW, et al. Recombinant human superoxide dismutase (h-SOD) fails to improve recovery of ventricular function in patients undergoing coronary angioplasty for acute myocardial infarction. Circulation 1994;89:1982–1991.
61. Zhang Y, Patel AA, Juergens C, et al. N-Acetylcysteine improves myocardial salvage after reperfusion therapy in humans [abstract]. Circulation 1999;100(Suppl I):I-371.
62. Oliver MF, Opie LH. Effects of glucose and fatty acids on myocardial ischemia and arrhythmias. Lancet 1994;343:155–158.
63. Eberli FR, Weinberg EO, Grice WN, et al. Protective effects of increased glycolytic substrate against systolic and diastolic dysfunction and increased coronary resistance from prolonged global underperfusion and reperfusion in isolated rabbit hearts perfused with erythrocytes suspensions. Circ Res 1991;68:466–481.
64. Apstein CS, Taegtmeyer H. Glucose-insulin-potassium in acute myocardial infarction: the time has come for a large, prospective trial [editorial]. Circulation 1997;96:1074–1077.
65. Díaz R, Paolasso EA, Piegas LS, et al. Metabolic modulation of acute myocardial infarction: the ECLA Glucose–Insulin–Potassium Pilot Trial. Circulation 1998;98:2227–2234.

6

Technical Approaches to Percutaneous Revascularization in the Patient with Cardiogenic Shock

David R. Holmes, Jr., MD

INTRODUCTION

Arrival of a patient with cardiogenic shock in the catheterization laboratory demands urgent attention. Vascular access sites must be evaluated and access obtained. Depending on the severity of the shock, the exact sequence of procedural performance may vary. Some aspects will be performed simultaneously and others sequentially, depending on personnel available and the specific clinical setting.

RIGHT-HEART CATHETERIZATION

Right-heart catheterization should be performed. The specific route and site used may vary. If possible, central venous access should be obtained from the neck. The reasons for this are twofold. First, central venous monitoring will probably be required for a longer period than arterial vascular access is required. That being the case, patient comfort and mobility will be improved if access is gained through the neck. Second, placement of arterial and venous access at the same femoral site has been associated with increased bleeding.

One of the goals of placement of right-heart catheterization is to assess the patient's fluid status. Fluid management will be dictated by the intracardiac pressures, which will be particularly important in patients with shock related to right ventricular infarction. The pressures obtained can also be used to risk stratify the patient. Hasdai et al. found, for example, that a pulmonary capillary wedge pressure of 20 mm/Hg was associated

From: *Contemporary Cardiology: Cardiogenic Shock: Diagnosis and Treatment*
Edited by: David Hasdai et al. © Humana Press Inc., Totowa, NJ

with a lower mortality rate, whereas values more or less were associated with an increased mortality rate *(1)*. Measurement of right-heart pressure and saturations can also ascertain the presence of a complication causing shock, such as a ventricular septal defect or acute papillary muscle rupture/dysfunction. (See Chapter 8.)

VASCULAR ACCESS

Vascular access should be obtained quickly, and both groins should be used if possible. Although radial access is possible, the patient will usually have vasoconstriction, making this approach more difficult; in addition, the size of the devices that can be used with a radial approach are usually limited to those that are 6 French-compatible.

Placement of a balloon pump is an important consideration (see Chapter 5). Although documentation of the isolated value of an intra-aortic balloon pump is lacking, circulatory support can improve the stability of the patient and the procedure *(2)*. This approach obviously works only if there is a baseline blood pressure; in cases of electromechanical dissociation or sustained refractory ventricular arrhythmia or asystole, an intra-aortic balloon pump is not effective. Continued development of more effective circulatory support devices will be important to improving outcome (see Chapter 20).

If possible, the intra-aortic balloon pump should be placed before or simultaneously with the start of the catheterization. If peripheral vascular disease is present, the intra-aortic balloon pump should be placed from the side with the least vascular compromise. In some settings, a hand injection of the aortoiliac tree is performed to assess the feasibility of placing a balloon pump. The delay required for this injection may not make this procedure widely used in the setting of myocardial infarction with shock.

Catheterization should be performed as quickly as possible. Some catheterization laboratories and operators first perform left ventricular angiography with minimal nonionic contrast to assess for potential mitral regurgitation and to evaluate left ventricular function. Other laboratories do not perform left ventricular angiography because of concern that further hemodynamic deterioration will ensue; in this setting, echocardiography is used later to assess left ventricular function. In general, we advocate the latter approach. A final intermediate approach is to proceed with the intervention and then at the end of the procedure to perform left ventricular angiography if hemodynamics are more stable.

The presumed non-infarct-related artery should be injected first. This allows the operator to assess any collaterals to the infarct-related artery. Following this, the infarct-related artery is engaged. To save time, a guiding catheter may be used to perform the diagnostic angiogram. Usually in patients with cardiogenic shock, the infarct-related arterial segment is proximal and supplies a large amount of myocardium. Because the patient has limited tolerance for any complications, the diagnostic angiogram needs to be very carefully considered.

One relatively common scenario is that of a very proximal left anterior descending occlusion. In this setting, the potential for withdrawing thrombus back into the left main coronary artery and embolizing it down to the circumflex must be kept in mind, as that may hasten a lethal outcome. Although the use of embolic protection devices or thrombectomy devices is attractive, in general they require a longer setup time and, when urgent revascularization is so important, they are not usually used. If evidence of distal embolization is seen following the intervention, it should be treated accordingly at that time. In general, if the vessel is of sufficient size (≥3.0 mm), a stent should be implanted. In this setting, we may proceed with direct stenting to decrease the trauma of repeated inflation of the infarct segment.

In general, treating only the infarct-related artery has been a basic tenet of acute percutaneous coronary intervention. With cardiogenic shock, however, that approach may be modified. If the patient's hemodynamic status remains marginal after treatment of the culprit lesion and if other major lesions appear suitable, they are often treated immediately to optimize total coronary flow. If the other lesions are critical and are not amenable to percutaneous coronary intervention, then urgent coronary bypass graft surgery should be considered.

ADJUNCTIVE THERAPY

Pharmacologic circulatory support is essential. Hypotension may beget further hypotension by worsening subendocardial ischemia, and pressor support to optimize the blood pressure to ≥90 mm Hg should therefore be used early. Other adjunctive therapy includes ventilatory support and a temporary pacemaker, as indicated. In the setting of cardiogenic shock and complete heart block, a temporary ventricular pacemaker may not result in any improvement in hemodynamics because of the presence of the V-A conduction and loss of AV synchrony. A temporary dual-chamber pacemaker may improve this situation.

The issue of antiplatelet/anticoagulant therapy is important. Aspirin should definitely be given as well as heparin. Use of a glycoprotein IIb/IIIa receptor inhibitor depends on the potential for urgent/emergency surgery. If, prior to intervention, surgery is considered likely (e.g., an occluded infarct-related artery in the circumflex, which is to be treated, but a critical left main coronary artery stenosis in addition), then a IIb/IIIa inhibitor should not be used. If surgery appears unlikely, as will usually be the case, a IIb/IIIa agent is indicated to improve outcome even though there are no specific data dealing with this shock situation. In this setting, a thienopyridine can be initiated immediately after the procedure.

Treatment of no reflow in the setting of cardiogenic shock is particularly difficult, as some of the drugs used (e.g., nitroprusside) can worsen or aggravate hypotension. The best approach is to make certain that the epicardial stenosis/stenoses are well treated and then deliver small incremental doses of drugs distally to reverse the situation as fully as possible.

POSTINTERVENTION CARE

Femoral arterial sheaths are usually removed as soon as possible following the procedure in an attempt to decrease vascular complications. If prolonged intra-arterial monitoring is required, a radial line can then be inserted. The balloon pump should be removed as soon as hemodynamics permit. As long as pressors are required, counterpulsation is maintained.

A relatively recent approach to management of the intra-aortic balloon pump is to put in a Perclose™ suture device prior to inserting the balloon pump, maintaining sterility of the sutures, and then use this device for closure when the balloon pump is withdrawn. Alternatively, the balloon pump can be removed while maintaining access with a guidewire and then a vascular closure device can be used. Great care must be taken to minimize the potential for local infection.

CONCLUSION

Cardiogenic shock results in multiple pathophysiologic abnormalities. Some of these abnormalities can be promptly corrected by restoration of flow. An aggressive approach has been proven in large well-controlled randomized studies of subsets of patients [e.g., the GUSTO *(3)* and SHOCK studies *(4)*]. Such an aggressive approach involves not only mechanical reperfusion but also treatment of the associated systemic abnormalities with appropriate ventilatory, circulatory, and adjunctive medical therapy.

REFERENCES

1. Hasdai D, Holmes DR Jr, Califf RM, et al. Cardiogenic shock complicating acute myocardial infarction: predictors of death. Am Heart J 1999;138:21–31.
2. Ohman EM, George BS, White CJ, et al. Use of aortic counterpulsation to improve sustained coronary artery patency during acute myocardial infarction. Results of a randomized trial. The Randomized IABP Study Group. Circulation 1994;90:792–799.
3. Berger PB, Holmes DR, Stebbins AL, Bates ER, Califf RM, Topol EJ. Impact of an aggressive invasive catheterization and revascularization strategy on mortality in patients with cardiogenic shock in the Global Utilization of Streptokinase and Tissue Plasminogen Activator for Occluded Coronary Arteries (GUSTO-I) trial. An observational study. Circulation 1997;96:122–127.
4. Webb JG, Sanborn TA, Sleeper LA, et al. Percutaneous coronary intervention for cardiogenic shock in the SHOCK Trial Registry. Am Heart J 2001;141:964–970.

7

Operative Strategies for Cardiogenic Shock Complicating Acute Coronary Syndromes

Ehud Raanani, MD,
Aharon Avramovich, MD,
David Hasdai, MD,
and Bernardo A. Vidne, MD

CONTENTS

INTRODUCTION

In a nonrandomized study, DeWood and colleagues *(1)* were the first to report improved results with surgical revascularization in patients in cardiogenic shock complicating acute myocardial infarction (MI). Shock patients were first stabilized with intra-aortic balloon pump (IABP) counterpulsation and then underwent emergent coronary artery bypass grafting (CABG) surgery, resulting in 75% survival. Later, others also reported encouraging results with surgical revascularization *(2,3)*. Only recently, the Should We Emergently Revascularize Occluded Coronaries for Cardiogenic Shock (SHOCK) Trial investigators conducted a prospective randomized study to compare early revascularization (angioplasty or CABG) versus medical treatment for patients with cardiogenic shock complicating MI *(4)*. Emergency revascularization did not significantly reduce overall mortality at 30 d, but there was a significant survival benefit after 6 mo. The investigators concluded that early revascularization should be strongly considered for this group of patients.

Unfortunately, there are no prospective randomized studies comparing the different operative strategies for these patients. In this chapter we will review and summarize the

From: *Contemporary Cardiology: Cardiogenic Shock: Diagnosis and Treatment*
Edited by: David Hasdai et al. © Humana Press Inc., Totowa, NJ

technical aspects of the surgical approach in cardiogenic shock, based on retrospective studies and reports, as well as our own experience. Mechanical complications of acute MI such as rupture of the ventricular septal, papillary muscle, or free wall are discussed elsewhere in this book (see Chapter 8).

PREOPERATIVE CONSIDERATIONS

The surgical treatment of acute coronary syndromes requires rapid and efficient coordination between the catheterization and surgical teams. Once coronary angiography is performed and the decision for emergency surgery is made, the patient should be quickly prepared. During this preparation time, placement of a pulmonary artery catheter should be given favorable consideration. If not already in place, an IABP should be inserted with fluoroscopic guidance, and the patient should be placed on inotropic support and vasodilators in order to maintain cardiac output and protect vital organs. Early use of IABP is preferable to overuse of inotropic agents, as IABP improves cardiac output and decreases end-organ failure in the early phase of cardiogenic shock. In the event of cardiovascular collapse in the catheterization laboratory before the operating room is ready, the use of percutaneous femoral bypass can provide sufficient flow rates (3.0–5.0 L/min) during the transition to the operating room. This approach has been useful when percutaneous bypass was achieved within 20 min *(5)*.

ANESTHESIA

Patients in cardiogenic shock referred for emergency cardiac surgery represent one of the greatest challenges in anesthesiology.

Preparing for Anesthesia

There are few situations in medicine in which time can be so crucial. Every minute lost means the death of more myocytes and the worsening of prognosis. Nevertheless, the anesthesiologist must remember that advanced planning for anesthesia is the key to operative success.

Patient History

The anesthesiologist should collect as much information as possible regarding the patient's past medical history in the very limited time before surgery begins. This can be elicited either from the patient or from another available source. Based on the collected data, the anesthesiologist should be able to prepare the anesthetic plan.

Preparing the Operating Room

The following anesthetic equipment should be checked in advance and be ready for use: anesthetic machine, laryngoscope, various kinds of laryngoscopic blades, and suction. Other items include the drugs to be administered, the equipment and catheters for measuring systemic blood pressure and inserting the pulmonary artery catheter, and the IABP and transesophageal echocardiography (TEE) equipment. Monitoring of the patient includes standard electrocardiographic leads V_2 and V_5, pulse oximetry, and invasive and noninvasive blood pressure measurements. If the patient arrives with a previously placed pulmonary artery catheter, then central venous pressure, pulmonary artery pressure, and thermodilution cardiac output should be measured before inducing anesthesia. Otherwise, the surgeon can insert the pulmonary artery catheter directly into the pulmonary artery at a later stage.

Theoretical Considerations

Cardiogenic shock can occur as a complication of unstable angina, non-ST-segment-elevation MI, and ST-segment-elevation MI *(6–8)*. When treating patients in cardiogenic shock presenting for emergency CABG, there are two goals: salvage as much myocardium as possible and minimize the adverse impact of the shock state on other organs. The anesthesiologist's goals are to minimize the oxygen demand of the myocardium and to improve the oxygen supply. Heart rate, myocardial contractility, and preload and afterload are factors that determine oxygen demand *(9–12)*. Tachycardia not only increases the work of the myocardium but also reduces the diastolic time, thus decreasing the coronary perfusion time and oxygen supply. Reducing preload and afterload can lessen the work of the heart by reducing the systolic and end-diastolic pressure.

Coronary flow and oxygen content of the blood determine the oxygen supply to the myocardium. The coronary flow depends on the coronary perfusion pressure (mean arterial flow minus left ventricular end-diastolic pressure) and resistance to flow. In the presence of a fixed occlusion in the coronary artery, normal autoregulation is lost and the flow may become dependent exclusively on the coronary perfusion pressure *(13)*. Reducing end-diastolic pressure not only decreases the oxygen demand but also increases the coronary flow. Therefore, reducing mean arterial pressure is problematic because this method can reduce the work of the heart but also reduce the coronary flow *(14–16)*. The best way to maintain adequate perfusion pressures and decrease oxygen demand is to place the patient on a cardiopulmonary bypass (CPB) machine. Until CPB is established, the anesthesiologist's objective is to induce anesthesia while optimizing the above-mentioned factors.

Inducing Anesthesia

The major steps and principles of induction for the shock patient are summarized in Fig. 1. This subsection discusses these steps in greater detail.

Determining the exact way to induce anesthesia depends on many different factors: patient's medical history, pathophysiology of cardiogenic shock, level of consciousness, whether the patient is already intubated, and degree of hemodynamic instability. Some patients are conscious and frightened and reassuring them can lower their anxiety. If the patient arrives already intubated and sedated, then a muscle relaxant should be administered and opioids, such as fentanyl, can be titrated based on the hemodynamic response. If the patient does not arrive intubated, the anesthesiologist should initiate intubation. Drugs should be given to keep the patient hemodynamically stable and to provide sufficient amnesia, analgesia, and immobility because laryngoscopy and intubation are very painful stimuli *(17)*.

No single anesthetic agent or combination of medications can be considered ideal for every situation. To complicate matters, we have to consider that a patient is "full stomach" until proven otherwise and is thus at risk for aspiration during intubation *(18)*. Two of the best ways to decrease the likelihood of a patient having an aspiration during intubation include using rapid-sequence induction or awake intubation. Rapid sequence induction indicates that the decision about the exact dose of the anesthetic agent and

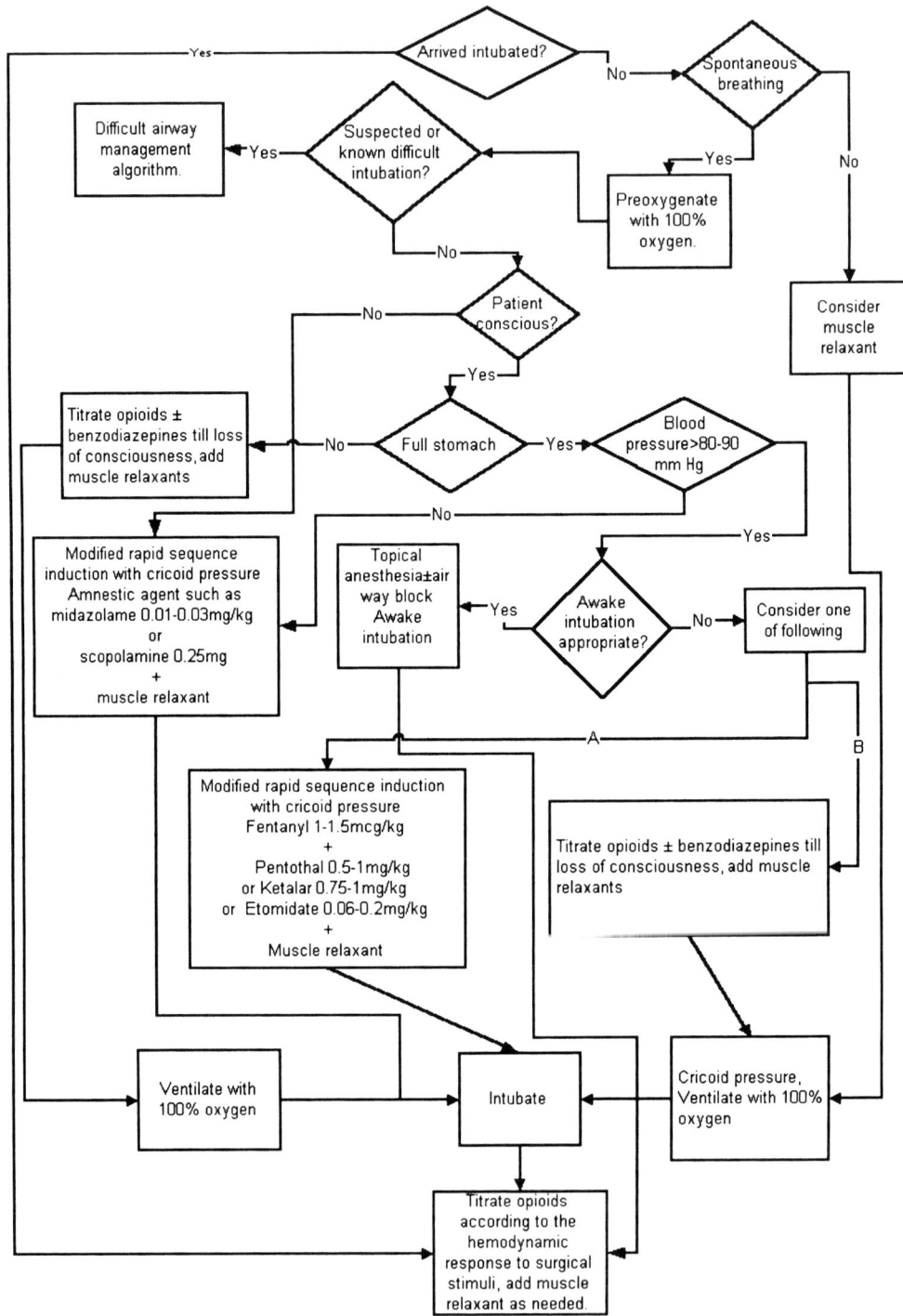

Fig. 1. Algorithm for anesthetic induction of the shock patient (of shock patients).

muscle relaxant to be delivered is made in advance. After a patient is preoxygenated for 3–5 min with pure oxygen, the anesthetic agent and the muscle relaxant are delivered in rapid sequence while cricoid pressure is applied. In the classic rapid-sequence induction, thiopental and succinylcholine are used. In some modifications of this technique, other anesthetic agents like propofol, etomidate, or ketamine in conjunction with succinylcholine or a high dose of nondepolarizing muscle relaxants are delivered (19,20). The drawback is that an overdose of medication before intubation can lead to cardiovascular collapse, whereas an underdose can cause tachycardia, a temporary rise in blood pressure, worsening of ischemia, and then cardiovascular collapse.

Awake intubation with topical anesthesia or upper airway block in experienced hands can be used as an alternative approach in a patient with full stomach. However, this is a stressful procedure that can worsen the ischemia. In addition, a patient with cardiogenic shock who is not fully alert may become combative, which can make the airway management more difficult.

Another method to consider is the titration approach, which entails delivering the anesthetic medication in small doses until the desired effect is achieved. Yet this approach cannot always ensure cardiovascular stability and may expose the patient to the risk of aspiration (18).

With whatever approach and whatever combination of anesthetic agents the anesthesiologist chooses, there will always be the risk that the patient will experience cardiovascular collapse during intubation. To be prepared for this complication, drugs for inotropic support should be ready for use in advance, an experienced cardiac surgeon should be present during induction of anesthesia, and the team should be ready for emergency sternotomy and connection to CPB.

Anesthetic Medication Choices

OPIOIDS

Morphine as a sole anesthetic agent for cardiac surgery was first introduced in the late 1960s and was popular in the 1970s. The need for prolonged mechanical ventilation after the surgery, cases of inadequate anesthesia (even with extremely high doses of 8–11 mg/kg), and the tendency for histamine release and hypotension led to the development of a new generation of opioids like fentanyl, sufentanil, remifentanil, and alfentanil (21). All of these agents were successfully tested as the sole anesthetic for cardiac surgery (22,23). Using an opioid as the sole anesthetic agent is advantageous because of the remarkable hemodynamic stability that occurs during the induction and maintenance of anesthesia. However, there have been occasional reports of awareness during surgery and the need for prolonged mechanical ventilation, as compared with anesthesia based on opioids in conjunction with nonopioid agents and volatile anesthetics (22–26).

NONOPIOID AGENTS

Many different nonopioids and inhalational agents were successfully investigated and are now used as supplements for opioids for induction and maintenance during CABG. It is beyond the scope of this chapter to describe all of them. The most common nonopioid agents, volatile anesthetics, and their cardiovascular effects are summarized in Table 1.

There are no prospective or retrospective reports in the literature that compare different anesthetic medications for intubating patients in cardiogenic shock and there are

Table 1
Hemodynamic Effects of Nonopiood Induction Agents

	Etomidate	Propofol	Ketamine	Thiopental	Diazepam	Midazolam
HR	–↑	↓–↑	–↑↑	–↑↑	↓–↑	↓–↑
MAP	–↓	–↓↓	–↑↑	↓–↑	–↓	↓↓
SVR	–↓	↓	–↑↑	–↑	↓–↑	–↓
PAP	–↑	↓–↑	↑↑	–	–↓	–
PVR	–↑		–↑↑	–	–↓	–
RAP	–↓	↓	↑↑	–↑↑	–	–
CI	–↑	↓	–↑↑	–↓	–	–↓
SV	–↓	↓	–↓	↓↓	–↓	–↓
LVSWI	–↓	↓↓	–↑	–↓	–↓↓	↓↓
dP/dT	–↓		–	↓	–	–↓

Abbreviations: HR = heart rate; MAP = mean arterial pressure; SVR = systemic vascular resistence; PVR = pulmonary vascular resistance; RAP = right atrial pressure; CI = cardiac index SV = stroke volume; LVSWI = left ventricular stroke work index; dP/dT = derivative of pressure; – = no effect; ↑ or ↓ = mild to moderate increase (less than 25%); ↑↑ or ↓↓ = moderate to marked increase (more than 25%).

Note: The effects of the drug may depend on many different factors such as dose, speed of injection, or the patient's characteristics (e.g., ventricular function, intravascular volume, medication the patient is receiving).

Sources: Modified from Reves JG, Berkowitz DE. In: Kaplan A, ed. Pharmacology of Intravenous Anesthetic Induction Drugs. Cardiac Anesthesia. 3rd ed. WB Saunders, Philadelphia, 1993, pp. 514,516,521; Rung GW, Conahan TJ. Induction of Anesthesia. In: Hensley FA Jr, Martin DE, eds. A Practical Approach to Cardiac Anesthesia. 2nd ed. Little Brown and Company, Boston, 1995, p. 152.

no universal recommendations for a specific anesthetic agent or combination of them. Maybe more important than the choice of specific agent for induction and intubation is the way this agent is used. The only current recommendation that can be given is to choose the agent with which one has experience and familiarity.

Maintenance of Anesthesia

After induction and tracheal intubation, the goal is to establish CPB as quickly as possible. During this period, the anesthesiologist should try to stabilize the hemodynamic parameters of the patient by using fluid infusion and inotropic support. The patient's response to surgical stimuli should be observed, with the addition of anesthetic agents as needed. A total dose of fentanyl 20–40 μg/kg/min usually will provide sufficient analgesia for skin incision and sternotomy, whereas 100–150 μg/kg/min is enough for the entire surgical procedure *(27,28)*. The addition of a nonopioid agent in conjunction with opioids in order to prevent awareness can cause severe hypotension and should be used cautiously or not at all until the patient is on CPB *(29)*. The activated coagulation time (ACT) should be checked before administering heparin, and a full dose of 300 U/kg should be given before CPB. The goal is to achieve an ACT of 400 s or longer *(30)*.

In our institution, we routinely require ACT to be longer than 480 s or above 700 s if aprotinin is used. Many patients receive heparin or thrombolytic therapy before

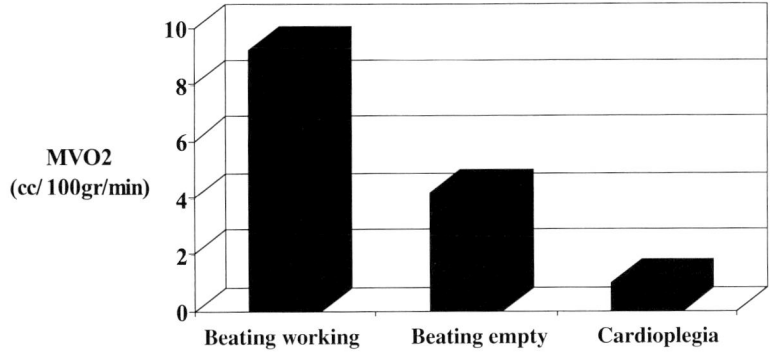

Fig. 2. Myocardial energy consumption. Modified from Allen BS, Rosenkranz ER, Buckberg GD, et al. High oxygen requirements of dyskinetic cardiac muscle. J Thorac Cardiovasc Surg 1986;92:543–552.

arriving at the operating room, and attempts to calculate the dose of heparin based on the treatment the patient received are unreliable. Because the consequence of under-dosing can be disastrous and titration of the heparin dose based on the ACT can be time-consuming, we prefer to use a full dose of heparin in advance. A patient who has received long-term therapy with heparin may need fresh frozen plasma, which should be ready in advance *(31)*.

As soon as the patient is on CPB, the full dose of the anesthetic agent can be delivered, and inotropic support can be discontinued. During the period of CPB, the acid–base and electrolyte status of the patient should be checked and corrected as needed. We routinely check electrolytes and blood gases every 30 min. TEE can greatly assist in the decision-making and should be favorably considered in these patients. Before terminating CPB, the surgeon should insert a pulmonary catheter and IABP, if not already in place.

INTRAOPERATIVE STRATEGIES

The major steps and principles for the operative treatment of the shock patient are summarized in Fig. 2. This protocol is based on the principles of the "Buckberg strategy" *(32)*. The following subsection discusses this protocol in greater detail.

Cardiopulmonary Bypass

Once a patient is in the operating room, CPB needs to be established as soon as possible. Only after CPB has been established should the heart be examined and the decision made regarding the number and type of bypass grafts. In the context of cardiogenic shock, most surgeons will use only saphenous vein grafts (SVG) because they can be harvested simultaneously with placing the patient on CPB. Once the culprit vessel is bypassed using a SVG, cardioplegia can be delivered through it. Others report the use of the internal mammary artery (IMA) to be safe and justifiable *(5,33)*. Taking into consideration the long-term benefits of IMA, we strongly believe that in the case of a young patient with large viable territory that can be bypassed with the IMA, one should consider this approach, provided it can be performed promptly and efficiently. The IMA should be harvested after placing the patient on CPB.

Myocardial Protection

Ventricular decompression reduces myocardial energy consumption by approx 60%. By avoiding the energy needed for myocardial contraction, diastolic arrest further reduces energy consumption by 30%. The final 10% of basal energy can be avoided by cooling the heart (Fig. 3) *(34)*. Once on CPB, the patient is cooled to a moderate level of hypothermia (25–28°C) to obtain a safety margin in protecting the heart and systemic vital organs. Prior to aortic cross-clamping, cardioplegia catheters are placed to allow immediate cardiac arrest once the aorta has been clamped.

Once cardioplegia is delivered, attention should be shifted to decompression of the heart. Venting the aortic root once antegrade cardioplegia is complete or preferably continuously venting the left ventricle through the right superior pulmonary vein can result in an empty flaccid heart throughout the operation. Directly venting the left ventricle is advantageous because this method can vent the heart during antegrade cardioplegia as well. As previously noted, there is no prospective randomized study demonstrating the best myocardial protection technique for the patient with acute coronary syndrome. Some authors reported good results using crystalloid cardioplegia or oxygenated crystalloid cardioplegia *(3,35)*. Blood cardioplegia is the most widely used and has been demonstrated to be superior over the crystalloid cardioplegia in patients with critical heart conditions *(35–37)*. Blood cardioplegia keeps the heart oxygenated while it is being arrested, minimizes hemodilution, and contains endogenous oxygen buffers, oxygen radical scavengers, and onconicity. In the setting of acute coronary occlusion, retrograde cardioplegia through the coronary sinus protects territories of the myocardium unreachable by the antegrade route.

Because the acutely ischemic myocardium is energy depleted and less tolerant to ischemia during aortic cross-clamping, a special myocardial protection protocol is to be followed.

WARM INDUCTION

The first step includes a 5-min induction of normothermic oxygenated blood as active resuscitation; normothermia facilitates the rate of cellular repair. Buckberg and colleagues *(32)* recommend adding to the warm induction substrates such as aspartate and glutamate because these amino acid precursors of the Krebs cycle improve ATP production and oxygen utilization. The normothermic induction is delivered both antegrade and retrograde to ensure maximal distribution.

GRAFTING SEQUENCE

Cardiogenic shock usually develops 24–72 h after acute MI or after an extending infarction. Because the acutely ischemic muscle stops contracting very early, cardiogenic shock can develop as a result of the progressive decline in the contractility of other myocardial territories at risk *(38–40)*. Thus, the operative strategy is to first ensure myocardial protection to the viable muscle territories. The grafts are placed first to the larger coronaries supplying the functioning muscle, and the vessel that supplies the infarcted territory is grafted last. In contrast, in the setting of an evolving MI, the territory at risk is still considered viable and the vessel supplying that area is grafted first.

DISTRIBUTING CARDIOPLEGIA

Cold blood cardioplegia is delivered to the critical regions by performing each proximal anastomosis immediately after the distal. This method prolongs the aortic cross-

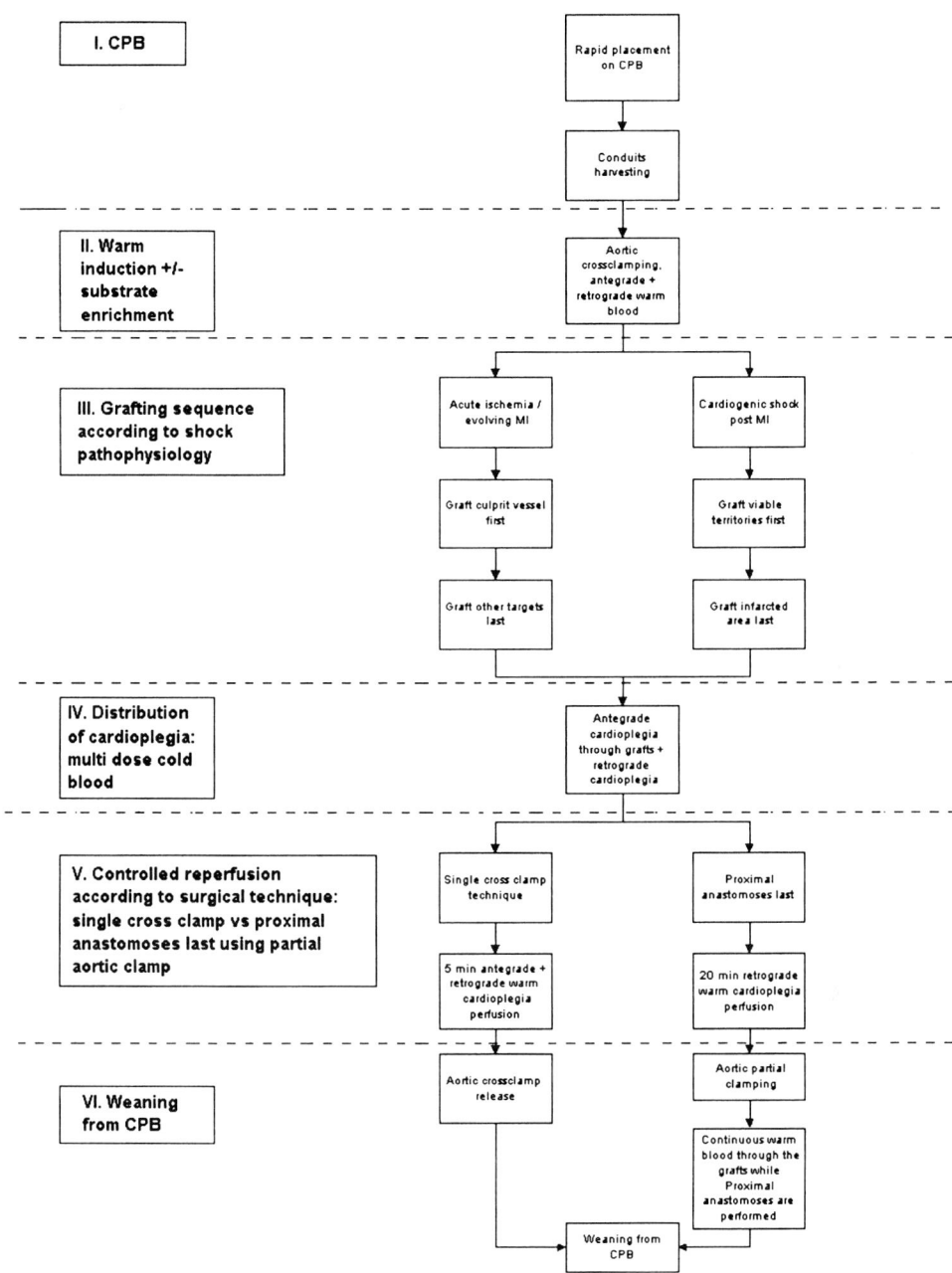

Fig. 3. Algorithm for the major steps and principles for the operative treatment of the shock patient.

clamping time, which may be problematic if complete revascularization is not achieved. Using retrograde cardioplegia partially circumvents this problem by protecting the obstructed nonvascularized areas. Multidose cold blood cardioplegia is delivered both antegrade and retrograde, and it is required because the low-level electrical activity precedes visible mechanical activity. Replenishments using 8–10 mg/L low-potassium limit systemic hyperkalemia.

CONTROLLED REPERFUSION

The final step is to minimize reperfusion injury once the aortic cross-clamp is released. Reperfusion injury is characterized by the inability to use delivered oxygen, the accumulation of intracellular calcium, and cell swelling that reduces blood flow and impairs ventricular compliance *(41)*. Byersdorf and others (36,42–44) studied the importance of controlled condition reperfusion in patients with an evolving MI. Their protocol includes an infusion (3–10 min) of normothermic blood cardioplegia prior to unclamping the aorta. In order to counteract the previously mentioned detrimental effects, several principles are followed. Reperfusion calcium is lowered (0.2–0.3 mmol) to limit calcium influx. In order to avoid cellular edema and endothelial damage, a hyperosmolar solution is used (360–400 mOsm) and infused by using gentle pressure (<50 mm Hg). In order to optimize metabolic function, buffers are used to counteract tissue acidosis. Reperfusion cardioplegia is delivered retrograde through the coronary sinus, into the aortic root, and through the grafts, if those have not yet been attached proximally to the aorta.

In a nonrandomized multicenter study, Allen and colleagues *(42)* demonstrated the superiority of controlled surgical reperfusion compared with reperfusion using percutaneous transluminal coronary angioplasty (PTCA). Controlled surgical reperfusion reduced mortality, and more patients achieved substantial regional wall motion recovery. If proximal anastomoses are not performed during the aortic cross-clamping period, warm blood cardioplegia is continuously delivered through the grafts while the proximal anastomoses are performed.

Weaning from Cardiopulmonary Bypass

Before the patient is weaned from CPB, the metabolic and hemodynamic status should be optimized. Increasing perfusion pressures and red blood cell mass can raise the subendocardial oxygen supply. Weaning from CPB is started after allowing the heart to recover in an empty beating state for at least 20–30 min. After that period, aerobic metabolism will support the return of myocardial contractility. In addition to the information obtained from the pulmonary catheter, we find it extremely useful to use TEE as a guide for determining the volume and contractile state of the heart during this stage. It is unlikely that one single approach will guarantee a successful result, but we have found that following the general concept with slight variations according to surgeons' preferences produces gratifying results.

Other Approaches

Several other approaches have been suggested in the surgical treatment of cardiogenic shock. Akins *(45,46)* continues to report excellent results using a hypothermic fibrillatory arrest technique for elective or emergency myocardial revascularization. With this technique, he avoids the deleterious affects of imposing a period of global ischemia on a heart that already has acute regional ischemia.

Mohr and colleagues *(47)* recently reported on surgical coronary revascularization without CPB in patients with acute MI. Of 57 patients, 8 were in a state of cardiogenic shock during the operation. The investigators reported excellent early outcomes with only one early death (1.7%). It is hoped that the off-pump coronary artery bypass techniques for patients in cardiogenic shock will be further investigated.

Perrault et al. *(48)* investigated on-pump beating heart coronary bypass in this group of patients because current cardioplegic techniques do not consistently avoid myocardial ischemic damage in high-risk patients. On the other hand, surgical revascularization without CPB is not always technically feasible. Of 37 patients who underwent this operation, 11 were in the state of evolving MI and 5 were in cardiogenic shock. There was a high operative mortality of 13.5% (5 of 37); however, it is difficult to draw conclusions because it was a small series with a small subgroup of patients in cardiogenic shock.

Ultrafiltration

Hemoultrafiltration during CPB and before a patient is weaned from bypass is an efficient method for fluid removal and concentration of red blood cells without the adverse effects on hemodynamics *(49,50)*. Moreover, compared with cell separator techniques, hemoultrafiltration does not adversely affect platelet aggregation function *(51)*. Cell-saver systems have been shown to effectively raise postoperative hemoglobin levels but may cause severe depletion of various plasma proteins (52–54). It is still debatable whether ultrafiltration is effective in removing myocardial depressant factors and reducing the postbypass inflammatory response *(55)*.

Bleeding

Emergency operation and cardiogenic shock are considered risk factors for excessive postoperative bleeding *(56)*. The combination of thromboxane A_2 released by CPB and cytokine release induced by blood product transfusion may stimulate pulmonary hypertension, a condition that in the setting of right-heart failure or ischemia may be catastrophic. It is therefore important to minimize postoperative bleeding. The use of aprotinin decreases post-CPB bleeding and reduces the need for blood product transfusions *(57,58)*. There are some case reports on the successful use of aprotinin during emergency CPB following thrombolytic therapy for acute MI *(59,60)*. The optimal dosage and timing of administering aprotinin is not completely clear yet because some investigators report low-dose results with similar success *(61)*. Giving aprotinin for high-risk cases such as emergency and reoperative surgery is routinely done in many cardiac centers. ε-Aminocaproic acid also has been shown to effectively reduce bleeding in routine CPB *(62,63)*, and this alternative should be considered for shock patients if bleeding ensues. A growing proportion of patients with acute coronary syndromes is treated with platelet glycoprotein IIb/IIIa inhibitors. Should such a patient develop shock, the drug should be stopped and transfusion of platelets be initiated.

POSTOPERATIVE MANAGEMENT

Maximal patient monitoring is required to optimize hemodynamics. By using a pulmonary artery catheter, it is possible to accurately optimize the patient's cardiac output and avoid overusing inotropic drugs. Overuse of inotropic agents causes unnecessary myocardial oxygen demand, excessive peripheral vasoconstriction, and, eventually, even multiorgan failure. A left atrial catheter left in by the surgeon at the end of the operation will provide some of the information required, in case a pulmonary artery catheter has not been placed.

In the event of unexpected instability or low cardiac output, TEE can rule out conditions such as excessive mediastinal fluid or an organized clot causing a cardiac tamponade effect. TEE also can provide important information regarding the volume and contractile status of the heart as well. Weaning from IABP is started once a patient is hemodynamically stable, and only small doses of inotropic drugs are required. It is important to assess how the patient is affected by being taken off the IABP through the use of hemodynamic monitoring or TEE. If weaning from IABP causes a reduction in the cardiac output or myocardial contractility, it should be left in place. In the event of limb ischemia resulting from the IABP catheter, the balloon needs to be removed earlier. An antibiotic protocol should be based on the individual institution.

RESULTS

Hospital mortality for patients undergoing surgery for acute coronary syndromes complicated by cardiogenic shock ranges between 12% and 60% *(42,64–68)*. Using warm substrate-enriched induction and controlled reperfusion yields lower mortality rates (13%) compared with uncontrolled reperfusion. Yet, a high rate (47%) of perioperative complications has been reported in patients in cardiogenic shock compared with that for elective procedures (13%) *(3,64–67)*. Complications include re-exploration for bleeding, respiratory failure, sepsis, and wound infection. Postoperative multiorgan failure is frequent, and this failure is usually a continuation of a preoperative state. Because preoperative multiorgan failure of more than 18 h is considered irreversible, it should be considered a relative contraindication for surgery *(65)*. Beyersdorf, Allen, and colleagues *(35,36,42)* demonstrated significant postoperative regional wall motion improvement in 87% of patients following a mean ischemic preoperative interval of 6 h. Perioperative MIs and postoperative wall motion abnormalities are associated with reduced late survival *(65)*. In 269 consecutive patients with evolving MIs, the 1-yr and 10-yr survival percentages after successful surgery were 77% and 66% for patients in cardiogenic shock compared with 98% and 77% for hemodynamically stable patients *(69)*. The long-term quality of life for patients surviving surgery is satisfactory, with 73% of the patients resuming work *(68,70)*.

REFERENCES

1. DeWood MA, Spores J, Berg R Jr, et al. Acute myocardial infarction: a decade of experience with surgical reperfusion in 701 patients. Circulation 1983;68(Suppl II):II-8–II-16.
2. Phillips SJ, Kongtahworn C, Skinner JR, Zeff RH. Emergency coronary artery reperfusion: a choice therapy for evolving myocardial infarction. Results in 339 patients. J Thorac Cardiovasc Surg 1983;86:679–688.
3. Guyton RA, Arcidi JM, Langford DA, Morris DC, Liberman HA, Hatcher CR. Emergency coronary bypass for cardiogenic shock. Circulation 1987;76(Suppl 5):V22–V27.
4. Hochman JS, Sleeper LA, Webb JG, et al. Early revascularization in acute myocardial infarction complicated by cardiogenic shock. SHOCK Investigators. Should we emergently revascularize occluded coronaries for cardiogenic shock. N Engl J Med 1999;341:625–634.
5. Lazar H. Methods of reducing myocardial necrosis after failed percutaneous transluminal coronary angioplasty in patients undergoing emergent coronary artery bypass surgery. In: Lazar H, ed. Current Therapy for Acute Coronary Ischemia. Futura, Mount Kisko, NY, 1993; pp. 167–186.
6. The Global Use of Strategies to Open Occluded Coronary Arteries (GUSTO) IIb Investigators. A comparison of recombinant hirudin with heparin for the treatment of acute coronary syndromes. N Engl J Med 1996;335:775–782.
7. Holmes DR Jr, Berger PB, Hochman JS, et al. Cardiogenic shock in patients with acute ischemic syndromes with and without ST-swegment elavation. Circulation 1999;100:2067–2073.
8. Hasdai D, Topol EJ, Califf RM, Berger PB, Holmes DR. Cardiogenic shock complicating acute coronary syndromes. Lancet 2000;356:749–756.

 9. Indolfi C, Ross J. The role of heart rate in myocardial ischemia and infarction: implications of myocardial perfusion-contraction matching. Prog Cardiovasc Dis 1993;36:61–74.
10. Merin RG. Physiology, pathophysiology and pharmacology of the coronary circulation with particular emphasis on anesthetics. Anaesthesiol Reanim 1992;17:5–26.
11. Suga H, Yasumura Y, Nozawa T, Futaki S, Tanaka N, Uenishi M. Ventricular systolic pressure-volume area (PVA) and contractile state (Emax) determine myocardial oxygen demand. Adv Exp Med Biol 1988;222:421–430.
12. Carlson RE, Kavanaugh KM, Buda AJ. The effect of different mechanisms of myocardial ischemia on left ventricular function. Am Heart J 1988;116(2 Pt 1):536–545.
13. Epstein SE, Cannon RO, Talbot TL. Hemodynamic principles in the control of coronary blood flow. Am J Cardiol 1985;56:4E–10E.
14. Bellamy RF. Diastolic coronary artery pressure-flow relations in the dog. Circ Res 1978;43:92–101.
15. Buffington CW: Hemodynamic determinants of ischemic myocardial dysfunction in the presence of coronary stenosis in dogs. Anesthesiology 1985;63:651–662.
16. Brazier J, Cooper N, Buckberg GD. The adequacy of subendocardial oxygen delivery: the interaction of determinants of flow, arterial oxygen content and myocardial oxygen need. Circulation 1974;49:968–977.
17. Hassan HG, el-Sharkawy TY, Renck H, Mansour G, Fouda A. Hemodynamic and catecholamine responses to laryngoscopy with vs. without endotracheal intubation. Acta Anaesthesiol Scand 1991;35:442–447.
18. Thibodeau LG, Verdile VP, Bartfield JM. Incidence of aspiration after urgent intubation. Am J Emerg Med 1997;15:562–565.
19. Andrews JI, Kumar N, van den Brom RH, Olkkola KT, Roest GJ, Wright PM. A large simple randomized trial of rocuronium versus succinylcholine in rapid-sequence induction of anesthesia along with propofol. Acta Anaesthesiol Scand 1999;43:4–8.
20. Sivilotti ML, Ducharme J. Randomized, double-blind study on sedatives and hemodynamics during rapid-sequence intubation in the emergency department: The SHRED Study. Ann Emerg Med 1998;31:313–324.
21. Bovill JG, Boer F. Opioids in cardiac anesthesia. In: Kaplan, JA, ed. Cardiac Anesthesia. 3rd ed. Saunders, Philadelphia, 1993; pp. 490–491.
22. Howie MB, McSweeney TD, Lingam RP, Maschke SP. A comparison of fentanyl–O$_2$ and sufentanil–O$_2$ for cardiac anesthesia. Anest Analg 1985;64:877–887.
23. Bovill JG, Warren PJ, Schuller JL, van Wezel HB, Hoeneveld MH. Comparison of fentanyl, sufentanil, and alfentanil anesthesia in patients undergoing valvular heart surgery. Anesth Analg 1984;63:1081–1086.
24. Mainzer J. Awareness during fentanyl anesthesia. Anesthesiology 1982;56:331–332.
25. Mummaneni N, Rao TL, Montoya A. Awareness and recall with high-dose fentanyl-oxygen anesthesia. Anesth Analg 1980;59:948–949.
26. Hilgenberg JC. Intraoperative awareness during high-dose fentanyl–oxygen anesthesia. Anesthesiology 1981;54:341–343.
27. Cheng DC, Karski J, Peniston C, et al. Morbidity outcome in early versus conventional tracheal extubation after coronary artery bypass grafting: a prospective randomized controlled trial. J Thorac Cardiovasc Surg 1996;112:755–764.
28. Wynands JE, Townsend GE, Wong P, Whalley DG, Srikant CB, Patel YC. Blood pressure response and plasma fentanyl concentrations during high- and very high-dose fentanyl anesthesia for coronary artery surgery. Anesth Analg 1983;62:661–665.
29. Tomicheck RC, Rosow CE, Philbin DM, Moss J, Teplick RS, Schneider RC. Diazepam–fentanyl interaction—hemodynamic and hormonal effects in coronary artery surgery. Anesth Analg 1983;62:881–884.
30. Cardoso PF, Yamazaki F, Keshavjee S, et al. A reevaluation of heparin requirements for cardiopulmonary bypass. J Thorac Cardiovasc Surg 1991;101:153–160.
31. Sabbagh AH, Chung GK, Shuttleworth P, Applegate BJ, Gabrhel W. Fresh frozen plasma: a solution to heparin resistance during cardiopulmonary bypass. Ann Thorac Surg 1984;37:466–468.
32. Buckberg GD, Allen BS. Myocardial protection management during adult cardiac operations. In: Glenn's Thoracic and Cardiovascular Surgery. 6th ed. Baue AE, et al. (eds.). Appleton & Lange, Stamford, CT, 1996, pp. 1653–1687.
33. Ferguson TB, Muhlbaier LH, Salai DL, Wechsler AS. Coronary bypass grafting after failed elective and failed emergent percutaneous angioplasty. J Thorac Cardiovasc Surg 1988;95:761–772.
34. Allen BS, Rosenkranz ER, Buckberg GD, Vinten-Johansen J, Okamoto F, Leaf J. High oxygen requirements of dyskinetic cardiac muscle. J Thorac Cardiovasc Surg 1986;92:543–552.

35. Beyersdorf F, Mitrev Z, Sarai K, et al. Changing patterns of patients undergoing emergency surgical revascularization for acute coronary occlusion. Importance of myocardial protection techniques. J Thorac Cardiovasc Surg 1993;106:137–148.

36. Beyersdorf F, Sarai K, Maul FD, Wendt T, Satter P. Immediate functional benefits after controlled reperfusion during surgical revascularization for acute coronary occlusion. J Thorac Cardiovasc Surg 1991;102:856–866.

37. Rosenkranz ER, Buckberg GD, Laks H, Mulder GD. Warm induction of cardioplegia with glutamate-enriched blood in coronary patients with cardiogenic shock who are dependent on inotropic drugs and intraaortic balloon support. J Thorac Cardiovasc Surg 1983;86:507–518.

38. Beyersdorf F, Acar C, Bukberg GD, et al. Studies on prolonged regional ischemia. III. Early natural history of simulated single and multivessel disease with emphasis on remote myocardium. J Thorac Cardiovasc Surg 1989;98:368–380.

39. Kerber RE, Marcus ML, Ehrhardt J, Wilson R, Abboud FM. Correlation between echocardiographically demonstrated segmental dyskinesis and regional myocardial perfusion. Circulation 1975;52:1097–1104.

40. Beyersdorf F, Acar C, Buckberg GD, et al. Studies on prolonged regional ischemia. IV. Aggressive surgical treatment for intractable ventricular fibrillation after acute myocardial infarction. J Thorac Cardiovasc Surg 1989;98:557–566.

41. Buckley GD. Myocardial protection during adult cardiac operations. In: Baue AE, Geha AS, Hammond GL, et al., eds. Glenn's Thoracic and Cardiovascular Surgery. 5th ed. Baue AE, et al. (eds.). Appleton & Lange, Norwalk, CT, 1991, Vol. 2, pp. 1417–1441.

42. Allen BS, Buckberg GD, Fontan FM, et al. Superiority of controlled surgical reperfusion versus percutaneous transluminal coronary angioplasty in acute coronary occlusion. J Thorac Cardiovasc Surg 1993;105:864–884.

43. Beyersdorf F, Buckberg G. Principles of myocardial protection during acute myocardial ischemia and reperfusion. In: Lazar H, ed. Current Therapy for Acute Coronary Ischemia. Futura, Mount Kisko, NY; 1993, pp. 111–148.

44. Buckberg GD. Substrate enriched warm blood cardioplegia reperfusion: an alternate view. Ann Thorac Surg 2000;69:334–335.

45. Akins CW. Early and late results following emergency isolated myocardial revascularization during hypothermic fibrillatory arrest. Ann Thorac Surg 1987;43:131–137.

46. Akins CW. 1987: Early and late results following emergency isolated myocardial revascularization during hypothermic fibrillatory arrest. Updated in 1994 by Cary W. Akins, MD. Ann Thorac Surg 1994;58:1205–1206.

47. Mohr R, Moshkovitch Y, Shapira I, Amir G, Hod H, Gurevitch J. Coronary artery bypass without cardiopulmonary bypass for patients with acute myocardial infarction. J Thorac Cardiovasc Surg 1999;118:50–56.

48. Perrault LP, Menasche P, Peyent J, et al. On-pump, beating-heart coronary artery operations in high-risk patients: an acceptable trade-off? Ann Thorac Surg 1997;64:1368–1373.

49. Cimochowski GE, Harostock MD, Foldes PJ. Minimal operative mortality in patients undergoing coronary artery bypass with significant left ventricular dysfunction by maximization of metabolic and mechanical support. J Thorac Cardiovasc Surg 1997;113:655–664.

50. Walpoth BH, Amport T, Schmid R, et al. Hemofiltration during cardiopulmonary bypass: quality assessment of hemoconcentrated blood. Thorac Cardiovasc Surg 1994;42:162–169.

51. Boldt J, Zickmann B, Czeke A, Herold C, Dapper F, Hempelmann G. Blood conservation techniques and platelet function in cardiac surgery. Anesthesiology 1991;75:426–432.

52. Nakamura Y, Masuda M, Toshima Y, et al. Comparative study of cell saver and ultrafiltration nontransfusion in cardiac surgery. Ann Thorac Surg 1990;49:973–978.

53. Breyer RH, Engelman RM, Rousou JA, Lemeshow SA. A comparison of cell saver versus ultrafilter during coronary artery bypass operations. J Thorac Cardiovasc Surg 1985;90:736–740.

54. Boldt J, Kling D, von Bormann B, Zuge M, Scheld H, Hempelmann G. Blood conservation in cardiac operations. Cell separation versus hemofiltration. J Thorac Cardiovasc Surg 1989;97:832–840.

55. Boga M, Islamoglu, Badak I, et al. The effects of modified hemofiltration on inflammatory mediators and cardiac performance in coronary artery bypass grafting. Perfusion 2000;15:143–150.

56. Magovern JA, Sakert T, Benckart DH, et al. A model for predicting transfusion after coronary artery bypass grafting. Ann Thorac Surg 1996;61:27–32.

57. Lemmer JH, Stanford W, Bonney SL, et al. Aprotinin for coronary artery bypass operations: efficacy, safety, and influence on early saphenous vein patency. J Thorac Cardiovasc Surg 1994;107:543–551.

58. Murkin JM, Lux J, Shannon NA, et al. Aprotinin significantly decreases bleeding and transfusion requirements in patients receiving aspirin and undergoing cardiac operations. J Thorac Cardiovasc Surg 1994;107:554–561.

59. Efstratiadis T, Munsch C, Crossman D, Taylor K. Aprotinin used in emergency coronary operation after streptokinase treatment. Ann Thorac Surg 1991;52:1320–1321.

60. Alajmo F, Calamai G. High-dose aprotinin in emergency coronary artery bypass after thrombolysis. Ann Thorac Surg 1992;54:1022–1023.

61. Dignan RJ, Law DW, Seah PW, et al. Ultra-low dose aprotinin decreases transfusion requirements and is cost effective in coronary operations. Ann Thorac Surg 2001;71:158–164.

62. Arom KV, Emery RW. Decreased postoperative drainage with addition of epsilon-amincaproic acid before cardiopulmonary bypass. Ann Thorac Surg 1994;57:1108–1113.

63. DelRossi AJ, Cernaianu AC, Bostros S, Lemole GM, Moore R. Prophylactic treatment of postperfusion bleeding using EACA. Chest 1989;96:27–30.

64. Moosvi AR, Khaja F, Villanueva L, Gheorghiade M, Douthat L, Goldstein S. Early revascularization improves survival in cardiogenic shock complicating myocardial infarction. J Am Coll Cardiol 192;19:907–914.

65. Laks H, Rosenkranz E, Buckberg GD. Surgical treatment of cardiogenic shock after myocardial infarction. Circulation 1986;74(5 Pt 2):III11–III16.

66. Hines GL, Mohtashemi M. Delayed operative intervention in cardiogenic shock after myocardial infarction. Ann Thorac Surg 1982;33:132–138.

67. Miller MG, Hedley-White J, Weintraub RM, Restall DS, Alexander M. Surgery for cardigenic shock. Lancet 1974;2:1342–1345.

68. Buffet P, Danchin N, Villemot JP, et al. Early and long-term outcome after emergency coronary artery bypass surgery after failed coronary angioplasty. Circulation 1991;84(Suppl III):III-254–III-259.

69. Sergeant P, Blackstone E, Meyens B. Early and late outcome after CABG in patients with evolving myocardial infarction. Eur J Cardiothorac Surg 1997;11:848–856.

70. Subramanian VA, Roberts AJ, Zema MJ, et al. Cardiogenic shock following myocardial infarction: late functional results after emergency cardiac surgery. NY State J Med 1980;80:947–952.

IV

MECHANICAL COMPLICATIONS OF ACUTE MYOCARDIAL INFARCTION CAUSING CARDIOGENIC SHOCK

8

Mechanical Complications
of Acute Myocardial Infarction
Causing Cardiogenic Shock

Yochai Birnbaum, MD,
and Robert J. Siegel, MD

CONTENTS

INTRODUCTION

Heart failure and hemodynamic deterioration in the course of acute myocardial infarction (MI) may be caused by several cardiac and noncardiac mechanisms (Table 1) *(1)*. In this chapter, we will discuss the following three mechanical complications of acute MI: ventricular septal rupture, left ventricular free wall rupture, and acute mitral regurgitation.

VENTRICULAR SEPTAL RUPTURE

Ventricular septal rupture (VSR) is a rare complication of acute MI that has not been adequately investigated. Most studies of VSR complicating MI have been retrospective, lacked a comparison group of acute MI patients without VSR, or included only a small number of patients or autopsy cases. In addition, many trial investigators combined patients with VSR with those who had left ventricular free wall rupture (VFWR). As a result, the specific role of VSR in complicating anterior and inferior acute MI has not been distinguished. Because of the weakness of the majority of these studies, the findings of VSR are often inconsistent and lack conclusive data.

Incidence

In the prethrombolytic era, the incidence of VSR was reported to be 1–3% *(2–8)*. Then, the Global Utilization of Streptokinase and TPA for Occluded Coronary Arteries (GUSTO-I) trial demonstrated that the VSR incidence rate was lower in acute MI

From: *Contemporary Cardiology: Cardiogenic Shock: Diagnosis and Treatment*
Edited by: David Hasdai et al. © Humana Press Inc., Totowa, NJ

Table 1
Differential Diagnosis of Acute Heart Failure and Hemodynamic Deterioration
in Acute Myocardial Infarction

Cardiac	Noncardiac
Large acute MI[a]	Anaphylaxis (streptokinase, etc.)
Previous MI, extensive coronary artery disease, concomitant left main coronary artery stenosis, cardiomyopathy, etc.	Hemorrhage (especially in patients receiving thrombolytics or undergoing invasive procedures)
Acute ventricular septal rupture	Drug-induced cardiac dysfunction and/or hypotensive drugs (β-blockers, nitrates, morphine, etc.)
Acute mitral regurgitation	
Acute left ventricular free wall rupture	Pulmonary emboli
	Infection, sepsis
Acute tamponade	
Reduced left ventricular reserve	
Right ventricular infarction	
Arrhythmia	

[a] MI=myocardial infarction.

patients undergoing thrombolytic therapy *(9)*. To date, GUSTO-I is the only study to specifically assess the incidence of VSR in the thrombolytic era. The trial included 41,021 patients, and VSR was suspected in 140 patients (0.34%) but later confirmed in 84 (0.2%) by retrospective ancillary questionnaires. Thus, the true incidence of VSR among the patients enrolled ranged from 0.2% to 0.34%, as some of the cases may have gone unsuspected *(9)*. However, among patients with cardiogenic shock, the incidence of VSR is higher: 3.9% of 1422 patients with cardiogenic shock had VSR in the SHOCK (SHould we emergently revascularize Occluded Coronaries for cardiogenic shocK) Trial and Registry *(1)*.

Risk Factors

In the prethrombolytic era, VSR occurred more frequently in anterior rather than nonanterior acute MI, and other risk factors include advanced age and female gender *(4,10–17)* (Table 2). Hypertension was found to be a risk factor for early VSR but not late VSR *(17)*. Notably, the absence of prior angina or MI was also a risk factor *(3,4,18–20)*. Previous angina or MI may precondition the myocardium and aid in developing collaterals, both of which may be protective against VSR *(20)*.

In patients undergoing thrombolytic therapy, VSR is still more commonly reported in anterior rather than nonanterior acute MI *(9)* (Table 2). Among the 10,927 patients with anterior acute MI enrolled in the GUSTO-I trial, VSR was confirmed in 48 (0.4%) *(21)*. VSR also continues to be associated with advanced age and female gender *(9)*. Systemic hypertension and the absence of previous angina are not risk factors for patients undergoing thrombolytic therapy, but having had a previous MI or not having been a smoker are associated with increased risk of VSR *(9)*.

In the GUSTO-I trial, investigators found that blood pressure also influenced a patient's chances of having VSR because the relationship between the enrollment

Table 2
Risk Factors of Ventricular Septal Rupture, Ventricular Free Wall Rupture,
and Acute Mitral Regurgitation With and Without Papillary Muscle Rupture

Risk factor	VSR	VFWR	MR without PMR	MR with PMR
Advanced age	✓	✓	✓	✓
Female gender	✓	✓	✓	✓
Low body weight and short stature		✓		
Systemic hypertension	✓[a]			
Absence of elevated blood pressure		✓		
Absence of LVH in response to hypertension	✓			
Absence of previous angina	✓[a]	✓[b]		✓
Absence of previous MI	✓	✓[b]		
Prior MI	✓[c]		✓	
Anterior location of MI	✓			
Inferoposterior MI				✓
Right ventricular involvement in inferior MI	✓			
Large infarct size			✓	
Recurrent myocardial ischemia			✓	
Multivessel coronary artery disease			✓	
Single vessel disease		✓[b]		✓
Absence of smoking history	✓	✓		
Absence of diabetes mellitus		✓		✓
Absence of peripheral vascular disease		✓		
Enrollment systolic blood pressure	✓[d]			
Enrollment diastolic blood pressure	✓[d]			
New right bundle-branch block	✓			
Heart failure on admission			✓	
Absence of previous CHF		✓		
Left ventricular lateral wall involvement		✓		
New interventricular conduction defect on EKG		✓		
High CRP levels		✓		

Abbreviations: VSR = ventricular septal rupture; VFWR = ventricular free wall rupture; MR = mitral regurgitation; PMR = papillary muscle rupture; LVH = left ventricular hypertrophy; MI = myocardial infarction; CHF = congestive heart failure; CRP = C-reactive protein.

[a] In the prethrombolytic era only.

[b] Other reports show presence of the variables to be risk factors.

[c] Thrombolytic era only.

[d] Nonlinear relationship.

systolic and diastolic blood pressures and VSR was significant. The likelihood of VSR decreased when systolic pressure increased to about 130 mm Hg. As the systolic pressure became >130 mm Hg, the risk of VSR increased. Similarly, the likelihood of VSR decreased when diastolic blood pressure increased to about 75 mm Hg, then the risk increased when diastolic pressure exceeded 75 mm Hg. The rise in the incidence of VSR as systolic blood pressure increased above 130 mm Hg and the diastolic blood pressure above 75 mm Hg may reflect the association between hypertension and VSR.

On the other hand, the negative correlations between VSR incidence and enrollment systolic blood pressure (≤130 mm Hg) and diastolic blood pressure (≤75 mm Hg) may relate to the occurrence of hemodynamic compromise associated with extensive MI or right ventricular infarction, both of which are established risk factors for VSR *(9)*. The presence of right bundle-branch block with or without fascicular block, advanced atrioventricular block, or atrial fibrillation may occur more frequently in patients with VSR than in patients with free wall rupture *(19,21,22)*.

Pathophysiology

After an MI, VSR generally develops at the margins of the necrotic and non-necrotic myocardium. The size of VSR ranges from a few millimeters to several centimeters. The septal tissue adjacent to the defect is often thin and necrotic, whereas the septum may be fibrotic in patients who die several weeks after the development of the VSR. Some patients develop a septal aneurysm adjacent to the rupture site. In addition, the rupture of other cardiac structures such as papillary muscles and the free wall of the left and/or right ventricles may occur concomitantly *(10,19,23,24)*.

Morphologically, VSR can be categorized into simple and complex forms. Simple VSR is a discrete hole with a direct through-and-through communication across the septum. The ventricular openings are located at the same level on both sides of the septum. Complex VSR is characterized by extensive hemorrhage around irregular serpiginous tracts extending in different directions within extensive necrotic tissue *(10,18)*. Complex ruptures are more likely to affect associated structures such as the right ventricle *(10)*. VSRs in anterior acute MI tend to be apical and simple, whereas in inferior acute MI, they involve the inferobasal septum and are usually complex *(6,10,18)*. Most patients with VSR complicating both anterior and inferior MI have evidence of right ventricular infarction *(16)*.

Ventricular septal rupture is complicated by left-to-right shunting, which results in right ventricular volume overload, increased pulmonary blood flow, as well as volume overload of the left atrium and left ventricle. As the left ventricular systolic function deteriorates and forward flow declines, compensatory vasoconstriction triggers an increase in systemic vascular resistance and in the magnitude of left-to-right shunt. The severity of the left-to-right shunt is determined by the size of the VSR, relative changes in the pulmonary and systemic vascular resistances and pressure, and left ventricular performance *(14)*.

Another pathophysiologic characteristic of VSR is that the condition may coexist with mitral regurgitation (MR). Ten to 20% of patients with VSR also have severe MR *(25,26)*, which may be the result of concomitant papillary muscle ischemia or infarction, dilatation of the mitral annulus, or deformation of the left ventricle with alteration of the geometry of the mitral apparatus *(13,22)*.

Angiographic Findings

In studies using angiographic data, investigators have consistently demonstrated that patients with VSR are more likely to have total occlusion of the infarct-related artery *(6,9,13,27)*. In patients who underwent angiography in the GUSTO-I study, total occlusion of the infarct-related artery was documented in 57% of patients with VSR and

18% of patients without VSR. However, reports vary as to the angiographic extent of coronary artery disease in patients with VSR *(4,10,13)*. Some investigators have found that VSR patients almost always have multivessel coronary artery disease *(4,10)*, whereas others have documented single-vessel disease more often than multivessel disease *(13,21)*. Lemery et al. reported that among 77 patients with VSR in whom the extent of coronary artery disease was evaluated by angiography or autopsy, 54% had single-vessel disease, 13% had two-vessel disease, and only 24% had three-vessel disease *(28)*. Investigators with the GUSTO-I study did not find a significant difference in the prevalence of two-vessel (40% vs 28%) or three-vessel disease (11% vs 18%) between patients with and without VSR *(9)*. In addition, most *(4,13,20)* but not all investigators *(22)* have reported that collaterals were less often identified by angiography in patients with VSR. This is consistent with the assumption that collateral circulation may prevent rupture of the interventricular septum *(2,20)*.

Time of Occurrence

In the prethrombolytic era, VSR typically occurred in patients during the first week after infarction with a mean time of 3–5 d from symptoms' onset *(6,8,10,28,29)*. The rupture rarely occurred after 2 wk. Lemery et al. demonstrated that the mean ± standard deviation (SD) time interval was 2.2 ± 2.1 d in patients with inferior acute MI and 6.2 ± 11 d in patients with anterior acute MI ($p < 0.01$) *(28)*.

The majority of studies involving thrombolytic therapy demonstrated an accelerated timing of occurrence for patients who received thrombolytics *(9,30,31)*. For example, Westaby et al. reported that the median interval from symptoms' onset of the index MI to the development of VSR was 24 h for patients receiving streptokinase compared to 6 d for those who did not receive thrombolysis *(30)*. Similarly, in the GUSTO-I Trial and the SHOCK Trial, the median time from onset of MI to VSR was 24 and16 h, respectively. However, Oskoui et al. reported that the time interval from symptoms' onset of MI to VSR was comparable between patients who had received thrombolytic therapy (115 ± 86 h) and those who had not (117 ± 106 h) *(17)*.

Thus, thrombolytic therapy may accelerate VSR by causing myocardial hemorrhage early after thrombolytic administration. However, thrombolytic therapy appears to reduce the incidence of VSR. This is probably because the therapy may prevent extensive transmural myocardial necrosis, a prerequisite for VSR.

Clinical Manifestations

Chest pain is a common clinical manifestation that often precedes VSR, particularly late VSR (>48 h after the onset of symptoms) *(4,19)*. For example, Oskoui et al. reported chest pain to occur prior to VSR in 67% of patients with late VSR versus only 35% of those with early VSR (≤48 h after symptoms' onset) *(17)*. Similarly, Figueras et al. found that 72% of patients with late VSR reported chest pain *(19)*. VSR is also characterized by a harsh holosystolic murmur often to the right or the left sternal border and radiating toward the base and the apex. The VSR murmur is accompanied by a thrill in about half of the patients *(28,32)*. In many cases, a right and left ventricular S3 gallop and accentuation of the pulmonic component of the second heart sound can be heard. Signs of tricuspid regurgitation may also be present. Acute biventricular heart failure including pulmonary edema and shock with severe right-heart failure generally ensues within hours to days.

It is sometimes difficult to distinguish between an acute intraventricular rupture and acute mitral regurgitation (MR). The clinical distinction between the two can often be made on the basis of the characteristics and intensity of the murmur, as the VSR murmur is louder and more often associated with the presence of a thrill, which is uncommon in papillary muscle rupture. In addition, right-heart failure is more common in the setting of VSR. The chest radiograph will more frequently show pulmonary edema in patients with severe MR. Nonetheless, physical findings may be unreliable, especially in those with extensive MI and low cardiac output.

Diagnosis

ECHOCARDIOGRAPHY

Doppler echocardiography has emerged as the main tool for the diagnosis of VSR because the exact site and approximate size of the VSR, as well as estimates of left-to-right shunt size, left and right ventricular function, and right ventricular systolic pressure can be obtained *(9,33–35)*. The sensitivity and specificity of two-dimensional (2D) transthoracic echocardiography combined with color Doppler has been reported to be 100% *(33,34)*. However, in severely ill patients on mechanical ventilators, the image quality of transthoracic echocardiography may be too poor for an accurate diagnosis or localization. Consequently, transesophageal echocardiography should be used in those cases with suboptimal or non diagnostic transthoracic studies *(36–38)*. Radionuclide scintigraphy is another noninvasive technique that can be used for diagnosing VSR, assessing left ventricular and right ventricular function, and calculating the magnitude of the shunt *(39)*. However, transesophageal echocardiography is probably the optimal technique for precise anatomic localization and sizing of the VSD.

INVASIVE TECHNIQUES

Although less accurate than Doppler echocardiography, pulmonary artery catheterization (Swan Ganz Catheter®, Baxter's Cardio Vascular Group, Irvine, CA) is an invasive technique that is helpful in diagnosing VSR. A step-up in oxygen saturation should be present within both the right ventricle and pulmonary artery in order for VSR to be diagnosed. However, the pressure waveforms in the pulmonary capillary wedge position cannot reliably distinguish between VSR and acute MR. This is because "V" waves are not specific for acute MR and may occur with VSR as well as the fact that both conditions may coexist. Because of this disadvantage and others, pulmonary artery catheterization is now primarily used for monitoring therapy and for patient follow-up rather than as a diagnostic modality *(40,41)*. Left-heart catheterization and left ventriculography are two invasive techniques that may also confirm the diagnosis of VSR. These two methods are employed if the patient is hemodynamically stable and if the coronary anatomy needs to be identified because concomitant coronary artery bypass surgery is an option.

Management of Patients

The initial management of those with VSR includes a rapid and aggressive approach to hemodynamically stabilize the patients, pending angiography and mechanical closure of the VSR. Initial stabilization with medical therapy usually provides only temporary relief because most patients with VSR deteriorate rapidly and die. Only those few who do not develop clinical and hemodynamic deterioration can be managed solely with medical therapy *(42)*. Medical therapy consists of afterload reduction, diuretics, and inotropic agents, in addition to mechanical support with intra-aortic balloon pump counterpulsation and intermittent positive-pressure mechanical ventilation *(43)*. Intravenous nitroprusside also reduces the left-to-right shunt and improves forward cardiac output, but this agent can cause severe hypotension and may be contraindicated in patients with acute renal failure, which frequently accompanies acute VSR. An infusion of inotropic and vasopressor agents is sometimes used in hypotensive patients to sustain arterial blood pressure, but these agents also can increase the left-to-right shunt as well as increase myocardial ischemia and possible infarct size.

The mortality of patients with VSR who are treated conservatively without mechanical closure has been reported to be 24% within 24 h, 46% within the first week, and 67–82% at 2 mo *(44,45)*. In the GUSTO-I study, 30-d mortality and 1-yr mortality in the 35 VSR patients who did not undergo surgery was 94% and 97%; patients who were selected for surgery had a better outcome, with 47% and 53% mortality ($p < 0.001$), respectively *(9)*.

Mechanical Closure of VSR

Despite the fact that patients who do not undergo surgical repair are often older and more critically ill, mechanical closure of VSR either by surgical repair or by use of percutaneous transcatheter techniques is generally mandated for most symptomatic patients *(28,46–48)*. However, the timing of surgical intervention remains unresolved. Previously, most cardiologists and cardiovascular surgeons claimed that the myocardial tissue was too fragile to allow for safe repair of the VSR shortly after an MI, so a waiting period of 3–6 wk before surgery was recommended to allow for myocardial healing and scar formation *(49)*. However, many patients died awaiting surgery or underwent emergency operations after sudden decompensation *(28,43,50)*. In 1977, this approach was questioned when investigators demonstrated an increase in the survival rate of 43 patients with VSR after acute MI following early surgical repair, and other studies have continued to confirm this finding *(3,51,52)*.

On the other hand, some still argue that a waiting period is beneficial for patients. Recent studies have shown that a short interval between VSR development and surgical repair is associated with early mortality *(53–55)*. For example, Lemery et al. reported a lower 30-d survival rate for patients who underwent surgical repair ≤48 h after the onset of symptoms (59%) compared with those operated 2–14 d after onset (84%) *(28)*. In those surgically treated >14 d after VSR, however, the 30-d mortality was only 33%. This finding supports the theory that the outcome after surgery is better for those who are stable enough to be treated medically for at least 2 wk *(28)*.

Percutaneous transcatheter closure of VSR is slowly emerging as an alternative to surgical repair in selected patients *(46–48)*. Although only a few cases have been reported, the following points should be considered when choosing this option: (1) VSR after acute MI is surrounded by fragile necrotic tissue and may increase in size during attempts to pass the sealing device; (2) VSR in anterior MI is located near the apex of the left ventricle, whereas the rupture is found near the origin of the right and left ventricular free wall in inferior MI. Thus, completely opening the wings of a device such as the Amplatzer® (AGA Medical Corporation, Golden Valley, MN) may distort the anatomy of the right or left ventricles; (3) VSR in inferior MI is usually basal and thus close to the tricuspid and mitral valve apparatus. Therefore, positioning and opening the sealing devices may damage or alter the function of these valvular structures.

Prognosis

In the prethrombolytic era, outcomes for patients with VSR were extremely poor with an in-hospital mortality of about 45% in surgically treated patients and 90% in those managed medically *(6,52,56,57)*. Despite the advances in therapy, like thrombolysis and surgical revascularization or balloon angioplasty, in-hospital mortality for patients with VSR has not improved *(9,54)*. In the SHOCK Trial registry, in-hospital mortality was significantly higher for patients in cardiogenic shock resulting from VSR than in all other categories of shock: 87.3% of the 55 patients with VSR died compared with 59.2% of those with pure left ventricular failure and 55.1% with acute MR *(1)*. However, the long-term prognosis is relatively good for patients who survive long enough to undergo surgery *(9)*. For example, Davies et al. reported that among 60 patients who survived surgical repair, the 5-, 10-, and 14-yr survival rates were 69%, 50%, and 37%, respectively *(57)*.

A number of possible determinants of outcome have been studied in patients with VSR *(6,22,29,52)*. One major determinant for postoperative outcome is the immediate preoperative hemodynamic status of the patient *(4,43)*. In the GUSTO-I trial, all 8 patients with VSR who were in Killip class III or IV at presentation died, compared with 53 out of 74 patients in Killip class I or II at presentation *(9)*. Patients with VSR complicating inferior MI have a worse outcome than those with VSR complicating anterior MI *(4,8,29,52)*.

Right ventricular function and the presence of renal failure are also important predictors of survival. Among patients who undergo surgical repair, prognosis is influenced by the duration of cardiopulmonary bypass, systolic blood pressure, and right atrial pressure *(4,8,29,53)*.

VENTRICULAR FREE WALL RUPTURE

Ventricular free wall rupture (VFWR) generally manifests as sudden cardiovascular collapse, electromechanical dissociation, and early death. However, VFWR is not always fatal; many patients who have subacute VFWR or a sealed rupture with a pseudoaneurysm of the left ventricle survive *(58–62)*. Although left VFWR is a rare catastrophic complication of acute MI, it is reported to be the cause of death in 15–30% of patients with a fatal acute MI. Right VFWR may also complicate right ventricular acute MI *(58,63)*. The pathophysiology, clinical manifestations, diagnosis, and management of left and right VFWR are indistinguishable, and the two entities will be discussed together.

Most studies on VFWR complicating acute MI have been retrospective, have combined patients with VFWR and VSR, and have not always confirmed the diagnosis of VFWR because most patients die suddenly and autopsies are not routinely performed. In the majority of studies, patients with sudden hemodynamic collapse, evidence of electromechanical dissociation, and cardiac tamponade are considered as having VFWR. However, cardiac tamponade may occur without VFWR in patients with acute MI, especially among patients who receive thrombolytic therapy (64–67). In addition, there are patients with VFWR who have also rupture of a papillary muscle and/or VSR *(24–26,68–70)*.

Table 3
Incidence of Cardiac Rupture/Electromechanical Dissociation
in Patients with Myocardial Infarction

Study	Trial	Publication year	% with VFWR	N	Type	% of VFWR confirmed by autopsy	% of in-hospital mortality
National Registry of MI *(71)*		1996	0.8	350,755	CR/ED		7.3[a]
Dellborg et al. *(72)*		1985	3.2	1,746	CR		
Shapira et al. *(15)*		1987	2.3	1,737	ED	40	15.7
Pohjola-Sintonen et al. *(3)*	MILIS	1989	1.3	845	ED	69	
Honan et al. *(73)*		1990	3.5	1,638	CR		
López-Sendón et al. *(58)*		1992	6.2	1,457	VFWR	32[a]	
Pollak et al. *(74)*		1993	3.13	2,608	VFWR	All were fatal	16.3
Purcaro et al. *(70)*		1997	6.56[b]		VFWR		
Becker et al. *(75)*	LATE	1995	1.6	5,711	CR/ED	All were fatal[c]	29.1[d]
Becker et al. *(76)*	TIMI 9	1999	1.7	3,759	VFWR		

Abbreviations: MI=myocardial infarction; MILIS=Multicenter Investigation of Limitation of Infarct Size; LATE=Late Assessment of Thrombolytic Efficacy; TIMI=Thrombolysis and Thrombin Inhibition in Myocardial Infarction; CR=cardiac rupture; ED=electromechanical dissociation; VFWR=ventricular free wall rupture.

[a] Diagnoses of VFWR were made because of sudden electromechanical dissociation followed by death.

[b] 4.1% acute VFWR and 2.5% subacute VFWR.

[c] 56% were confirmed VFWR.

[d] Confirmed rupture accounted for 29.1% of all deaths at 35 d; including cases with electromechanical dissociation, cardiac rupture accounted for 53.1% of all deaths at 35 d.

Incidence

The reported incidence of VFWR ranges from 0.8% to 6.2% (Table 3). Although the prevalence is low, VFWR accounts for a large portion of in-hospital mortality, especially within the first 24 h of presentation and in patients undergoing thrombolytic therapy *(71–79)*. For example, in a postmortem retrospective study of 125 patients with VFWR (prior to the thrombolytic era), 33% died on the first hospital day (Siegel and Fishbein, unpublished data). In the Thrombolysis in Myocardial Infarction II (TIMI-II) Trial, cardiac rupture was the cause of death in 16% of patients who died within the first 18 h of therapy *(78)*. Because rates of death from arrhythmias have decreased in intensive care units, the relative contribution of cardiac rupture to mortality after MI has increased, making it the second most common cause of death after left ventricular failure *(80)*.

Risk Factors

Risk factors for VFWR include female gender, advanced age, low body weight, short stature, strenuous activities during recovery phases, and large myocardial infarct size *(3,58,68,71,72,74–76,81–83)* (Table 2). Some studies indicate that women aged 60–69 y are especially at risk *(15,72)*, although this finding is controversial *(3,68)*. Warning signs for VFWR may include intraventricular conduction defect on an electrocardiogram (ECG), echocardiographic signs of lateral wall involvement, and high serum C-reactive proteins *(74,82,84–86)*. Resuscitation measures, such as external cardiac massage and intracardiac injections, have also been suggested as possible causes of cardiac rupture *(87)*.

Some factors that are normally considered high risk for serious cardiac diseases may not be risk factors for cardiac rupture. For example, there are two studies in which patients who are active smokers are less likely to have a cardiac rupture *(75,76)*, whereas the study of Pollak et al. reported no difference between smokers and non-smokers *(74)*. Additionally, in patients with cardiogenic shock, those who develop VWFR are less likely to have peripheral vascular disease or diabetes mellitus *(81)*.

In patients with hypertension, left ventricular hypertrophy appears to be protective against cardiac rupture *(82,88)*. Mann and Roberts found the mean heart weights were lower (although not significantly lower) in patients with hypertension who developed cardiac rupture *(84)*. Thus, failure to develop left ventricular hypertrophy in response to hypertension could be a risk factor for VFWR.

A history of hypertension is not considered to be a risk factor for or an independent predictor of VFWR *(3,72,76,84,89)*. However, some studies show significantly more hypertension among patients with cardiac rupture than among surviving patients with no rupture *(71,74)*. VFWR may be associated with acute or sustained hypotension related to severe heart failure caused by a large infarct *(15,72,83)*. Indeed, Pohjola-Sintonen et al. found that cardiac rupture was more prevalent in patients with systolic blood pressure <150 mm Hg than in those with systolic blood pressure >150 mm Hg *(3)*.

Most studies indicate that patients with a history of angina pectoris, prior MI, three-vessel coronary artery disease, or congestive heart failure are also less likely to develop VFWR *(3,72,74,81,84,90)*. Prior angina suggests the presence of chronic obstructive coronary artery disease, which is associated with the development of coronary artery collaterals that may reduce the incidence of both free wall and septal rupture. In addition, previous angina may precondition the myocardium and be protective against ventricular septal *(20)* and free wall rupture. Scar formation resulting from a previous MI or pericardial thickening resulting from previous inflammation may also offer protection against VFWR *(81,82)*.

However, there are conflicting data indicating that prior angina, prior MI, or three-vessel coronary artery disease may not be protective against cardiac rupture. Becker et al. found prior angina to be an independent risk factor for cardiac rupture *(76)*. In the National Registry of Myocardial Infarction (NRMI), prior MI was independently associated with cardiac rupture *(71)*. Other reports indicate a higher incidence of three-vessel coronary artery disease in patients with cardiac rupture *(68,82)*.

Pathophysiology

Left VFWR usually occurs on the anterior or lateral wall of the left ventricle at the mid-papillary muscle level *(91,92)*. Veinot et al. found that in 20 of 25 patients (80%), the endocardial tear associated with LVFWR was within 1 cm of the base of a papillary muscle where it inserted in the left ventricular free wall *(91).* This location suggests that the increased stress at the site of papillary muscle insertion facilitates cardiac rupture because of the different arrangement of muscle fibers.

Becker et al. *(93),* Perigao et al. (94), and Pucaro et al. (70) have described the many pathologic varieties of cardiac rupture (Table 4). In a study of 50 patients, Becker described three types of VFWR: an abrupt slitlike tear (Type I), an erosion of the infarcted myocardium at the border between the infarcted and viable myocardium (Type II), and an early aneurysm formation that is correlated with older, severely expanded infarctions (Type III) *(93,95).* Because reperfusion therapy inhibits myocardial expansion *(96)* and thrombolytic therapy reduces the incidence of late rupture *(75,97),* the incidence of Type III may be reduced with reperfusion therapy, and patients who undergo reperfusion therapy and develop a rupture may be more likely to have Type I or II VFWR.

Perdigao et al. described four types of VFWR in 42 patients (Table 4). The ruptures were characterized by little dissection (Type I), widespread myocardial dissection (Type II), protection by an intraventricular thrombus or a pericardial symphysis (Type III), or an incomplete epicardial, endocardial, or intramyocardial rupture that was not transmural (Type IV) (94).

Finally, Purcaro et al. described six pathophysiologic varieties of VFWR in 28 patients: through-and-through rupture of the infarcted area in the presence of normal wall thickness (Type I), expansion of softened necrotic zone and rupture(s) of the wall (Type II), numerous small perforations within an area of myomalacia (Type III), rupture of the outer layers of the infarcted area in the presence of normal wall thickness (Type IV), large epicardial hematoma under pressure (Type V), and hemorrhagic infarcts with grossly intact, abraded, and leaking epicardial surfaces *(70)* (Table 4).

Pseudoaneurysm is another pathophysiologic variety of subacute or chronic myocardial rupture *(98–104).* In these cases, the myocardial rupture is sealed by the pericardium. A discrete space develops and connects to the left ventricle through a narrow neck. In contrast to a true left ventricular aneurysm, the wall of a pseudoaneurysm is composed of pericardium and not myocardium or scar tissue. The neck of a pseudoaneurysm is typically (but not always) narrower than that of a true aneurysm.

Time of Occurrence

Ventricular free wall rupture generally occurs between 1 and 7 d after MI *(15,68,75,82,88,90,105).* In the prethrombolytic era, among 100 consecutive autopsies of patients with postinfarction left VFWR, 13% occurred during the first day, 58% within 5 d, and 80% within 7 d *(82).* In another report, VFWR occurred within 24 h of the onset of myocardial infarction in 15 patients (54%), within 7 d in 12 patients (43%), and by 12 d in 1 patient (4%) *(70).*

Reperfusion therapy is used to restore blood flow in MI patients. There are two major types of reperfusion therapy — thrombolytic therapy and primary angioplasty — and both can impact the incidence and timing of cardiac rupture.

Thrombolytic therapy reduces infarct size and prevents expansion but has not reduced the incidence rate for all cardiac ruptures *(71,75,76).* It has, however, reduced the incidence of a few specific types of rupture, such as those associated with severely expanded

Table 4
Classifications of VFWR

	Becker (93)	Perdigao et al. (94)	Purcaro et al. (70)
Type I	• An abrupt, slitlike tear • Acute and early presentation • More common in anterior MI • Associated with single-vessel disease.	• An almost direct trajectory with little dissection and bloody infiltration of the myocardium	• Through-and-through rupture of the infarcted area in the presence of normal thickness of the wall
Type II	• An "erosion" of the infarcted myocardium, usually at the border between infarcted and viable myocardium • Subacute presentation and longer time interval between onset of symptoms and development of tamponade • More common in posterior MI • Associated with multivessel disease	• A multicanalicular trajectory, widespread myocardial dissection, and bloody infiltration	• Expansion of softened necrotic zone with rupture(s) of the wall
Type III	• Early aneurysm formation, which correlates clinically with older infarctions • Usually late presentation • More common in large anterior MI (expansion) • Associated with single-vessel disease	• The orifice of rupture is protected by an intraventricular thrombus or a pericardial symphysis	• Numerous small perforations within an area of myomalacia • Subacute presentation
Type IV	—	• Incomplete epicardial, endocardial, or intramyocardial rupture	• Rupture of the outer layers of the infarcted area in the presence of normal thickness of the wall
Type V	—	—	• Large epicardial hematoma under pressure (covert rupture) • Subacute presentation
Type VI	—	—	• Bleeding infarcts: hemorrhagic infarct with grossly intact, but abraded and leaking epicardial surface

infarctions (Becker's Type III), expansion of a necrotic zone (Purcaro's Type II), or small perforations in an area of morbid softening (Purcaro's Type III). On the other hand, it has been suggested that thrombolytic therapy accelerates cardiac ruptures associated with an abrupt tear or an erosion of infarcted myocardium (Becker's Type I and II) *(71)*.

In the thrombolytic era, although the incidence rate of rupture has not changed *(75,76)* or has declined *(71)*, the onset of rupture has accelerated *(71,75,76)*. For example, Becker et al. reported a mean onset time of 3.7 d in the prethrombolytic era and 2.7 d in the thrombolytic era *(71)*. There are many potential reasons for this acceleration. Thrombolytic therapy increases the incidence of intramyocardial hemorrhage *(106,107)*, and intramyocardial hemorrhages may weaken the supporting framework of the necrotic zone and lead to cardiac rupture. Plasmin, a nonspecific proteolytic enzyme generated by all thrombolytic agents, increases collagen breakdown *(108)*, which can accelerate rupture. In addition, according to NRMI, those who receive thrombolytic therapy and have a cardiac rupture account for a larger percentage of the in-hospital mortality (12.1%) than patients who do not receive thrombolytic therapy and have a cardiac rupture (6.1%; $p < 0.001$) *(71)*.

The studies that have evaluated the impact of thrombolytic therapy on the incidence and timing of VFWR have shown that early treatment (within approximately the first 6–7 h of symptomatic onset) reduces the risk. However, late treatment (after approx 11 h) increases the risk for VFWR *(73,75)*.

As opposed to reperfusion therapy with thrombolytics, primary angioplasty consistently reduces the risk of cardiac rupture *(83,109)*. For example, Solodky et al. reported that among 2377 consecutive patients with acute MI, cardiac rupture (VFWR or VSR) occurred in 2.8%, 0%, and 2.4% of the patients who received thrombolytic therapy ($n = 1162$), primary percutaneous transluminal coronary angioplasty (PTCA) ($n = 103$), and those who did not undergo reperfusion therapy ($n = 1112$) *(83)*. Primary angioplasty may be associated with a lower risk of cardiac rupture than thrombolytic therapy because it causes less hemorrhagic transformation and does not activate proteolytic enzymes.

Clinical Manifestations

One clinical manifestation of VFWR is cardiac tamponade, which can result from acute or subacute VFWR. When cardiac tamponade results from acute VFWR (usually Becker's Type I), the clinical presentation is sudden, with abrupt development of electromechanical dissociation or asystole *(110,111)*. In some patients, severe chest pain briefly precedes hemodynamic collapse. Most patients show pericardial effusion with tamponade on an echocardiogram and die shortly after onset of rupture.

Subacute VFWR can also lead to cardiac tamponade. Marked distention of the jugular veins and pulsus paradoxus (inspiratory drop of >10 mm Hg in systemic arterial pressure) are classical signs of cardiac tamponade. However, marked jugular vein distention has been found in only 29% of patients who develop tamponade after cardiac rupture *(74)*, and pulsus paradoxus in only 46–48% of these patients *(58,70)*.

In about one-third of the patients with VFWR, the course is subacute *(58,74)*. The clinical presentations of these patients include transient, prolonged, or recurrent chest pain, syncope, hypotension, shock, arrhythmia, and transient electromechanical dissociation *(58,61,74,112–114)*. Pleuritic or pericardial pain may also occur *(70)*. In addition, transient bradycardia, nausea, repetitive emesis, and restlessness may precede cardiac rupture *(70,113,115)*.

In some cases, the patient may have tamponade resulting from pericarditis and not VFWR. The electrocardiographic findings of pericarditis include persistent or new ST-segment elevations, persistently positive T-waves, or inverted T-waves becoming positive *(74,115,116)*. These findings are insensitive and nonspecific, and the ECG cannot be considered a useful tool for the diagnosis *(58,70)*. However, echocardiography showing a >5 mm pericardial effusion in a patient with acute MI and transient hypotension, electromechanical dissociation, or syncope is highly indicative of VFWR *(58,114)*.

Ventricular free wall rupture may be the presenting manifestation of acute MI *(117)*, especially in diabetic patients *(118)*. In others, the acute MI might be silent or subclinical, and the first episode of chest pain may be related to the cardiac rupture *(88)*.

Diagnosis

Ventricular free wall rupture must be suspected in any patient with shock or chest pain suggestive of infarct extension or severe arrhythmias followed by shock *(74)*. The abrupt development of electromechanical dissociation in patients without preceding heart failure is highly predictive of VFWR *(110)*, but this association is less strong in patients with preceding heart failure.

ECHOCARDIOGRAPHY

Echocardiography is the most widely used tool for diagnosing VFWR *(88,92,119,120)*, yet pericardial effusion is often found in patients after acute MI (up to 28%) even without cardiac rupture *(58,121)*. López-Sendón et al. found pericardial effusion in patients with and without ruptures and concluded that the absence of pericardial effusion excludes VFWR, but the presence of effusion does not prove the existence of VFWR *(58)*. In contrast, in the SHOCK trial, only 15 of the 20 patients with VFWR who underwent echocardiography had pericardial effusion *(81)*.

Echocardiographic signs of increased intrapericardial pressure and tamponade are frequently seen in patients with acute MI and pericardial effusion associated with VFWR *(58)*. In addition, high acoustic echoes within the pericardial effusion are indicative of blood clots in the pericardial cavity and have been described in patients with subacute VFWR *(58,70,88,122–126)*. However, these high acoustic echoes can also be found in patients with fibrinous pericarditis who may have acute MI without VFWR *(127)*. In some patients, pericardial fat can be misdiagnosed as thrombus because of high acoustic echoes on an echocardiogram. However, compared with fat, pericardial thrombus has a layered appearance and a higher echodensity *(128)*.

In some cases, direct visualization of the myocardial tear is possible *(63,70,81,88,92,122,129,130)*. Recent improvements in echocardiographic imaging allow identification of myocardial tears in a larger percentage of patients with VFWR. For example, intravenous injections of echocardiographic contrast agents result in the contrast agent appearing in the pericardial space or pseudoaneurysm *(131)*. Echocardiography is also useful to identify acquired VSR and acute MR that may mimic or be associated with VFWR. In patients who have poor transthoracic echocardiographic images that are often found in those being treated with mechanical ventilation, transesophageal echocardiography may be needed for diagnosing VFWR and identifying the exact site of the myocardial tear *(132,133)*.

Following echocardiographic documentation of pericardial effusion and tamponade, pericardiocentesis should be performed emergently to relieve pericardial tamponade and hemodynamically stabilize the patient. In addition, if pericardiocentesis yields serous fluid, the diagnosis of VFWR can be excluded *(88)*.

VENTRICULOGRAPHY AND RIGHT-HEART CATHETERIZATION

The diagnosis of VFWR with ventriculography is insensitive because it requires an ongoing leak through the ventricular wall, which is an unusual finding in patients who are stable enough to undergo cardiac catheterization *(88)*. Diagnosis with right-heart catheterization may also be insensitive for two potential reasons: (1) the classic equalization of diastolic pressures between the cardiac chambers that results in tamponade may not occur because pericardial clots are usually bound to the rupture and may cause selective chamber compression and (2) a significantly increased left ventricular end-diastolic pressure (LVEDP) may result in severe right-sided tamponade or compression before equalization of the right atrial, left atrial, or pulmonary capillary wedge pressures can occur.

ANGIOGRAPHY

In patients with VFWR, the benefit of routine coronary angiography before surgery versus immediate cardiac surgery has not been resolved. For example, only 9 of the reported 87 long-term survivors of VFWR had coronary artery bypass grafting as part of their surgery *(88)*. Compared with patients with shock unrelated to cardiac rupture in the SHOCK registry, in the 19 patients with shock or tamponade related to VFWR who underwent cardiac catheterization, the infarct-related artery was more often the left anterior descending or the left circumflex and, less often, the right coronary or the left main coronary artery *(81)*.

Management of Patients

MEDICAL THERAPY

Medical therapy should be viewed only as a temporizing approach prior to surgical correction. The first objective of therapy is resuscitation of the patient to achieve hemodynamic stability. Occasionally, this can be achieved by rapid intravenous infusion of fluids and administration of inotropic agents *(134,135)*.

PERICARDIOCENTESIS

Pericardiocentesis, which is preferentially done under echocardiographic guidance, decreases the threat of tamponade *(135)*. However, pericardiocentesis may give only temporary relief because bleeding usually recurs rapidly and blood clotting inside the drainage tubing may prevent further evacuation of pericardial fluid *(70)*. Mechanical ventilation may be needed *(135)*. Intra-aortic balloon pumping is recommended to decrease afterload and to improve perfusion *(136)*. After an initial stabilization, treatment with prolonged bed rest and β-blockers is recommended, whereas heparin should be withheld *(135)*.

MECHANICAL CLOSURE OF VFWR

Although there have been a few case reports of long-term survival without surgical repair *(135,137,138)*, almost all patients need to be referred for surgery as soon as the diagnosis is made. Several different surgical approaches have been used, including infarctectomy and use of the prosthetic patch *(58,117,139)*, pledgeted sutures without infarctectomy *(92,113,140,141)*, pericardial patch adhered with biologic glue *(142)* or sutures *(143)*, and a Dacron or Teflon patch adhered with biologic glue or sutures *(58,62,123,139,140,144,145)*. (See Chapter 10.)

When the defect is on the anterior or lateral surface of the heart, simple closure can be achieved without resorting to cardiopulmonary bypass *(92,144)*. In addition, adhering pericardial or Teflon patches with biologic glue can be performed without cardiopulmonary bypass *(145)*. López-Sendón et al. reported that 33 patients with subacute VFWR (30 left, 3 right) were operated on 30 min to 24 h after the diagnosis was suspected *(59)*. A Teflon patch was sutured or adhered with biologic glue to the epicardial surface of the ruptured wall. Twenty-five (76%) of the 33 patients survived the operation and 16 (48.5%) were alive after a mean follow-up of 30 mo *(59)*.

Recently, Murata et al. reported on a novel approach to therapy. In two patients, fibrin glue was percutaneously injected into the pericardial space after pericardiocentesis *(146)*. After the procedure, there was no detectable pericardial effusion on echocardiography, and the patients became hemodynamically stable.

Prognosis

The reported survival rate varies depending on the study, but it is usually low. Pollak et al. reported that only 1 of 24 patients with subacute VFWR survived. Survival time (from critical event to death) was 45 min to 6.5 wk (median survival 8 h) *(74)*. In another series, the immediate operative mortality was reported to be 24% (8 out of 33 patients) *(58)*.

However, the prognosis of patients with subacute rupture who survive surgical repair is excellent *(147)*. For example, study investigators reported that of 28 patients with subacute left VFWR, 4 patients died after initial resuscitation (including pericardiocentesis) while awaiting surgery and 8 died during or shortly after surgery (average hospital stay of 15 d). After 30 mo, three more patients died. However, 11 of those who survived surgical repair were asymptomatic at moderate levels of activity after 30 mo *(70)*. There are rare cases of subacute rupture with long-term survival even without surgical or transcatheter repair *(135,137,138)*. Isolated case reports of patients with pseudoaneurysm and extremely long survival (up to 12 yr after MI) also have been reported *(148–150)*. Thus, prognosis is highly variable, ranging from sudden and inevitable death in patients with acute rupture to long-term survival among patients with subacute rupture who survive surgery or medical therapy or among those with pseudoaneurysm detected late after the index MI.

Hemopericardium with Cardiac Tamponade

As mentioned previously, cardiac tamponade resulting from hemopericardium (a bloody pericardial effusion) without evidence of acute or subacute VFWR may occur after intravenous thrombolysis for acute MI *(64–67)*. In addition, patients who receive thrombolytic therapy because they present with ST-segment elevation may develop cardiac tamponade if they actually have pericarditis *(151,152)* or aortic dissection *(152)* instead of acute MI. For example, Renkin et al. reported early hemorrhagic pericardial effusion in 4 out of 392 patients (1%) who received thrombolytic therapy. These patients developed cardiogenic shock as a result of tamponade within 24 h of administration of thrombolytic therapy *(64)*.

Cardiac tamponade usually occurs within the first 24–48 h after administration of thrombolytic therapy. This complication, although uncommon, may occur more frequently with the increasing use of aggressive anticoagulant and antiplatelet regimens following thrombolytic therapy. Thus, a patient who received thrombolytic therapy and developed tamponade and whose reported death was because of cardiogenic shock or suspected VFWR may actually have had cardiac tamponade without VFWR. Prompt echocardiographic examination in every patient with hemodynamic deterioration following thrombolytic therapy is mandatory for diagnosing this rare complication and differentiating it from other mechanical causes of acute heart failure after acute MI. Immediate percutaneous pericardiocentesis followed by continuous drainage usually results in rapid recovery in most patients with hemorrhagic cardiac tamponade without VFWR.

ACUTE MITRAL REGURGITATION

Mitral valve regurgitation (MR) is frequently detected in patients with acute MI. During the early phase of acute MI, transient MR is common and rarely causes hemodynamic compromise. However, when one of the chordae tendineae or papillary muscles ruptures, the left atrium and ventricle are overloaded with blood. This can cause sudden and severe left ventricular failure, which results in abrupt hemodynamic deterioration with cardiogenic shock. Unless rapidly diagnosed and treated, acute MR is associated with high morbidity and mortality.

Incidence

The incidence rate of MR is high among patients with acute MI *(153–167)* (Table 5). In studying the incidence of MR, investigators have focused on how different therapies affect the incidence rate. In the GUSTO-I trial, the incidence rate was reported to be 1.73% among patients receiving thrombolytic therapy. Kinn et al. found that primary angioplasty was associated with an 82% risk reduction for acute MR compared with thrombolytic therapy (0.31% vs 1.73%, $p < 0.001$) *(109)*.

In another comparison, Lehmann et al. reported that MR occurs independent of coronary artery patency (both early and late) after thrombolysis and, therefore, cannot be reliably treated by improving arterial perfusion with thrombolytic agents *(161)*. However, other investigators demonstrated that the incidence of successful recanalization was higher in MR patients who improved during follow-up compared with those whose conditions did not change or worsened during follow-up *(163)*. They concluded that successful reperfusion after acute MI reduces the incidence of MR by preventing left ventricular remodeling *(109,163,168,169)*.

Risk Factors

Common risk factors for MR include advanced age, prior MI, infarct extension, and recurrent ischemia *(153–155,158,165–168,170–172)* (Table 2). Compared to patients without MR, those with MR more frequently have multivessel coronary artery disease *(158,165,173)*, a higher admission Killip class *(153,155,165–167,168,171)*, and higher peak creatine kinase *(165,171)*. Some debatable risk factors include the prevalence of MR in specific sites of the MI (inferior or posterior wall) and whether acute MR is more prevalent in non–Q-wave MI than in Q-wave MI *(153,154,163,164,166,171,172,174–176)*. Interestingly, MR caused by papillary muscle rupture has different risk factors than MR from other mechanisms (Table 2).

Table 5
Incidence of Acute Mitral Regurgitation in Patients with Acute Myocardial Infarction

Study (ref.)	Auscultation	Ventriculography	Doppler echocardiography
Hochman et al. *(1)*			98/1422 (6.9%)[a]
Maisel et al. *(153)*	283/1653 (17%)		
Barzilai et al. *(154)*	10/59 (17%)		23/59 (39%)
Barzilai et al. *(155)*	76/849 (8%)		
Bhatnagar et al. *(156)*			15/186 (8%)
Lehmann et al. *(157)*		26/206 (13%)	
Tcheng et al. *(158)*		50/1480 (3.4%)[a]	
O'Connor et al. *(159)*		(1.6%)[b]	
Lamas et al. *(160)*		141/727 (19.4%)	
Lehmann et al. *(161)*		21/132 (16%)	
Vicente et al. *(162)*			55/108 (51%)
Ma et al. *(163)*			47/223 (21%)[c]
Alam et al. *(164)*			45/61 (74%)
Neskovic et al. *(165)*			50/131 (38%)
Van Dantzig et al. *(166)*			25/188 (13%)[a]
Feinberg et al. *(167)*			121/417 (29%)[d]
			25/417 (6%)[a]

[a] Moderate to severe mitral regurgitation.

[b] 1.6% in patients with congestive heart failure; 0.21% in patients without congestive heart failure.

[c] 21% at onset, 18% at follow-up.

[d] Mild mitral regurgitation.

Pathophysiology

In patients with acute MI, several different mechanisms can cause MR *(166,177–193)* (Table 6). One mechanism that has been heavily investigated is papillary muscle rupture. Papillary muscle rupture occurs in approx 1% of patients with acute MI and, more frequently, involves the posteromedial papillary muscle rather than the anterolateral papillary muscle *(45,173–175,177,194–197)*. Rupture of the papillary muscle may be partial or complete, but either condition results in severe MR. Rupture of other cardiac structures, including the free wall of the left and right ventricles and the interventricular septum, may occur concomitantly *(10,19,23)*. MR can also occur when the global geometry of the left ventricle changes and/or becomes spherical. A spherical shape to the LV leads to lateral migration of the papillary muscle that results in poor coaptation of the mitral leaflets *(166,183–187)*.

The pathophysiologic characteristics of MR can differ according to how and when they occur in the development of MI. For example, MR is usually caused by ischemia in the acute phase of MI rather than in the subacute or chronic phases *(179)*. This ischemia results in transient papillary muscle dysfunction as well as regional wall motion abnormalities in the left ventricular segments adjacent to the papillary muscles, resulting in poor coaptation of the leaflets *(169,180–184)*. Large posterior infarctions produce acute MR because of asymmetric annular dilatation and alteration of papillary muscle geom-

Table 6
Major Causes of Mitral Regurgitation in Myocardial Infarction

- Papillary muscle rupture
- Change in the global geometry of the left ventricle
- Mitral annulus dilatation
- Alteration of the alignment of the mitral apparatus and leaflets
- Ischemia/scar of the papillary muscle
- Rupture of a head of a chordae tendineae
- Pre-existing MR

etry and function. With small posterior infarctions that include the posterior papillary muscle, MR occurs in the subacute phase *(177,178,181,193)*. In the subacute and chronic phases of MI, MR may disappear, remain the same, or become more severe.

Time of Occurrence

Different factors can affect the time of occurrence of MR, including the therapy a patient receives. For example, Leor et al. used transthoracic echocardiography to detect MR and found MR within the first 24 h of admission in 4% of the patients who received thrombolytic therapy and in 16% of the patients who did not receive thrombolytic therapy; at 10 d, MR was found in 11% and 24%; by d 30, the condition was detected in 7% and 15%, respectively. Calvo et al. found that MR related to papillary muscle rupture occurred at a median of 1 d (range of 1–14 d) after onset of the index infarction, whereas acute MR unrelated to papillary muscle rupture was detected at a median of 7 d (range of 5–45 d) after the index infarction ($p < 0.02$) *(170,174)*.

Clinical Manifestations

Depending on the severity of acute MR, clinical manifestations range from an incidental finding of a new systolic murmur to the abrupt development of flash pulmonary edema and shock *(153,173)*. The systolic murmur is usually holosystolic and apical and may occur early or late after the onset of symptoms. In many patients, S3 and S4 gallops can be heard.

An acute papillary muscle rupture usually results in an abrupt onset of severe pulmonary edema. The regurgitant orifice with acute MR due to papillary muscle rupture is large, and thus the turbulence is less than with other murmurs. In contrast to VSR, a thrill rarely accompanies the systolic murmur. In some patients, the murmur may seem inconsequential because it may be masked by the auscultatory features of severe pulmonary edema or because of a reduced pressure gradient between the left ventricle and atrium due to a rapid increase of pressure in the noncompliant left atrium *(198,199)*.

Diagnosis

Mitral regurgitation should be suspected in all patients with pulmonary edema or cardiogenic shock, especially if there is well-preserved or even hyperdynamic left ventricular systolic function. Auscultation may be useful to identify acute MR, which may present as a new systolic murmur *(153–156)*. As with VSR, transthoracic and transesophageal color Doppler echocardiography have become the main diagnostic tools for detecting MR *(120,199–201)*. Transthoracic echocardiography often cannot delineate the severity and exact mechanism of acute MR, especially when a papillary muscle rupture needs to be differentiated from other mechanisms of acute MR. In these cases, transesophageal echocardiography is useful *(202,203)*. Other tools that can assist in diagnosis as well as achieving hemodynamic stabilization in patients include pulmonary artery catheterization with monitoring of the right atrial and pulmonary capillary wedge pressures *(40,41)*.

Study investigators who use echocardiography with color Doppler mapping report a higher incidence of MR than those using other diagnostic methods, particularly in patients with first-time mild to moderate MI *(1,154,162–167)*.

Presently, bedside right-heart catheterization (Swan–Ganz catheter) is less often used for diagnosis then it was in the past. However, with right-heart catheterization, an oxygen step-up from the right atrium to the right ventricle, suggesting VSR, can be excluded. It should be remembered that in rare cases with severe acute MR, a step-up in oxygen saturation in the peripheral pulmonary arteries might occur *(39)*. The pressure waveforms in the pulmonary capillary wedge position cannot distinguish between acute MR and VSR, as both conditions may coexist, especially in inferior acute MI, and the presence of large V-waves is a nonspecific finding indicating poor left ventricular compliance and not necessarily acute MR *(40)*. Currently, pulmonary artery catheterization is mainly used for guiding and monitoring therapy. Right atrial and capillary wedge pressure monitoring, along with repeated measurement of cardiac output, may assist to guide therapy to achieve hemodynamic stabilization of the patient.

Management of Patients

The initial management of patients with MR is twofold: aggressively attempt to hemodynamically stabilize the patient and diagnose the exact mechanism of acute MR. Patients can be stabilized with medical therapy (consisting of afterload reduction, diuretics, and inotropic agents) and by use of mechanical support with an intra-aortic balloon counterpulsation pump and intermittent positive-pressure mechanical ventilation. Intravenous nitroprusside may improve forward cardiac output, but this agent can also cause severe hypotension and be contraindicated in patients with acute renal failure, which frequently accompanies acute MR.

Even if medical therapy results in initial stabilization, patients with chordal or papillary muscle rupture (partial or complete) have a poor prognosis without surgical repair *(194)*. Sudden hemodynamic deterioration is frequent; therefore, prompt surgical intervention is needed (see Chapter 10). When MR is the result of the rupture of a single papillary muscle head and the surrounding muscle is not extensively infarcted, it is possible to suture the papillary muscle head in place with pledget sutures or to use other repair techniques such as chordal transfer or replacement *(204)*. When MR is caused by extensive necrosis of the papillary muscle and the ventricular wall, mitral valve replacement is more reliable than repair. Nonetheless, the mitral chordae tendineae should be preserved for optimal conservation of LV function. Correcting MR by means of valve repair in patients with a healed MI is often possible once the cause of MR is determined by color Doppler echocardiography *(191)*. However, when the acute MR is episodic, successful myocardial revascularization either by angioplasty or by coronary artery bypass grafting may effectively resolve the MR without the need for mitral valve replacement or repair *(191,205)*.

REFERENCES

1. Hochman JS, Buller CE, Sleeper LA, et al. Cardiogenic shock complicating acute myocardial infarction—etiologies, management and outcome: a report from the SHOCK Trial Registry. SHould we emergently revascularize Occluded Coronaries for cardiogenic shocK? J Am Coll Cardiol 2000;36:1063–1070.
2. Madsen JC, Daggett WM Jr. Postinfarction ventricular septal rupture. In: Baue AE, ed. Glenn's Thoracic and Cardiovascular Surgery. Prentice-Hall International, Englewood Cliffs, NJ, 1996, pp. 2115–2129.
3. Pohjola-Sintonen S, Muller JE, Stone PH, et al. and the MILLS Study Group. Ventricular septal and free wall rupture complicating acute myocardial infarction: experience in the Multicenter Investigation of Limitation of Infarct Size. Am Heart J 1989;117:809–818.
4. Radford MJ, Johnson RA, Daggett WMJ, et al. Ventricular septal defect: a review of clinical and physiologic features and an analysis of survival. Circulation 1981;64:545–553.
5. Edmondson HA, Hoxie HJ. Hypertension and cardiac rupture: clinical and pathological study of 72 cases, in 13 of which rupture of the interventricular septum occurred. Am Heart J 1942;24:719–733.
6. Topaz O, Taylor AL. Interventricular septal rupture complicating acute myocardial infarction: from pathophysiologic features to the role of invasive and noninvasive diagnostic modalities in current management. Am J Med 1992;93:683–688.
7. Hutchins GM. Rupture of the interventricular septum complicating myocardial infarction: pathological analysis of 10 patients with clinically diagnosed perforations. Am Heart J 1979;97:165–173.
8. Moore CA, Nygaard TW, Kaiser DL, Cooper AA, Gibson RS. Postinfarction ventricular septal rupture: the importance of location of infarction and right ventricular function in determining survival. Circulation 1986;74:45–55.
9. Crenshaw BS, Granger CB, Birnbaum Y, et al. Risk factors, angiographic patterns, and outcomes in patients with ventricular septal defect complicating acute myocardial infarction. GUSTO-I (Global Utilization of Streptokinase and TPA for Occluded Coronary Arteries) Trial Investigators. Circulation 2000;101:27–32.
10. Edwards BS, Edwards WD, Edwards JE. Ventricular septal rupture complicating acute myocardial infarction: identification of simple and complex types in 53 autopsied hearts. Am J Cardiol 1984;54:1201–1205.
11. Vlodaver Z, Edwards JE. Rupture of ventricular septum or papillary muscle complicating myocardial infarction. Circulation 1977;55:815–822.
12. Parry G, Goudevenos J, Adams PC, Reid DS. Septal rupture after myocardial infarction: is very early surgery really worthwhile? Eur Heart J 1992;13:373–382.
13. Skehan JD, Carey C, Norrell MS, de Belder M, Balcon R, Mills PG. Patterns of coronary artery disease in post-infarction ventricular septal rupture. Br Heart J 1989;62:268–272.
14. Feneley MP, Chang VP, O'Rourke MF. Myocardial rupture after acute myocardial infarction. Ten year review. Br Heart J 1983;49:550–556.
15. Shapira I, Isakov A, Burke M, Almog CH. Cardiac rupture in patients with acute myocardial infarction. Chest 1987;92:219–223.
16. Cummings RG, Reimer KA, Califf R, Hackel D, Boswick J, Lowe JE. Quantitative analysis of right and left ventricular infarction in the presence of postinfarction ventricular septal defect. Circulation 1988;77:33–42.
17. Oskoui R, Van Voorhees LB, DiBianco R, Kiernan JM, Lee F, Lindsay J, Jr. Timing of ventricular septal rupture after acute myocardial infarction and its relation to thrombolytic therapy. Am J Cardiol 1996;78:953–955.
18. Mann JM, Roberts WC. Acquired ventricular septal defect during acute myocardial infarction: analysis of 38 unoperated necropsy patients and comparison with 50 unoperated necropsy patients without rupture. Am J Cardiol 1988;62:8–19.
19. Figueras J, Cortadellas J, Soler-Soler J. Comparison of ventricular septal and left ventricular free wall rupture in acute myocardial infarction. Am J Cardiol 1998;81:495–497.
20. Pretre R, Rickli H, Ye Q, Benedikt P, Turina MI. Frequency of collateral blood flow in the infarct-related coronary artery in rupture of the ventricular septum after acute myocardial infarction. Am J Cardiol 2000;85:497–499.

21. Birnbaum Y, Wagner GS, Gates KB, et al. Clinical and electrocardiographic variables associated with increased risk of ventricular septal defect in acute anterior myocardial infarction. Am J Cardiol 2000;86:830–834.
22. Topaz O, Mallon SM, Chahine RA, Sequeira RF, Myerburg RJ. Acute ventricular septal rupture. Angiographic-morphologic features and clinical assessment. Chest 1989;95:292–298.
23. Mann JM, Roberts WC. Fatal rupture of both left ventricular free wall and ventricular septum (double rupture) during acute myocardial infarction: analysis of seven patients studied at necropsy. Am J Cardiol 1987;60:722–724.
24. Aravot DJ, Dhalla N, Banner NR, Mitchell A, Rees A. Combined septal perforation and cardiac rupture after myocardial infarction. Clinical features and surgical considerations of a correctable condition. J Thorac Cardiovasc Surg 1989;97:815–820.
25. Gowda KS, Loh CW, Roberts R. The simultaneous occurrence of a ventricular septal defect and mitral insufficiency after myocardial infarction. Am Heart J 1976;92:234–236.
26. Amico A, Iliceto S, Rizzo A, Cascella V, Rizzon P. Color Doppler findings in ventricular septal dissection following myocardial infarction. Am Heart J 1989;117:195–198.
27. Cheriex EC, de Swart H, Dijkman LW, et al. Myocardial rupture after myocardial infarction is related to the perfusion status of the infarct-related coronary artery. Am Heart J 1995;129:644–650.
28. Lemery R, Smith HC, Giuliani ER, Gersh BJ. Prognosis in rupture of the ventricular septum after acute myocardial infarction and role of early surgical intervention. Am J Cardiol 1992;70:147–151.
29. Loisance DY, Lordez JM, Deleuze PH, Dubois-Rande JL, Lellouche D, Cachera JP. Acute postinfarction septal rupture: long-term results. Ann Thorac Surg 1991;52:474–478.
30. Westaby S, Parry A, Ormerod O, Gooneratne P, Pillai R. Thrombolysis and postinfarction ventricular septal rupture. J Thorac Cardiovasc Surg 1992;104:1506–1509.
31. Menon V, Webb JG, Hillis LD, et al. Outcome and profile of ventricular septal rupture with cardiogenic shock after myocardial infarction: a report from the SHOCK Trial Registry. SHould we emergently revascularize Occluded Coronaries in cardiogenic shocK? J Am Coll Cardiol 2000;36:1110–1116.
32. Perloff JK, Talano JV, Ronan JA Jr. Noninvasive techniques in acute myocardial infarction. Prog Cardiovasc Dis 1971;13:437–464.
33. Smyllie JH, Sutherland GR, Geuskens R, Dawkins K, Conway N, Roelandt JR. Doppler color flow mapping in the diagnosis of ventricular septal rupture and acute mitral regurgitation after myocardial infarction. J Am Coll Cardiol 1990;15:1449–1455.
34. Fortin DF, Sheikh KH, Kisslo J. The utility of echocardiography in the diagnostic strategy of postinfarction ventricular septal rupture: a comparison of two-dimensional echocardiography versus Doppler color flow imaging. Am Heart J 1991;121:25–32.
35. Vargas Barron J, Sahn DJ, Valdes-Cruz LM, et al. Clinical utility of two-dimensional doppler echocardiographic techniques for estimating pulmonary to systemic blood flow ratios in children with left to right shunting atrial septal defect, ventricular septal defect or patent ductus arteriosus. J Am Coll Cardiol 1984;3:169–178.
36. Obarski TP, Rogers PJ, Debaets DL, Murcko LG, Jennings MR. Assessment of postinfarction ventricular septal ruptures by transesophageal Doppler echocardiography. J Am Soc Echocardiogr 1995;8:728–734.
37. Ballal RS, Sanyal RS, Nanda NC, Mahan EFD. Usefulness of transesophageal echocardiography in the diagnosis of ventricular septal rupture secondary to acute myocardial infarction. Am J Cardiol 1993;71:367–370.
38. Harpaz D, Shah P, Bezante GP, Meltzer RS. Ventricular septal rupture after myocardial infarction. Detection by transesophageal echocardiography. Chest 1993;103:1884–1885.
39. Wynne J, Fishbein MC, Holman BL, Alpert JS. Radionuclide scintigraphy in the evaluation of ventricular septal defect complicating acute myocardial infarction. Cathet Cardiovasc Diagn 1978;4:189–197.
40. Tatooles CJ, Gault JH, Mason DT, Ross J Jr. Reflux of oxygenated blood into the pulmonary artery in severe mitral regurgitation. Am Heart J 1968;75:102–106.
41. Fuchs RM, Heuser RR, Yin FC, Brinker JA. Limitations of pulmonary wedge V waves in diagnosing mitral regurgitation. Am J Cardiol 1982;49:849–854.
42. Kamishirado H, Inoue T, Sakai Y, Matsunaga R, Morooka S. Six-year survival of unoperated ventricular septal rupture following myocardial infarction. Tex Heart Inst J 1999;26:315–317.
43. Daggett WM, Guyton RA, Mundth ED, et al. Surgery for post-myocardial infarct ventricular septal defect. Ann Surg 1977;186:260–271.

44. Gray RJ, Sethna D, Matloff JM. The role of cardiac surgery in acute myocardial infarction. I. With mechanical complications. Am Heart J 1983;106:723–728.
45. Fox AC, Glassman E, Isom OW. Surgically remediable complications of myocardial infarction. Prog Cardiovasc Dis 1979;21:461–484.
46. Lee EM, Roberts DH, Walsh KP. Transcatheter closure of a residual postmyocardial infarction ventricular septal defect with the Amplatzer septal occluder. Heart 1998;80:522–524.
47. Landzberg MJ, Lock JE. Transcatheter management of ventricular septal rupture after myocardial infarction. Semin Thorac Cardiovasc Surg 1998;10:128–132.
48. Pesonen E, Thilen U, Sandstrom S, et al. Transcatheter closure of post-infarction ventricular septal defect with the Amplatzer Septal Occluder device. Scand Cardiovasc J 2000;34:446–448.
49. Giuliani ER, Danielson GK, Pluth JR, Odyniec NA, Wallace RB. Postinfarction ventricular septal rupture: surgical considerations and results. Circulation 1974;49:455–459.
50. Montoya A, McKeever L, Scanlon P, Sullivan HJ, Gunnar RM, Pifarre R. Early repair of ventricular septal rupture after infarction. Am J Cardiol 1980;45:345–348.
51. Scanlon PJ, Montoya A, Johnson SA, et al. Urgent surgery for ventricular septal rupture complicating acute myocardial infarction. Circulation 1985;72:II-185–II-190.
52. Jones MT, Schofield PM, Dark JF, et al. Surgical repair of acquired ventricular septal defect. Determinants of early and late outcome. J Thorac Cardiovasc Surg 1987;93:680–686.
53. Held AC, Cole PL, Lipton B, et al. Rupture of the interventricular septum complicating acute myocardial infarction: a multicenter analysis of clinical findings and outcome. Am Heart J 1988;116:1330–1336.
54. Pretre R, Ye Q, Grunenfelder J, Lachat M, Vogt PR, Turina MI. Operative results of "repair" of ventricular septal rupture after acute myocardial infraction. Am J Cardiol 1999;84:785–788.
55. Massetti M, Babatasi G, Le Page O, Bhoyroo S, Saloux E, Khayat A. Postinfarction ventricular septal rupture: early repair through the right atrial approach. J Thorac Cardiovasc Surg 2000;119:784–789.
56. Heitmiller R, Jacobs ML, Daggett WM. Surgical management of postinfarction ventricular septal rupture. Ann Thorac Surg 1986;41:683–691.
57. Davies RH, Dawkins KD, Skillington PD, et al. Late functional results after surgical closure of acquired ventricular septal defect. J Thorac Cardiovasc Surg 1993;106:592–598.
58. Lopez-Sendon J, Gonzalez A, Lopez de Sa E, et al. Diagnosis of subacute ventricular wall rupture after acute myocardial infarction: sensitivity and specificity of clinical, hemodynamic and echocardiographic criteria. J Am Coll Cardiol 1992;19:1145–1153.
59. Nunez L, de la Llana R, Lopez Sendon J, Coma I, Gil Aguado M, Larrea JL. Diagnosis and treatment of subacute free wall ventricular rupture after infarction. Ann Thorac Surg 1983;35:525–529.
60. Windsor HM, O'Rourke MF, Feneley MP. Subacute heart rupture and hemopericardium following acute myocardial infarction: report of successful treatment and ten year follow-up. Aust NZ J Med 1984;14:47–49.
61. O'Rourke MF. Subacute heart rupture following myocardial infarction. Clinical features of a correctable condition. Lancet 1973;2:124–126.
62. Coma-Canella I, Lopez-Sendon J, Nunez Gonzalez L, Ferrufino O. Subacute left ventricular free wall rupture following acute myocardial infarction: bedside hemodynamics, differential diagnosis, and treatment. Am Heart J 1983;106:278–284.
63. Commeau P, Grollier G, Pelouze GA, et al. Diagnostic echocardiographique d'une complication mechanique rare de l'infarctus biventriculaire: la rupture de la paroi libre du ventricule droit. Ann Cardiol Angeiol (Paris) 1985;34:425–429.
64. Renkin J, de Bruyne B, Benit E, Joris JM, Carlier M, Col J. Cardiac tamponade early after thrombolysis for acute myocardial infarction: a rare but not reported hemorrhagic complication. J Am Coll Cardiol 1991;17:280–285.
65. Valeix B, Labrunie P, Jahjah F, et al. Hemopericardium after coronary recanalization with streptokinase in the acute phase of myocardial infarction. Drainage and early aortocoronary bypass on the 4th day. Arch Mal Coeur Vaiss 1983;76:1081–1084.
66. Mohammad S, Austin SM. Hemopericardium with cardiac tamponade after intravenous thrombolysis for acute myocardial infarction. Clin Cardiol 1996;19:432–434.
67. Barrington WW, Smith JE, Himmelstein SI. Cardiac tamponade following treatment with tissue plasminogen activator: an atypical hemodynamic response to pericardiocentesis. Am Heart J 1991;121:1227–1229.
68. Salem BI, Lagos JA, Haikal M, Gowda S. The potential impact of the thrombolytic era on cardiac rupture complicating acute myocardial infarction. Angiology 1994;45:931–936.

69. Ballet-Mechain M, Gayet C, Perret T, et al. Double postinfarction cardiac rupture of left ventricular free wall and papillary muscle documented by transthoracic echocardiography. J Am Soc Echocardiogr 1998;11:1084–1086.

70. Purcaro A, Costantini C, Ciampani N, et al. Diagnostic criteria and management of subacute ventricular free wall rupture complicating acute myocardial infarction. Am J Cardiol 1997;80:397–405.

71. Becker RC, Gore JM, Lambrew C, et al. A composite view of cardiac rupture in the United States National Registry of Myocardial Infarction. J Am Coll Cardiol 1996;27:1321–1326.

72. Dellborg M, Held P, Swedberg K, Vedin A. Rupture of the myocardium. Occurrence and risk factors. Br Heart J 1985;54:11–16.

73. Honan MB, Harrell FE, Jr., Reimer KA, et al. Cardiac rupture, mortality and the timing of thrombolytic therapy: a meta-analysis. J Am Coll Cardiol 1990;16:359–367.

74. Pollak H, Diez W, Spiel R, Enenkel W, Mlczoch J. Early diagnosis of subacute free wall rupture complicating acute myocardial infarction. Eur Heart J 1993;14:640–648.

75. Becker RC, Charlesworth A, Wilcox RG, et al. Cardiac rupture associated with thrombolytic therapy: impact of time to treatment in the Late Assessment of Thrombolytic Efficacy (LATE) study. J Am Coll Cardiol 1995;25:1063–1068.

76. Becker RC, Hochman JS, Cannon CP, et al. Fatal cardiac rupture among patients treated with thrombolytic agents and adjunctive thrombin antagonists: observations from the Thrombolysis and Thrombin Inhibition in Myocardial Infarction 9 Study. J Am Coll Cardiol 1999;33:479–487.

77. Reeder GS. Identification and treatment of complications of myocardial infarction. Mayo Clin Proc 1995;70:880–884.

78. Kleiman NS, Terrin M, Mueller H, et al. Mechanisms of early death despite thrombolytic therapy: experience from the Thrombolysis in Myocardial Infarction Phase II (TIMI II) study. J Am Coll Cardiol 1992;19:1129–1135.

79. Kleiman NS, White HD, Ohman EM, et al. Mortality within 24 hours of thrombolysis for myocardial infarction. The importance of early reperfusion. The GUSTO Investigators, Global Utilization of Streptokinase and Tissue Plasminogen Activator for Occluded Coronary Arteries. Circulation 1994;90:2658–2665.

80. Reddy SG, Roberts WC. Frequency of rupture of the left ventricular free wall or ventricular septum among necropsy cases of fatal acute myocardial infarction since introduction of coronary care units. Am J Cardiol 1989;63:906–911.

81. Slater J, Brown RJ, Antonelli TA, Menon V, et al. Cardiogenic shock due to cardiac free-wall rupture or tamponade after acute myocardial infarction: a report from the SHOCK Trial Registry. Should we emergently revascularize occluded coronaries for cardiogenic shock? J Am Coll Cardiol 2000;36:1117–1122.

82. Batts KP, Ackermann DM, Edwards WD. Postinfarction rupture of the left ventricular free wall: clinicopathologic correlates in 100 consecutive autopsy cases. Hum Pathol 1990;21:530–535.

83. Solodky A, Behar S, Herz I, et al. Comparison of incidence of cardiac rupture among patients with acute myocardial infarction treated by thrombolysis-vs-percutaneous transluminal coronary angioplasty. Am J Cardiol 2001;87:1105–1108.

84. Mann JM, Roberts WC. Rupture of the left ventricular free wall during acute myocardial infarction: analysis of 138 necropsy patients and comparison with 50 necropsy patients with acute myocardial infaction without rupture. Am J Cardiol 1988;62:847–859.

85. Bodi V, Monmeneu JV, Marin F. Acute cardiac rupture complicating pre-discharge exercise testing. A case report with complete echocardiographic follow-up. Int J Cardiol 1999;68:333–335.

86. Ueda S, Ikeda U, Yamamoto K, et al. C-Reactive protein as a predictor of cardiac rupture after acute myocardial infarction. Am Heart J 1996;131:857–860.

87. Hashell WK. Physical activity after myocardial infarction. Am J Cardiol 1974;33:776–781.

88. Raitt MH, Kraft CD, Gardner CJ, Pearlman AS, Otto CM. Subacute ventricular free wall rupture complicating myocardial infarction. Am Heart J 1993;126:946–955.

89. Christensen DJ, Ford M, Reading J, Castle CH. Effect of hypertension on myocardial rupture after acute myocardial infarction. Chest 1977;72:618–622.

90. Bates RJ, Beutler S, Resnekov L, Anagnostopoulos CE. Cardiac rupture—challenge in diagnosis and management. Am J Cardiol 1977;40:429–437.

91. Veinot JP, Walley VM, Wolfsohn AL, et al. Postinfarct cardiac free wall rupture: the relationship of rupture site to papillary muscle insertion. Mod Pathol 1995;8:609–613.

92. Sutherland FW, Guell FJ, Pathi VL, Naik SK. Postinfarction ventricular free wall rupture: strategies for diagnosis and treatment. Ann Thorac Surg 1996;61:1281–5.

93. Becker AE, van Mantgem JP. Cardiac tamponade. A study of 50 hearts. Eur J Cardiol 1975;3:349–358.

94. Perdigao C, Andrade A, Ribeiro C. Cardiac rupture in acute myocardial infarction. Various clinico-anatomical types in 42 recent cases observed over a period of 30 months. Arch Mal Coeur Vaiss 1987;80:336–344.

95. Schuster EH, Bulkley BH. Expansion of transmural myocardial infarction: a pathophysiologic factor in cardiac rupture. Circulation 1979;60:1532–1538.

96. Hochman JS, Choo H. Limitation of myocardial infarct expansion by reperfusion independent of myocardial salvage. Circulation 1987;75:299–306.

97. The ISIS-2 Collaborative Group. Randomised trial of intravenous streptokinase, oral aspirin, both, or neither among 17,187 cases of suspected acute myocardial infarction: ISIS-2. Lancet 1988;2:349–460.

98. Chesler E, Korns ME, Semba T, Edwards JE. False aneurysms of the left ventricle following myocardial infarction. Am J Cardiol 1969;23:76–82.

99. Rittenhouse EA, Sauvage LR, Mansfield PB, Smith JC, Davis CC, Hall DG. False aneurysm of the left ventricle. Report of four cases and review of surgical management. Ann Surg 1979;189:409–415.

100. Tirilomis T, Mahmoud FO, Von der Emde J. Left ventricular false aneurysm. Acta Cardiol 2000;55:269–270.

101. Pretre R, Linka A, Jenni R, Turina MI. Surgical treatment of acquired left ventricular pseudoaneurysms. Ann Thorac Surg 2000;70:553–557.

102. Hung MJ, Wang CH, Cherng WJ. Unruptured left ventricular pseudoaneurysm following myocardial infarction. Heart 1998;80:94–97.

103. Csapo K, Voith L, Szuk T, Edes I, Kereiakes DJ. Postinfarction left ventricular pseudoaneurysm. Clin Cardiol 1997;20:898–903.

104. Brown SL, Gropler RJ, Harris KM. Distinguishing left ventricular aneurysm from pseudoaneurysm. A review of the literature. Chest 1997;111:1403–1409.

105. Proli J, Laufer N. Left ventricular rupture following myocardial infarction treated with streptokinase: successful resuscitation in the cardiac catheterization laboratory using pericardiocentesis and auto-transfusion. Cathet Cardiovasc Diagn 1993;29:257–260.

106. Yasuno M, Endo S, Takahashi M, et al. Angiographic and pathologic evidence of hemorrhage into the myocardium after coronary reperfusion. Angiology 1984;35:797–801.

107. Richardson SG, Allen DC, Morton P, Murtagh JG, Scott ME, O'Keeffe DB. Pathological changes after intravenous streptokinase treatment in eight patients with acute myocardial infarction. Br Heart J 1989;61:390–395.

108. Peuhkurinen KJ, Risteli L, Melkko JT, Linnaluoto M, Jounela A, Risteli J. Thrombolytic therapy with streptokinase stimulates collagen breakdown. Circulation 1991;83:1969–1975.

109. Kinn JW, O'Neill WW, Benzuly KH, Jones DE, Grines CL. Primary angioplasty reduces risk of myocardial rupture compared to thrombolysis for acute myocardial infarction. Cathet Cardiovasc Diagn 1997;42:151–157.

110. Figueras J, Curos A, Cortadellas J, Soler-Soler J. Reliability of electromechanical dissociation in the diagnosis of left ventricular free wall rupture in acute myocardial infarction. Am Heart J 1996;131:861–864.

111. Lavie CJ, Gersh BJ. Mechanical and electrical complications of acute myocardial infarction. Mayo Clin Proc 1990;65:709–730.

112. Ennix CL, Jr., Ecker RR, Iverson LI, et al. Early detection and management of left ventricular free wall rupture during acute myocardial infarction. Am J Cardiol 1989;63:151–152.

113. Kendall RW, DeWood MA. Postinfarction cardiac rupture: surgical success and review of the literature. Ann Thorac Surg 1978;25:311–315.

114. Carey JS, Cukingnan RA, Eugene J. Myocardial rupture in expanded infarcts: repair using pericardial patch. Clin Cardiol 1989;12:157–160.

115. Oliva PB, Hammill SC, Edwards WD. Cardiac rupture, a clinically predictable complication of acute myocardial infarction: report of 70 cases with clinicopathologic correlations. J Am Coll Cardiol 1993;22:720–726.

116. Oliva PB, Hammill SC, Edwards WD. The electrocardiographic diagnosis of regional pericarditis in acute inferior myocardial infarction. Eur Heart J 1993;14:1683–1691.

117. Reardon MJ, Carr CL, Diamond A, et al. Ischemic left ventricular free wall rupture: prediction, diagnosis, and treatment. Ann Thorac Surg 1997;64:1509–1513.

118. Zahger D, Milgalter E, Pollak A, et al. Left ventricular free wall rupture as the presenting manifestation of acute myocardial infarction in diabetic patients. Am J Cardiol 1996;78:681–682.

119. Lindower P, Embrey R, Vandenberg B. Echocardiographic diagnosis of mechanical complications in acute myocardial infarction. Clin Intensive Care 1993;4:276–283.

120. Buda AJ. The role of echocardiography in the evaluation of mechanical complications of acute myocardial infarction. Circulation 1991;84:I109–I121.

121. Galve E, Garcia-Del-Castillo H, Evangelista A, Batlle J, Permanyer-Miralda G, Soler-Soler J. Pericardial effusion in the course of myocardial infarction: incidence, natural history, and clinical relevance. Circulation 1986;73:294–299.

122. Desoutter P, Halphen C, Haiat R. Two-dimensional echographic visualization of free ventricular wall rupture in acute anterior myocardial infarction. Am Heart J 1984;108:1360–1361.

123. Pappas PJ, Cernaianu AC, Baldino WA, Cilley JH, Jr., DelRossi AJ. Ventricular free-wall rupture after myocardial infarction. Treatment and outcome. Chest 1991;99:892–895.

124. Knopf WD, Talley JD, Murphy DA. An echo-dense mass in the pericardial space as a sign of left ventricular free wall rupture during acute myocardial infarction. Am J Cardiol 1987;59:1202.

125. Garcia-Fernandez MA, Moreno M, Rossi PN, Lopez-Sendon JL, Banuelos F. Echocardiographic features of hemopericardium. Am Heart J 1984;107:1035–1036.

126. Pierli C, Lisi G, Mezzacapo B. Subacute left ventricular free wall rupture. Surgical repair prompted by echocardiographic diagnosis. Chest 1991;100:1174–1176.

127. Martin RP, Bowden R, Filly K, Popp RL. Intrapericardial abnormalities in patients with pericardial effusion. Findings by two-dimensional echocardiography. Circulation 1980;61:568–572.

128. Brack M, Asinger RW, Sharkey SW, Herzog CA, Hodges M. Two-dimensional echocardiographic characteristics of pericardial hematoma secondary to left ventricular free wall rupture complicating acute myocardial infarction. Am J Cardiol 1991;68:961–964.

129. Kawai J, Yoshikawa J, Yoshida K, et al. Pseudoaneurysm and ventricular septal rupture complicated with inferior myocardial infarction diagnosed by two-dimensional and Doppler echocardiography: case report. J Cardiol 1996;27:77–83.

130. Taylor DA, Chan KL, Higginson L. Complementary role of two-dimensional and Doppler echocardiography in the diagnosis of left ventricular free-wall rupture. J Am Soc Echocardiogr 1992;5:93–95.

131. Waggoner AD, Williams GA, Gaffron D, Schwarze M. Potential utility of left heart contrast agents in diagnosis of myocardial rupture by 2-dimensional echocardiography. J Am Soc Echocardiogr 1999;12:272–274.

132. Delgado C, Duran RM, Serra E, Barturen F. Left ventricular pseudoaneurysm with left atrium tamponade: a rare postinfarction complication. J Am Soc Echocardiogr 1997;10:582–587.

133. Deshmukh HG, Khosla S, Jefferson KK. Direct visualization of left ventricular free wall rupture by transesophageal echocardiography in acute myocardial infarction: Am Heart J 1993;126:475–477.

134. Hoit BD, Gabel M, Fowler NO. Hemodynamic efficacy of rapid saline infusion and dobutamine versus saline infusion alone in a model of cardiac rupture. J Am Coll Cardiol 1990;16:1745–1749.

135. Figueras J, Cortadellas J, Evangelista A, Soler-Soler J. Medical management of selected patients with left ventricular free wall rupture during acute myocardial infarction. J Am Coll Cardiol 1997;29:512–518.

136. Pifarre R, Sullivan HJ, Grieco J, et al. Management of left ventricular rupture complicating myocardial infarction. J Thorac Cardiovasc Surg 1983;86:441–443.

137. Blinc A, Noc M, Pohar B, Cernic N, Horvat M. Subacute rupture of the left ventricular free wall after acute myocardial infarction. Three cases of long-term survival without emergency surgical repair. Chest 1996;109:565–567.

138. Sherer Y, Levy Y, Shahar A, Leibovich L, Konen E, Shoenfeld Y. Survival without surgical repair of acute rupture of the right ventricular free wall. Clin Cardiol 1999;22:319–320.

139. Yamazaki Y, Eguchi S, Miyamura H, et al. Replacement of myocardium with a Dacron prosthesis for complications of acute myocardial infarction. J Cardiovasc Surg (Torino) 1989;30:277–280.

140. Stryjer D, Friedensohn A, Hendler A. Myocardial rupture in acute myocardial infarction: urgent management. Br Heart J 1988;59:73–74.

141. Chemnitius JM, Schmidt T, Wojcik J, Ruschewski W, Kreuzer H, Tebbe U. Successful surgical management of left ventricular free wall rupture in the course of myocardial infarction. Eur J Cardiothorac Surg 1991;5:51–55.

142. Almdahl SM, Hotvedt R, Larsen U, Sorlie DG. Postinfarction rupture of left ventricular free wall repaired with a glued-on pericardial patch. Case report. Scand J Thorac Cardiovasc Surg 1993;27:105–107.

143. Coletti G, Torracca L, Zogno M, et al. Surgical management of left ventricular free wall rupture after acute myocardial infarction. Cardiovasc Surg 1995;3:181–186.

144. Padro JM, Caralps JM, Montoya JD, Camara ML, Garcia Picart J, Aris A. Sutureless repair of postinfarction cardiac rupture. J Card Surg 1988;3:491–493.

145. Padro JM, Mesa JM, Silvestre J, et al. Subacute cardiac rupture: repair with a sutureless technique. Ann Thorac Surg 1993;55:20–23.

146. Murata H, Masuo M, Yoshimoto H, et al. Oozing type cardiac rupture repaired with percutaneous injection of fibrin-glue into the pericardial space: case report. Jpn Circ J 2000;64:312–315.

147. Guron CW, Hagman M, Hartford M, Svensson S, Caidahl K. Echocardiography allows early detection and long-term survival after infarct free wall rupture. J Am Soc Echocardiogr 1998;11:307–309.

148. Bolognesi R, Cucchini F, Lettieri C, Manca C, Visioli O. Left ventricular false aneurysm: an unusually prolonged natural history. Cathet Cardiovasc Diagn 1995;36:46–50.

149. Fazia RB, Lewis JF, Mills RM, Jr, Normann S, Conti CR. Prolonged survival of a patient with left ventricular pseudoaneurysm following myocardial infarction and mitral valve replacement. Chest 1996;109:577–579.

150. Natarajan MK, Salerno TA, Burke B, Chiu B, Armstrong PW. Chronic false aneurysms of the left ventricle: management revisited. Can J Cardiol 1994;10:927–931.

151. Heymann TD, Culling W. Cardiac tamponade after thrombolysis. Postgrad Med J 1994;70:455–456.

152. Blankenship JC, Almquist AK. Cardiovascular complications of thrombolytic therapy in patients with a mistaken diagnosis of acute myocardial infarction. J Am Coll Cardiol 1989;14:1579–1582.

153. Maisel AS, Gilpin EA, Klein L, Le Winter M, Henning H, Collins D. The murmur of papillary muscle dysfunction in acute myocardial infarction: clinical features and prognostic implications. Am Heart J 1986;112:705–711.

154. Barzilai B, Gessler C, Jr, Perez JE, Schaab C, Jaffe AS. Significance of Doppler-detected mitral regurgitation in acute myocardial infarction. Am J Cardiol 1988;61:220–223.

155. Barzilai B, Davis VG, Stone PH, Jaffe AS. Prognostic significance of mitral regurgitation in acute myocardial infarction. The MILIS Study Group. Am J Cardiol 1990;65:1169–1175.

156. Bhatnagar SK, al Yusuf AR. Significance of a mitral regurgitation systolic murmur complicating a first acute myocardial infarction in the coronary care unit—assessment by colour Doppler flow imaging. Eur Heart J 1991;12:1311–1315.

157. Lehmann KG, Francis CK, Dodge HT. Mitral regurgitation in early myocardial infarction. Incidence, clinical detection, and prognostic implications. TIMI Study Group. Ann Intern Med 1992;117:10–17.

158. Tcheng JE, Jackman JD, Jr, Nelson CL, et al. Outcome of patients sustaining acute ischemic mitral regurgitation during myocardial infarction. Ann Intern Med 1992;117:18–24.

159. O'Connor CM, Hathaway WR, Bates ER, et al. Clinical characteristics and long-term outcome of patients in whom congestive heart failure develops after thrombolytic therapy for acute myocardial infarction: development of a predictive model. Am Heart J 1997;133:663–673.

160. Lamas GA, Mitchell GF, Flaker GC, et al. Clinical significance of mitral regurgitation after acute myocardial infarction. Survival and Ventricular Enlargement Investigators. Circulation 1997;96:827–833.

161. Lehmann KG, Francis CK, Sheehan FH, Dodge HT. Effect of thrombolysis on acute mitral regurgitation during evolving myocardial infarction. Experience from the Thrombolysis in Myocardial Infarction (TIMI) Trial. J Am Coll Cardiol 1993;22:714–719.

162. Vicente Vera T, Valdes Chavarri M, Garcia Alberola A, et al. Mitral valve insufficiency in acute myocardial infarction. Assessment with pulsed and coded Doppler color. Arch Inst Cardiol Mex 1991;61:117–121.

163. Ma HH, Honma H, Munakata K, Hayakawa H. Mitral insufficiency as a complication of acute myocardial infarction and left ventricular remodeling. Jpn Circ J 1997;61:912–920.

164. Alam M, Thorstrand C, Rosenhamer G. Mitral regurgitation following first-time acute myocardial infarction—early and late findings by Doppler echocardiography. Clin Cardiol 1993;16:30–34.

165. Neskovic AN, Marinkovic J, Bojic M, Popovic AD. Early predictors of mitral regurgitation after acute myocardial infarction. Am J Cardiol 1999;84:329–332.

166. Van Dantzig JM, Delemarre BJ, Koster RW, Bot H, Visser CA. Pathogenesis of mitral regurgitation in acute myocardial infarction: importance of changes in left ventricular shape and regional function. Am Heart J 1996;131:865–871.

167. Feinberg MS, Schwammenthal E, Shlizerman L, et al. Prognostic significance of mild mitral regurgitation by color Doppler echocardiography in acute myocardial infarction. Am J Cardiol 2000;86:903–907.

168. Leor J, Feinberg MS, Vered Z, et al. Effect of thrombolytic therapy on the evolution of significant mitral regurgitation in patients with a first inferior myocardial infarction. J Am Coll Cardiol 1993;21:1661–1666.

169. Tenenbaum A, Leor J, Motro M, et al. Improved posterobasal segment function after thrombolysis is associated with decreased incidence of significant mitral regurgitation in a first inferior myocardial infarction. J Am Coll Cardiol 1995;25:1558–1563.

170. Calvo FE, Figueras J, Cortadellas J, Soler-Soler J. Severe mitral regurgitation complicating acute myocardial infarction. Clinical and angiographic differences between patients with and without papillary muscle rupture. Eur Heart J 1997;18:1606–1610.

171. De Servi S, Vaccari L, Assandri J, et al. Clinical significance of mitral regurgitation in patients with recent myocardial infarction. Eur Heart J 1988;9(Suppl F):5–9.

172. Thompson CR, Buller CE, Sleeper LA, et al. Cardiogenic shock due to acute severe mitral regurgitation complicating acute myocardial infarction: a report from the SHOCK Trial Registry. SHould we use emergently revascularize Occluded Coronaries in cardiogenic shocK? J Am Coll Cardiol 2000;36:1104–1109.

173. Sharma SK, Seckler J, Israel DH, Borrico S, Ambrose JA. Clinical, angiographic and anatomic findings in acute severe ischemic mitral regurgitation. Am J Cardiol 1992;70:277–280.

174. Nishimura RA, Schaff HV, Shub C, Gersh BJ, Edwards WD, Tajik AJ. Papillary muscle rupture complicating acute myocardial infarction: analysis of 17 patients. Am J Cardiol 1983;51:373–377.

175. Coma-Canella I, Gamallo C, Onsurbe PM, Jadraque LM. Anatomic findings in acute papillary muscle necrosis. Am Heart J 1989;118:1188–1192.

176. Bordalo e Sa AL, Gonzalez DS, Leon MG, et al. The clinical significance of mitral insufficiency detected by Doppler echocardiography in acute myocardial infarct. Rev Port Cardiol 1993;12:15–21.

177. Gorman JH, 3rd, Jackson BM, Gorman RC, Kelley ST, Gikakis N, Edmunds LH, Jr. Papillary muscle discoordination rather than increased annular area facilitates mitral regurgitation after acute posterior myocardial infarction. Circulation 1997;96:II-124–II-127.

178. Gorman JH, 3rd, Gorman RC, Jackson BM, et al. Distortions of the mitral valve in acute ischemic mitral regurgitation. Ann Thorac Surg 1997;64:1026–1031.

179. Ballester M, Tasca R, Marin L, Rees S, Rickards A, McDonald L. Different mechanisms of mitral regurgitation in acute and chronic forms of coronary heart disease. Eur Heart J 1983;4:557–565.

180. Kono T, Sabbah HN, Rosman H, et al. Mechanism of functional mitral regurgitation during acute myocardial ischemia. J Am Coll Cardiol 1992;19:1101–1105.

181. Gorman RC, McCaughan JS, Ratcliffe MB, et al. Pathogenesis of acute ischemic mitral regurgitation in three dimensions. J Thorac Cardiovasc Surg 1995;109:684–693.

182. Kinney EL, Frangi MJ. Value of two-dimensional echocardiographic detection of incomplete mitral leaflet closure. Am Heart J 1985;109:87–90.

183. Becker AE, Anderson RH. Mitral insufficiency complicating acute myocardial infarction. Eur J Cardiol 1975;2:351–359.

184. Burch GE, DePasquale NP, Phillips JH. The syndrome of papillary muscle dysfunction. Am Heart J 1968;75:399–415.

185. Sabbah HN, Kono T, Rosman H, Jafri S, Stein PD, Goldstein S. Left ventricular shape: a factor in the etiology of functional mitral regurgitation in heart failure. Am Heart J 1992;123:961–966.

186. Kono T, Sabbah HN, Rosman H, Alam M, Jafri S, Goldstein S. Left ventricular shape is the primary determinant of functional mitral regurgitation in heart failure. J Am Coll Cardiol 1992;20:1594–1598.

187. Perloff JK, Roberts WC. The mitral apparatus. Functional anatomy of mitral regurgitation. Circulation 1972;46:227–239.

188. Mittal AK, Langston M, Jr, Cohn KE, Selzer A, Kerth WJ. Combined papillary muscle and left ventricular wall dysfunction as a cause of mitral regurgitation. An experimental study. Circulation 1971;44:174–180.

189. Llaneras MR, Nance ML, Streicher JT, et al. Pathogenesis of ischemic mitral insufficiency. J Thorac Cardiovasc Surg 1993;105:439–442.

190. Kaul S, Spotnitz WD, Glasheen WP, Touchstone DA. Mechanism of ischemic mitral regurgitation. An experimental evaluation. Circulation 1991;84:2167–2180.

191. David TE. Techniques and results of mitral valve repair for ischemic mitral regurgitation. J Card Surg 1994;9:274–277.

192. Loisance DY, Deleuze P, Hillion ML, Cachera JP. Are there indications for reconstructive surgery in severe mitral regurgitation after acute myocardial infarction? Eur J Cardiothorac Surg 1990;4:394–397.
193. Gorman JH, 3rd, Gorman RC, Plappert T, et al. Infarct size and location determine development of mitral regurgitation in the sheep model. J Thorac Cardiovasc Surg 1998;115:615–622.
194. Wei JY, Hutchins GM, Bulkley BH. Papillary muscle rupture in fatal acute myocardial infarction: a potentially treatable form of cardiogenic shock. Ann Intern Med 1979;90:149–152.
195. Barbour DJ, Roberts WC. Rupture of a left ventricular papillary muscle during acute myocardial infarction: analysis of 22 necropsy patients. J Am Coll Cardiol 1986;8:558–565.
196. Estes EH, Jr, Dalton FM, Entman ML, Dixon HBD, Hackel DB. The anatomy and blood supply of the papillary muscles of the left ventricle. Am Heart J 1966;71:356–362.
197. Voci P, Bilotta F, Caretta Q, Mercanti C, Marino B. Papillary muscle perfusion pattern. A hypothesis for ischemic papillary muscle dysfunction. Circulation 1995;91:1714–1718.
198. Schreiber TL, Fisher J, Mangla A, Miller D. Severe "silent" mitral regurgitation. A potentially reversible cause of refractory heart failure. Chest 1989;96:242–246.
199. Goldman AP, Glover MU, Mick W, et al. Role of echocardiography/Doppler in cardiogenic shock: silent mitral regurgitation. Ann Thorac Surg 1991;52:296–299.
200. Mintz GS, Victor MF, Kotler MN, Parry WR, Segal BL. Two-dimensional echocardiographic identification of surgically correctable complications of acute myocardial infarction. Circulation 1981;64:91–96.
201. Alam M. The role of echocardiography in acute myocardial infarction. Henry Ford Hosp Med J 1991;39:165–169.
202. Moursi MH, Bhatnagar SK, Vilacosta I, San Roman JA, Espinal MA, Nanda NC. Transesophageal echocardiographic assessment of papillary muscle rupture. Circulation 1996;94:1003–1009.
203. Herrera CJ, Gurevicius J, Stecy P, Dahodwala M, Tummala A, Nemickas R. The clinical utility of transesophageal echocardiography in ischemic papillary muscle rupture. Am J Card Imaging 1995;9:226–228.
204. Yamanishi H, Izumoto H, Kitahara H, Kamata J, Tasai K, Kawazoe K. Clinical experiences of surgical repair for mitral regurgitation secondary to papillary muscle rupture complicating acute myocardial infarction. Ann Thorac Cardiovasc Surg 1998;4:83–86.
205. Heuser RR, Maddoux GL, Goss JE, Ramo BW, Raff GL, Shadoff N. Coronary angioplasty for acute mitral regurgitation due to myocardial infarction. A nonsurgical treatment preserving mitral valve integrity. Ann Intern Med 1987;107:852–855.

9 Percutaneous Treatment of Acute Mechanical Complications of Myocardial Infarction

Elchanan Bruckheimer, MBBS, and Kevin P. Walsh, MD

CONTENTS

INTRODUCTION
ANATOMY
EQUIPMENT AND STAFF
METHODS
DEVICES
CLINICAL EXPERIENCE
CONCLUSION
REFERENCES

INTRODUCTION

Acute myocardial infarction (AMI) often results in significant impairment to contractility, which can be further compounded by tearing of the damaged myocardium *(1–3)*. Ventricular septal rupture (VSR) presents the failing left ventricle with increased preload, and a vicious cycle of hemodynamic deterioration ensues with a dismal outcome of greater than 90% mortality if untreated *(2–4)*. Surgery has been the only recourse for these patients who are unfavorable candidates because of their perioperative hemodynamic instability *(3–5)*. Earlier intervention, improved surgical technique, and aggressive perioperative management have resulted in a hospital survival approaching 60–70% in recent reports *(4–7)*.

Advances in interventional cardiac catheterization have made possible the transcatheter closure of ventricular septal defects *(8–10)*. This procedure is generally reserved for patients with congenital heart disease with residual defects following surgical repair or with muscular defects, which would require a left ventriculotomy *(11–13)*. The encouraging results of this approach have increased its use and led to the development of specific devices for ventricular septal defect closure *(11–13)*. The transcatheter approach is appealing in the setting of myocardial rupture because this method is minimally invasive for the unstable patient *(14–16)*. However, there has been

From: *Contemporary Cardiology: Cardiogenic Shock: Diagnosis and Treatment*
Edited by: David Hasdai et al. © Humana Press Inc., Totowa, NJ

only scarce reporting of transcatheter closure of VSR because of the technical complexity of the procedure, the restricted availability of appropriate devices, and the infrequent occurrence of this complication *(3,14–17)*. There have been no reports of transcatheter interventions for treating other forms of myocardial rupture such as papillary muscle tearing, as no appropriate methods or devices are currently available.

An uncommon complication of AMI is hypoxemia resulting from right-to-left shunting across a patent foramen ovale (PFO) *(18,19)*. This has been reported in right ventricular infarction and the use of left ventricular assist devices *(18,19)*. Temporary and permanent closure of the foramen has been reported *(20,21)*. Transcatheter techniques for device closure of PFO have been well described elsewhere and therefore will not be discussed further *(22,23)*.

In this chapter, we review the previous reports of transcatheter closure of VSR *(14,16,17)*, report on our experience with Amplatzer septal closure devices, discuss the relationship between the anatomy of VSR and choice of device/technique, and detail the various catheterization techniques that can be employed. Transcatheter methods for cardiac support (e.g., intra-aortic balloon pumps and revascularization procedures) are discussed in other chapters of this book (see Chapters 4 and 5 for discussions of intra-aortic balloon pumps; in addition, Holmes [Chapter 6] discusses percutaneous revascularization and Raanani et al. [Chapter 7] discuss surgical revascularization for shock).

ANATOMY

The site of septal rupture has more than anatomical importance and often defines the severity of clinical status, presence of coexistent lesions, suitability of intervention, and overall prognosis *(24–26)*. Anterior, or anterior-apical, lesions are typically the result of complete occlusion of the left anterior descending artery *(24)*. These are usually solitary well-defined lesions, left ventricular dysfunction is common, and, most often, there is single-vessel coronary artery disease *(24,25)*. In contrast, posterior defects involve the more proximal portion of the septum and are associated with occlusion of the posterior descending artery (dominance from right or circumflex) *(24,26)*. These can be serpiginous tracklike lesions and are associated with either right ventricular dysfunction or papillary muscle damage with mitral regurgitation *(25–27)*. The defect may grow in size because it commonly lies in a "necrotic lake" of tissue of questionable viability *(14)*. A collateral circulation is of paramount importance and, therefore, a previous history of coronary artery disease is, incongruously, a good prognostic sign *(28,29)*.

Transcatheter closure of VSR is becoming more prevalent because, unlike surgery, the techniques of defect closure are similar to those employed in congenital heart disease *(8–13)*. However, the unique anatomy and pathophysiology of septal rupture pose additional specific challenges *(14,16,17)*. The possibility of delayed extension of the myocardial tear or the appearance of additional defects is of major concern, especially in the transcatheter approach, in which the infarcted area is not excluded from the functioning ventricular septum *(14)*. The "necrotic lake" presents a weak and unpredictable border for the selected device, which requires considerable tissue overlap for stable deployment *(14,16)*. In addition, the immediate reduction of the hemodynamic disturbance imposed by the shunt is limited in transcatheter VSR closure by significant leaking through the device prior to its endothelialization *(14)*.

EQUIPMENT AND STAFF

Transcatheter VSR closure requires an experienced team. This includes interventional cardiologists, a transesophageal echocardiographer, a cardiac anesthesiologist, catheterization laboratory technicians, and nurses. Single-plane fluoroscopic imaging is usually sufficient because the definition of the defect size and location and relationship of device to defect is best achieved by color-Doppler transesophageal echocardiography *(30)*. General anesthesia with endotracheal intubation is recommended to ensure a more stable patient especially because transesophageal echocardiography is required. A counterpulsation intra-aortic balloon pump is often required in the critical patient and does not interfere with the procedure.

METHODS

Two types of device have been used in VSR closure: the Bard Septal Clamshell double umbrella and its more recent modification, the cardioseal device *(14),* and the Amplatzer atrial or ventricular septal occluder devices *(16,17).* Both devices, in essence, are composed of cojoined disks made of synthetic fabric and a metal skeleton *(31,32).* These disks can be folded/collapsed into an 11Fr or smaller delivery sheath. When extruded from the sheath, the disks reform their shape as a result of their inherent elastic or shape memory properties. The devices are placed so that each disk overlies the defect on either side of the ventricular septum. For successful implantation of the device, there needs to be a concentric rim of tissue around the defect that will allow the device to have sufficient purchase to maintain position and prevent embolization *(8,12).* All implantation techniques require crossing of the central area of the defect with a guidewire over which the delivery sheath is subsequently advanced. This can be achieved from either a systemic venous or arterial approach *(8,10,12).*

Our approach has been to induce general anesthesia and then percutaneously place sheaths in the right internal jugular vein and right femoral artery and vein. Heparin (50–100 IU/kg) is administered intravenously to maintain an activated coagulation time (ACT)>200 s. Intravenous antibiotics, appropriate to the patient's condition and according to the hospital's current practice, are administered prior to device deployment. Initially, a hemodynamic study is performed to measure the shunt and filling pressures. Left ventricular angiography in an angled lateral projection is then performed.

DELIVERY SHEATH PLACEMENT

The most commonly used approach is the establishment of an arteriovenous wire loop across the defect (Fig. 1) *(8–13).* This technique is employed because right ventricular trabeculation makes it easier to cross the defect from the left side. Device delivery is preferable from the venous side to accommodate the design, size, and length of the device and the delivery sheath required. A visceral or right coronary catheter is placed retrogradely into the left ventricle and advanced directly or with a guidewire across the defect. The guidewire is then advanced into the pulmonary artery or looped in the right ventricle and prolapsed across the tricuspid valve into the right atrium. Both methods attempt to avoid wire entanglement in tricuspid valve chordae. The catheter is advanced over the wire and the guidewire is exchanged for a stiffer wire to advance the delivery sheath. The tip of the guidewire is caught in a snare advanced from the right internal jugular or femoral vein and

A

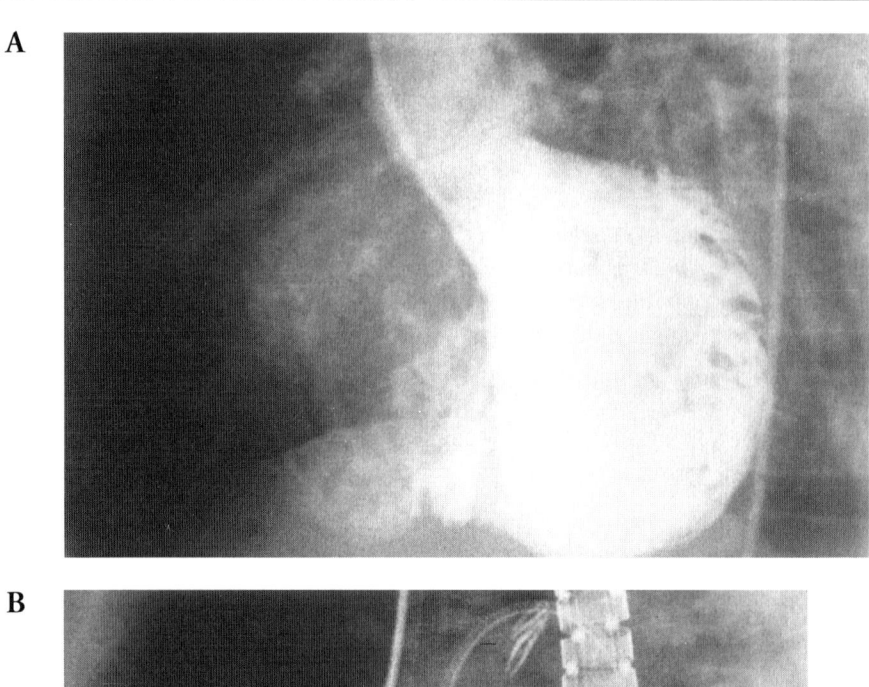

B

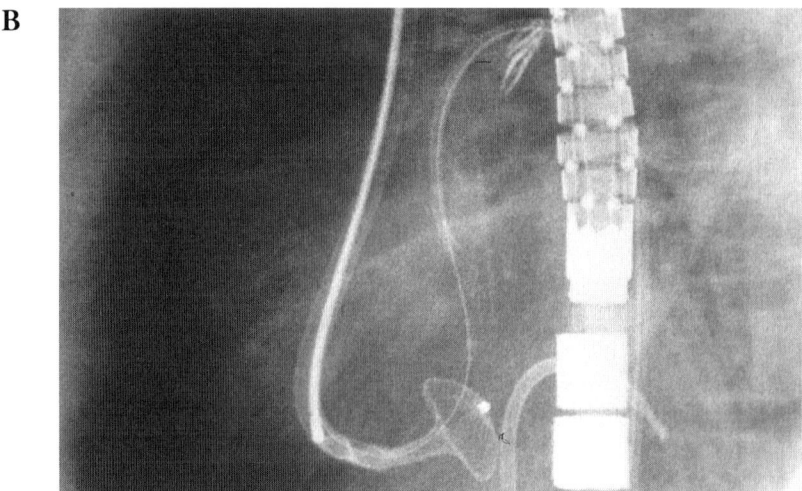

Fig. 1. Technique of VSD closure with an Amplatzer septal occluder. An apical muscular VSD (**A**) is traversed by a delivery sheath advanced from the right ventricle. The left ventricular disk is delivered and opposed to the septum (**B**) while the right disk remains collapsed in the sheath. The right disk is then delivered (**C**) and left ventricular angiography demonstrates device position and defect closure (**D**). A coronary guidewire can be seen passing through the device to maintain position and prevent sheath kinking.

exteriorized establishing the arteriovenous loop. The systemic vein chosen is the one that will allow the delivery sheath to be advanced to the defect with minimal bends to avoid sheath kinking. An alternative method is by advancing a balloon-tipped end-hole catheter transseptally to the left ventricle from the right femoral vein. Inflation of the balloon or the use of a guidewire facilitates crossing of the defect *(8,10)*.

The establishment of an arteriovenous wire loop can be time-consuming and we have recently attempted crossing defects from the right ventricular side as our initial approach.

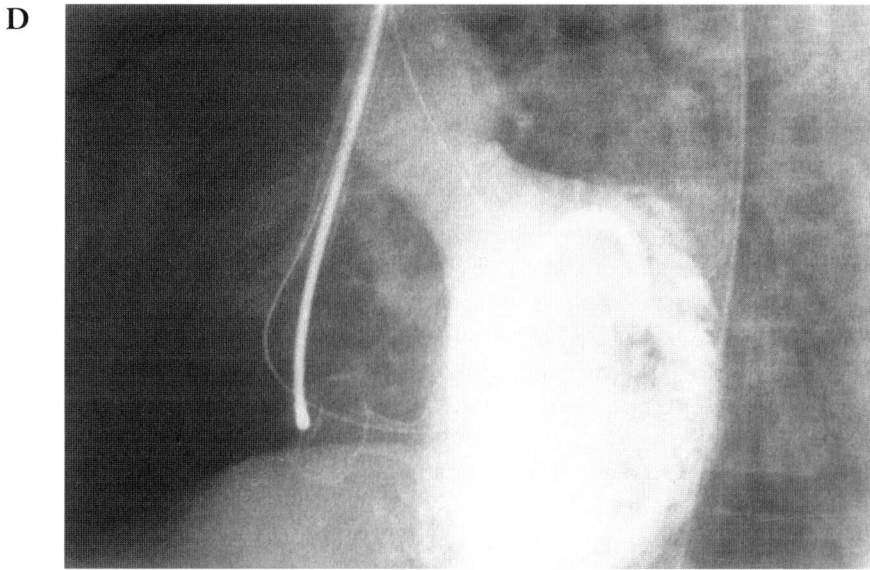

Fig. 1. *(Continued).*

Most anterior-apical defects were relatively easily crossed from the right internal jugular vein, although some antero-superior defects may be better approached from the right femoral vein. This approach is not recommended for posterior defects because of their proximity to the tricuspid valve; they should be approached from the left ventricular side.

Once a guidewire has been placed, the position and size of the defect are carefully evaluated by color-Doppler transesophageal echocardiography (TEE). Color-Doppler imaging is helpful in defining defect borders, ruling out additional defects, and assessing atrioventricular valve regurgitation *(30)*. The guidewire can usually be identified and gentle tension on both ends allows for verification that it passes through the center of the defect and that atrioventricular valve tissue is not entangled. Defect size is measured from the two-dimensional image in diastole. A compliant contrast-filled sizing balloon advanced over the wire and gently inflated or pulled through the defect can assess defects that are less well defined. Over-the-wire angiography is not usually helpful.

Following sizing, an appropriate device and delivery sheath are selected. The delivery sheath and dilator are advanced over the wire so that the tip of the delivery sheath just traverses the defect and is then "milked" forward over the dilator as the dilator is removed. If the sheath is advanced too far, it tends to buckle and kink, especially when the device is advanced. A number of methods are available to prevent sheath kinking. First, the straightest route should be chosen. The delivery sheath and dilator can be appropriately curved by hand after warming with steam. Armored sheaths can avoid kinking and it is essential that they have a Teflon inner coating to reduce friction with the device (Flexor sheath, Cook, Bloomington, IN). We have occasionally placed a stiff 0.014-in. coronary guidewire through the sheath in parallel to the device. The stiff wire gives a "backbone" to the sheath maintaining the curves. When using an arteriovenous wire loop, we occasionally replace the wire loop with a stiff coronary guidewire and pierce the Amplatzer device with the guidewire to maintain the loop while advancing the device. This has been extremely useful in cases where maintaining sheath position has been difficult during device delivery.

DEVICES

To date, there are no specifically designed devices for transcatheter closure of post-AMI VSR. Only two types of transcatheter device have been used consistently for closure of ventricular septal rupture. The first device is the Bard Clamshell double umbrella, and its modification — the cardioseal — which consists of two opposing umbrellas attached at their centers. The umbrellas are made of metal alloy arms that support a Dacron mesh *(14,32)*. The arms have a spring mechanism so that when extruded from the delivery sheath, the umbrellas are opened and their edges are held against the septum. The connector between the umbrellas is narrow and therefore does not center the device in the defect *(14,32)*. Its final position is dependent on the relationship of the umbrellas to the surrounding structures. (A later version of the device, the Starflex, is similar to the cardioseal but has a centering mechanism of nitinol springs draped between opposing umbrella arms.) The devices are manufactured in five sizes, but for the purpose of VSR only, the larger 33-mm- and 40-mm-diameter devices are useful *(14)*. In residual defects, the smaller devices may be appropriate. These devices have the advantages of being compliant with a lack of centering and large overlap of the tissue surrounding the defect, which is particularly useful when a large area of necrotic tissue surrounds the defect or small additional "satellite" defects need to be occluded *(14)*. The major disadvantage of this device is that the proximal umbrella, once released, cannot be fully collapsed back into the delivery sheath; thus, device retrieval or repositioning is limited.

Alternative devices are the series of Amplatzer septal occluders made of superelastic nitinol wires that are woven and crimped to form two disks with a cylindrical central stent *(31)*. The disks overlap the central stent by 7 mm in the atrial version and 3 mm in the ventricular version of the device. The diameter of the central stent increases in 2-mm increments from 6 mm to 24 mm in the ventricular version of the device and has a constant length of 7 mm *(31)*. The atrial version has a wider range of diameters from 4 mm to 38 mm and the central stent is short *(31)*. For VSR closure, we usually choose a device of a central stent diameter 2–3 mm greater than the diameter of the defect measured in diastole by TEE. However, the device size chosen is extremely dependent on the septal anatomy in proximity to the site of rupture. The size of the defect, both on the left and right ventricular aspects, has to be taken into consideration. The left ventricular aspect may be larger than that on the right ventricular aspect. The atrial version of the device is often more suitable for VSR closure because of its larger rim.

The Amplatzer devices are fully retrievable even when both disks have been deployed and can be easily repositioned. The positional relationship between the device and defect is well visualized by TEE. The disadvantages of the device include centering with only a small amount of overlap of surrounding tissue, especially with the VSD device. Distortion of the central stent of the device can deform the shape of the disks, particularly in serpiginous lesions, and this may lead to increased residual shunting.

CLINICAL EXPERIENCE

Temporary closure of VSR with a balloon catheter *(33,34)* has been reported and there are individual cases of successful transcatheter closure of VSR with a Rashkind umbrella *(35)* and an Amplatzer septal occluder device *(16,17)*. Landzberg and Lock *(14)* reported the only series of transcatheter closure of VSR and they used a Bard Septal Clamshell double umbrella. In their series of 18 patients, 11 patients had undergone a surgical attempt at VSR closure, whereas 7 patients had had no previous intervention. In the post-surgical group with residual shunt, there were three deaths unrelated to the catheterization procedure, which was successful in closing the defects. However, in the nonsurgical group, four patients, despite initial improvement, were decompensated in the first week after catheterization and no further therapy was attempted and they died. This failure was consistent with enlargement of the defect resulting from continued necrosis and tissue retraction. The three remaining patients in this group underwent successful closure. The difference in these patients was that they presented some months after the initial VSR and necrosis and retraction were presumably complete *(14)*.

The Amplatzer septal occluder devices have been reported for closure of VSR in three patients *(16,17)*. These cases have been in patients in whom a surgical repair had been performed and there was a significant residual leak. Our experience with transcatheter VSR closure has also been with Amplatzer septal occluder devices. The procedure was attempted in six patients with VSR post-MI. The patients were all men, ranging in age from 50 to 85 yr. The location of the infarction and VSR was anterior in five patients and inferior in one; two patients had multiple defects. Three patients were catheterized soon after the AMI and were on inotropic support and intra-aortic balloon pump. Three patients had residual defects after surgical repair and were in heart failure. The procedure was performed under general anesthesia with transesophageal echocardiography. The VSD was crossed from the left ventricle and an arteriovenous guide wire-loop created. The transvenous route was used in all patients to implant an Amplatzer ASD device with sizes ranging from 10 to 26 mm. Procedure time ranged from 90 to 216 min. Device placement was successful in all cases. Two patients had complete closure, three patients had trivial or small residual leaks, and one patient had a large residual leak. The latter patient had a second device, a 14-mm Amplatzer Muscular VSD device, implanted but continued to have a large residual shunt. Successful surgical repair of the residual VSD was performed 1 mo after the acute infarction. Procedural complications included arrhythmia in three patients (transient complete heart block, two episodes of ventricular fibrillation and cardiac arrest) and avulsion of the tricuspid septal leaflet in one patient. All patients survived to hospital discharge and remain well at 6–36 mo follow-up.

Although clinical experience is limited, it appears that device closure of residual defects following surgical repair of VSR is successful and shows potential as an alternative to late reoperation. In this setting, the transcatheter approach probably has a lower risk and is similar to closure of congenital muscular ventricular septal defects with a defined size and border. It is important to note that in both our experience and that of others, device implantation was achieved in most, if not all, cases of post-AMI VSR in which it was attempted *(14,16,17)*.

The role of transcatheter closure for VSR in the immediate post-infarction period is less clear *(14)*. The inherent advantages of a minimally invasive approach in the acute unstable cardiac patient are obvious but are not necessarily borne out in the clinical setting. The devices that are currently available are inadequate for solving the unique problems posed by post-AMI VSR. Of particular concern are defect enlargement resulting from necrosis and tissue retraction, and the persistence of the shunt, despite accurate deployment of the device, resulting from flow through the device material. Landzberg and Lock found early transcatheter intervention for VSR in the nonoperated patient to be ineffective *(14)*. Our experience with the Amplatzer device in nonsurgical patients has been more encouraging, but the small number of patients may not be truly representative.

A major factor in the improvement of the results of surgery for post-AMI VSR has been a rapid and aggressive approach to minimize preoperative decompensation *(2–5)*. Such an approach for transcatheter closure of VSR may produce similar results and minimize the impact of the technical shortcomings of the devices. Primary catheter closure of post-AMI VSR may avoid surgery or serve as a bridge to subsequent elective, lower-risk surgery. However, prospective evaluation of transcatheter closure for post-AMI VSR is hampered by the infrequency of this condition.

CONCLUSION

In this chapter, we have reviewed the current status of transcatheter device closure of ventricular septal rupture following acute myocardial infarction. The rapidly progressing field of interventional cardiology will continue to provide new devices and methodologies. The development of transcatheter valves may afford solutions for papillary muscle rupture, and future septal closure devices may improve outcome. As with many therapeutic aspects of cardiology, a collaborative approach between the interventional cardiologist and cardiac surgeon is required to achieve the most favorable outcome in these uncommon but devastating complications.

REFERENCES

1. Figueras J, Cortadellas J, Calvo F, Soler-Soler J. Relevance of delayed hospital admission on development of cardiac rupture during acute myocardial infarction: study in 225 patients with free wall, septal or papillary muscle rupture. J Am Coll Cardiol 1998;32:135–139.
2. Menon V, Webb JG, Hillis LD, Sleeper LA, Abboud R, Dzavik V, et al. Outcome and profile of ventricular septal rupture with cardiogenic shock after myocardial infarction: a report from the SHOCK Trial Registry. SHould we emergently revascularize Occluded Coronaries in cardiogenic shocK? J Am Coll Cardiol 2000;36(Suppl A):1110–1116.

3. Crenshaw BS, Granger CB, Birnbaum Y, Pieper KS, Morris DC, Kleiman NS, et al. Risk factors, angiographic patterns, and outcomes in patients with ventricular septal defect complicating acute myocardial infarction. GUSTO-I (Global Utilization of Streptokinase and TPA for Occluded Coronary Arteries) Trial Investigators. Circulation 2000;101:27–32.

4. Madsen JC, Daggett WM. Repair of postinfarction ventricular septal defects. Semin Thorac Cardiovasc Surg 1998;10:117–127.

5. Massetti M, Babatasi G, Le Page O, Bhoyroo S, Saloux E, Khayat A. Postinfarction ventricular septal rupture: early repair through the right atrial approach. J Thorac Cardiovasc Surg 2000;119:784–789.

6. Pretre R, Ye Q, Grunenfelder J, Lachat M, Vogt PR, Turina MI. Operative results of "repair" of ventricular septal rupture after acute myocardial infarction. Am J Cardiol 1999;84:785–788.

7. Dalrymple-Hay MJ, Monro JL, Livesey SA, Lamb RK. Postinfarction ventricular septal rupture: the Wessex experience. Semin Thorac Cardiovasc Surg 1998;10:111–116.

8. Lock JE, Block PC, McKay RG, Baim DS, Keane JF. Transcatheter closure of ventricular septal defects. Circulation 1988;78:361–368.

9. O'Laughlin MP, Mullins CE. Transcatheter occlusion of ventricular septal defect. Cathet Cardiovasc Diagn 1989;17:175–179.

10. Bridges ND, Perry SB, Keane JF, et al. Preoperative transcatheter closure of congenital muscular ventricular septal defects. N Engl J Med 1991;324:1312–1317.

11. Tofeig M, Patel RG, Walsh KP. Transcatheter closure of a mid-muscular ventricular septal defect with an amplatzer VSD occluder device. Heart 1999;81:438–440.

12. Thanopoulos BD, Tsaousis GS, Konstadopoulou GN, Zarayelyan AG. Transcatheter closure of muscular ventricular septal defects with the amplatzer ventricular septal defect occluder: initial clinical applications in children. J Am Coll Cardiol 1999;33:1395–1399.

13. Hijazi ZM, Hakim F, Al-Fadley F, Abdelhamid J, Cao QL. Transcatheter closure of single muscular ventricular septal defects using the amplatzer muscular VSD occluder: initial results and technical considerations. Catheter Cardiovasc Interv 2000;49:167–172.

14. Landzberg MJ, Lock JE. Transcatheter management of ventricular septal rupture after myocardial infarction. Semin Thorac Cardiovasc Surg 1998;10:128–132.

15. Laussen PC, Hansen DD, Perry SB, et al. Transcatheter closure of ventricular septal defects: hemodynamic instability and anesthetic management. Anesth Analg 1995;80:1076–1082.

16. Lee EM, Roberts DH, Walsh KP. Transcatheter closure of a residual postmyocardial infarction ventricular septal defect with the Amplatzer septal occluder. Heart 1998;80:522–524.

17. Pesonen E, Thilen U, Sandstrom S, et al. Transcatheter closure of post-infarction ventricular septal defect with the Amplatzer Septal Occluder device. Scand Cardiovasc J 2000;34:446–448.

18. Bansal RC, Marsa RJ, Holland D, Beehler C, Gold PM. Severe hypoxemia due to shunting through a patent foramen ovale: a correctable complication of right ventricular infarction. J Am Coll Cardiol 1985;5:188–192.

19. Baldwin RT, Duncan JM, Frazier OH, Wilansky S. Patent foramen ovale: a cause of hypoxemia in patients on left ventricular support. Ann Thorac Surg 1991;52:865–867.

20. Krueger SK, Lappe DL. Right-to-left shunt through patent foramen ovale complicating right ventricular infarction. Successful percutaneous catheter closure. Chest 1988;94:1100–1101.

21. Nguyen DQ, Das GS, Grubbs BC, Bolman RM 3rd, Park SJ. Transcatheter closure of patent foramen ovale for hypoxemia during left ventricular assist device support. J Heart Lung Transplant 1999;18:1021–1023.

22. Bridges ND, Hellenbrand W, Latson L, Filiano J, Newburger JW, Lock JE. Transcatheter closure of patent foramen ovale after presumed paradoxical embolism. Circulation 1992;86:1902–1908.

23. Chan KC, Godman MJ, Walsh K, Wilson N, Redington A, Gibbs JL. Transcatheter closure of atrial septal defect and interatrial communications with a new self expanding nitinol double disc device (Amplatzer septal occluder): multicentre UK experience. Heart 1999;82:300–306.

24. Skehan JD, Carey C, Norrell MS, de Belder M, Balcon R, Mills PG. Patterns of coronary artery disease in post-infarction ventricular septal rupture. Br Heart J 1989;62:268–272.

25. Edwards BS, Edwards WD, Edwards JE. Ventricular septal rupture complicating acute myocardial infarction: identification of simple and complex types in 53 autopsied hearts. Am J Cardiol 1984;54:1201–1205.

26. Swithinbank JM. Perforation of the interventricular septum in myocardial infarction. N Engl J Med 1959;21:562–567.

27. Fananapazir L, Bray CL, Dark JF, Moussalli H, Deiraniya AK, Lawson RA. Right ventricular dysfunction and surgical outcome in postinfarction ventricular septal defect. Eur Heart J 1983;4:155–167.

28. Rubinstein P, Levinson DC. Acquired interventricular septal defects due to myocardial infarction and nonpenetrating trauma to the chest. Am J Cardiol 1961;7:277–282.

29. Chaux A, Blanche C, Matloff JM, DeRobertis MA, Miyamoto A. Postinfarction ventricular septal defect. Semin Thorac Cardiovasc Surg 1998;10:93–99.

30. van der Velde ME, Sanders SP, Keane JF, Perry SB, Lock JE. Transesophageal echocardiographic guidance of transcatheter ventricular septal defect closure. J Am Coll Cardiol 1994;23:1660–1665.

31. Walsh KP, Maadi IM. The Amplatzer septal occluder. Cardiol Young 2000;10:493–501.

32. Rome JJ, Keane JF, Perry SB, Spevak PJ, Lock JE. Double-umbrella closure of atrial defects. Initial clinical applications. Circulation 1990;82:751–758.

33. Abhyankar AD, Jagtap PM. Post-infarction ventricular septal defect: percutaneous transvenous temporary closure using a Swan-Ganz catheter. Catheter Cardiovasc Interv 1999;47:208–10.

34. Sochman J, Peregrin JH. Temporary balloon closure of a postinfarction interventricular septal rupture. Int J Cardiol 1993;42:302–306.

35. Benton JP, Barker KS. Transcatheter closure of ventricular septal defect: a nonsurgical approach to the care of the patient with acute ventricular septal rupture. Heart Lung 1992;21:356–364.

10

Surgical Management of Mechanical Complications of Acute Coronary Syndromes Causing Cardiogenic Shock

Harold M. Burkhart, MD,
and Joseph A. Dearani, MD

INTRODUCTION

Approximately 15% of all patients suffering a fatal myocardial infarction die of myocardial rupture. Eighty-five percent of these deaths are from ventricular free wall ruptures. Ventricular septal ruptures (VSDs) and papillary muscle ruptures account for 10% and 5%, respectively *(1,2)*. The natural history of these ruptures is dismal and, therefore, expeditious surgical repair is generally advocated. The focus of this chapter will be the surgical treatment of mechanical complications of acute coronary syndrome and myocardial infarction that result in cardiogenic shock. (An additional presentation of these mechanical complications is provided in Chapter 8. Chapter 7 contains discussions about anesthesia and surgical revascularization techniques.)

VENTRICULAR SEPTAL RUPTURE

Ventricular septal rupture complications occur in 1–2% of all myocardial infarctions *(3)*. The first surgical repair of this defect was performed by Cooley in 1957 *(4)*. This operation was done 9 wk after the acute myocardial infarction; unfortunately, the patient died 6 wk postoperatively. The first long-term survivor after surgical repair was a patient operated on at the Mayo Clinic by Kirklin in 1963.

From: *Contemporary Cardiology: Cardiogenic Shock: Diagnosis and Treatment*
Edited by: David Hasdai et al. © Humana Press Inc., Totowa, NJ

Anatomy

Ventricular septal ruptures can occur in the anterior or posterior septum. Approximately 60% of postinfarction ventricular septal ruptures occur in the anterior septum after a myocardial infarction secondary to occlusion of the left anterior descending artery *(5)*. In these patients, the defect is located in the distal half of the anterior septum. Posterior septal ruptures account for about 30% of septal ruptures. They usually occur in the proximal half of the posterior septum after occlusion of a dominant right coronary artery or, on occasion, a dominant circumflex artery *(5)*.

An autopsy study of 53 hearts with postinfarction VSDs performed by Edwards et al. *(6)* demonstrated the two types of septal rupture. They described both simple and complex ruptures. The simple defect was a direct interventricular connection, whereas the complex defect had an undulating or serpiginous route tracking through the septum. Both occurred with similar frequency. However, the complex rupture was most often associated with an inferior myocardial infarction.

Pathophysiology

Determinants of early outcome of the course of a postinfarction ventricular septal rupture are the development of congestive heart failure and cardiogenic shock, which are dependent on the magnitude of the infarction and the degree of left-to-right shunt. Anterior septal rupture is most commonly associated with extensive left ventricular necrosis and left ventricular dysfunction, whereas posterior septal ruptures are usually associated with right ventricular infarction *(7–9)*. The results of medical management are poor, with greater than 50% mortality at 2 wk and less than 10% surviving 3 mo *(5)*. Given these results, surgical repair of ventricular septal rupture is the standard of care.

Preoperative Strategy

The timing of surgical repair of a postinfarction VSD has changed over the past two decades. In the past, surgery was delayed to allow the infarct to heal. This was believed to make the repair easier because the surgeon would have scar tissue to suture to rather than the fresh, friable tissue of an acute ventricular infarct. Patients who survived this healing period had a lower operative mortality than those operated on earlier *(10,11)*. The problem with delayed surgical management is the dismal natural history of a ventricular septal rupture. Approximately 25% of patients die within 24 h, 50% within a week, and more than 80% within the first month. Therefore, the management strategy of delayed surgery seemed to select out the patients with smaller infarcts and less myocardial damage *(12)*.

Daggett et al. *(13)* reported their experience of early versus delayed surgical treatment of postinfarction VSDs. They had two groups of patients: Group 1 (before 1975), when operative intervention was delayed, and Group 2 (after 1975), when patients underwent early operation. Survival was 59% in Group 1 and 75% in Group 2. In addition, if cardiogenic shock was present preoperatively, an even greater survival advantage was seen in Group 2. Given these results, as well as others *(12,14)*, early surgical intervention has now become the standard approach.

Once the diagnosis of postinfarction ventricular septal rupture has been established, aggressive efforts are made to stabilize the patient in preparation for prompt surgical intervention. This includes standard pharmacologic therapy of inotropic agents, afterload reducing agents, and diuretic therapy *(15)*. In most patients, intra-aortic balloon pump (IABP) counterpulsation is initiated to decrease left ventricular afterload, thus decreasing the left-to-right shunt across the VSD and increasing systemic and coronary artery perfusion. This usually provides some hemodynamic improvement while preparation is being made for urgent surgery. It is important to note that the improvement seen with the IABP may be temporary and clinical deterioration may still rapidly ensue *(12)*.

The role of preoperative angiography is debatable. Because decreased left ventricular function and recurrent myocardial infarction are major causes of morbidity and mortality postoperatively, most advocate preoperative coronary angiography when possible *(10,12,15)*. Series have shown that more than one-half of patients who suffer a postinfarction ventricular septal rupture have significant coronary artery disease in at least one vessel other than the infarct vessel *(16,17)*. The main disadvantage of preoperative coronary angiography is that it delays the surgery; early surgical treatment cannot be overemphasized. Skillington et al. *(18)* reported a small number of patients who died during the coronary angiogram. Although they advised against preoperative angiography because it delayed surgery, most other series have not had mortality during angiography and advocate it as an important preoperative study *(16,19)*. In fact, Pretre et al. *(16)* showed similar early and late results in patients with coronary artery disease who underwent coronary artery bypass grafting at the time of ventricular septal rupture repair compared with patients without coronary artery disease. In our practice, a preoperative coronary angiogram is obtained routinely, except for unusual circumstances.

Surgical Technique

Repair is accomplished through median sternotomy using standard cardiopulmonary bypass techniques and cardioplegic arrest. Intraoperative transesophageal echocardiography is used routinely. Coronary revascularization, if necessary, is performed first using saphenous vein conduits. Depending on the stability and age of the patient, consideration is given to the use of the internal mammary artery conduit for anterior descending coronary grafting. (See also Chapter 7 on operative strategies for cardiogenic shock.)

Repair of the ventricular septal rupture is performed after coronary artery grafting. Different reparative techniques have been described *(5,15,20)* and will be reviewed later in this chapter. Defects can occur in the apical, anterior, or posterior septum. General principles of the classical surgical management include transinfarct left ventriculotomy, debridement of necrotic septum and free wall, patch closure of the VSD, and ventriculotomy closure with felt strips or patch closure as needed to minimize tension on the suture lines. Repair by infarction exclusion as described by David et al. *(9,20)* is also reviewed.

Apical

True apical defects are uncommon, but when they do occur, they can oftentimes be managed by amputation of the apex of the heart *(21)*. This involves opening the heart over the left ventricular infarct and excising and debriding all necrotic tissue from the left ventricle, right ventricle, and septum back to healthy myocardium. Repair is then accomplished by sandwiching the cut ventricular walls and septum together.

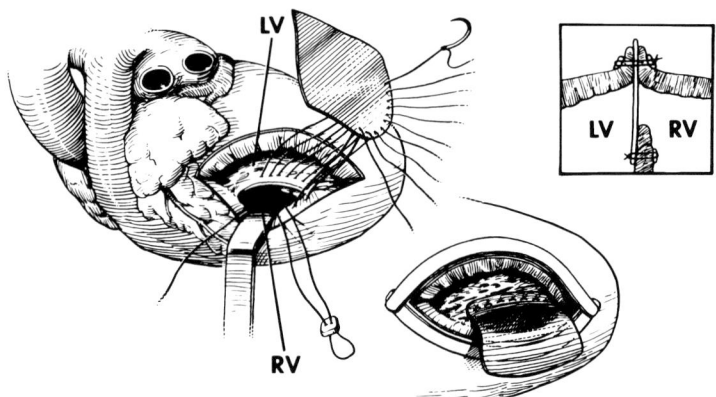

Fig. 1. Repair of a large anterior ventricular septal rupture using a prosthetic (Dacron) patch to provide a tension-free repair (RV; right ventricle, LV; left ventricle).

Anterior

The technique used for anterior VSDs depends on the size of the defect. If the defect is small, a plication technique can be used *(22,23)* and a prosthetic patch avoided as long as there is no tension on the repair. After a transinfarction left ventriculotomy and adequate necrotic tissue debridement, the free edge of the anterior septal defect is approximated to the right ventricular free wall. This is accomplished using mattress sutures and a felt strip on both the left ventricular side of the septum and the epicardial surface of the right ventricle. The transinfarct incision is then closed in a similar fashion using felt strips and mattress sutures.

Larger anterior ventricular septal ruptures require a synthetic patch in order to obtain a tension-free repair *(15)*. The patch is sutured to the left side of the free edge of the septal defect using pledgetted interrupted mattress sutures. The rest of the patch is either sutured in a similar fashion to the free wall of the right ventricle or incorporated into the left transinfarct ventriculotomy closure. After adequate infarct debridement, closure is performed using mattress sutures and felt strips on both sides of the closure (Fig. 1).

Posterior

Inferoposterior septal defects are the most difficult to repair *(15)*. Unlike anterior defects, the posterior defect usually requires a second patch for the infarctectomy defect in order to avoid undue tension on the suture lines. After initiation of cardiopulmonary bypass, the apex of the heart is retracted superiorly to gain access to the inferoposterior infarct. All necrotic tissue is debrided from both ventricles and septum. A prosthetic patch is sutured to the free edge of the left side of the septum with pledgetted mattress sutures. The rest of the patch is then sutured to the free wall of the right ventricle or to the second patch. The second patch is used to cover the infarctectomy defect. Again, pledgetted mattress sutures are used to prevent damage to the friable myocardium (Fig. 2).

Infarct Exclusion

An alternative approach for repair of postinfarction VSD is the infarct exclusion technique described by David et al. *(9,20)*. This technique excludes the healing infarct from

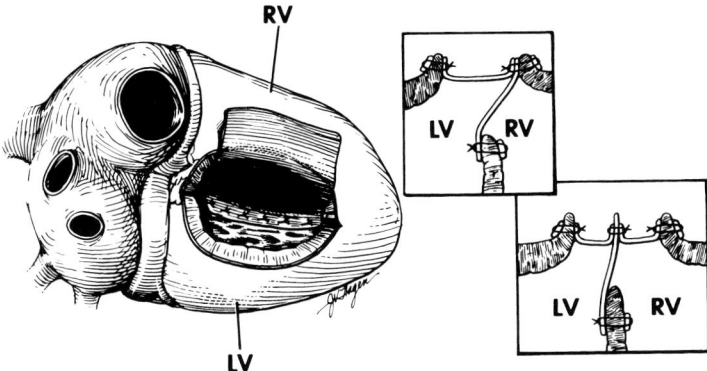

Fig. 2. View of a posterior ventricular septal rupture repair. Note that a second prosthetic (Dacron) patch is typically required to avoid tension on the repair.

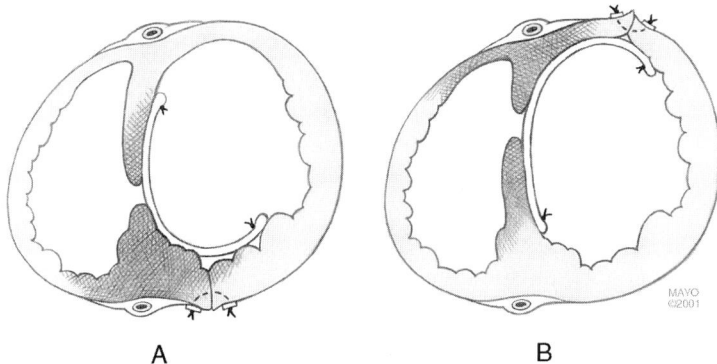

A   B

Fig. 3. Cross-sectional views of the infarct exclusion technique for anterior **(A)** and posterior **(B)** ventricular septal ruptures.

the high left ventricular pressures while attempting to preserve left ventricular geometry. In *anterior* septal defects, a left ventriculotomy is made across the infarcted tissue on the anterior surface of the heart. A large glutaraldehyde-fixed bovine pericardial patch or synthetic patch (approximately 4×6 cm) is sutured to the left side of the septum and to healthy endocardium away from the area of the infarct. The infarctotomy is then closed in two layers with felt strips to buttress the tissue (Fig. 3A). A *posterior* ventricular septal rupture is treated in a similar fashion. An incision is made through the infarct on the posterior left ventricular wall. A large triangular patch (4×7 cm) is then sutured to the mitral annulus, the endocardium of the left side of the septum, and, finally, the endocardium of the posterior wall left of the infarction. The ventriculotomy is then closed in two layers with felt strips (Fig. 3B). Note that with both of these repairs, by suturing the patch to healthy tissue away from the area of infarction, the friable tissues of the infarction are not directly exposed to the high left ventricular pressure. Because right ventricular dysfunction is often present with a posterior VSD (and usually concomitant right ventricular infarction), the infarction exclusion technique may be advantageous because it leaves the damaged right ventricle relatively undisturbed *(9)*.

Recovery

Postoperatively, IABP counterpulsation is generally continued for approximately 48–72 h. This allows maximum afterload reduction and maximum decrease in left ventricular wall stress that are important following repair where tissue quality is poor and chance for breakdown of the repair is greatest. Liberal use of transthoracic and transesophageal echocardiography should readily identify residual or recurrent defects if the clinical status is not improving or is worsening. A pulmonary artery catheter is also helpful in determining the presence of an oxygen-saturation step-up from the right atrium to the pulmonary artery and calculating the degree of a left-to-right shunt.

Results

Although progress has been made, the surgical repair of postinfarction ventricular septal rupture continues to be associated with significant morbidity and mortality. Skillington et al. *(18)* reported their experience with 101 patients undergoing surgical repair of postinfarction VSDs. Overall operative mortality was 20.8%. The presence of an inferior infarct, operation within the first week of myocardial infarction, and the presence of cardiogenic shock were all risk factors for early mortality. Daggett and colleagues *(24)* reported similar results in their series with a mortality rate of 25% since 1975. Their data also showed a worse prognosis with posterior versus anterior infarctions (15% mortality vs 34%, respectively).

A more recent study by Deja et al. *(25)* reported a 30-d mortality of 37%. Of note was that there was no difference in mortality based on infarct location. David and Armstrong *(20)* also reported that infarct location did not significantly influence outcome in their 52 patients repaired using the exclusion technique (19% mortality).

In summary, although early results with postinfarction VSD have improved with earlier surgical intervention, mortality continues to be high. Although results have indicated that there can be little difference in outcome with regard to VSD location, we have found repair of posterior infarctions with VSD, especially with concomitant right ventricular infarction, to be the most difficult to repair and obtain a satisfactory result.

PAPILLARY MUSCLE RUPTURE

Papillary muscle rupture after a myocardial infarction accounts for up to 5% of all deaths associated with acute myocardial infarctions *(26)*. Stevenson and Turner were the first to describe this postinfarction complication at autopsy in 1935 *(27)*. It was not until 1948 that the diagnosis was made antemortem by Davidson *(28)*. This complication was managed medically until 1965, when Austen and colleagues successfully treated severe mitral regurgitation resulting from papillary muscle rupture by replacing a mitral valve *(29)*.

Anatomy

Either the anterolateral or posteromedial papillary muscle may be involved in a postinfarction papillary muscle rupture. The coronary blood supply to the anterolateral papillary muscle is usually a dual system composed of the left anterior descending

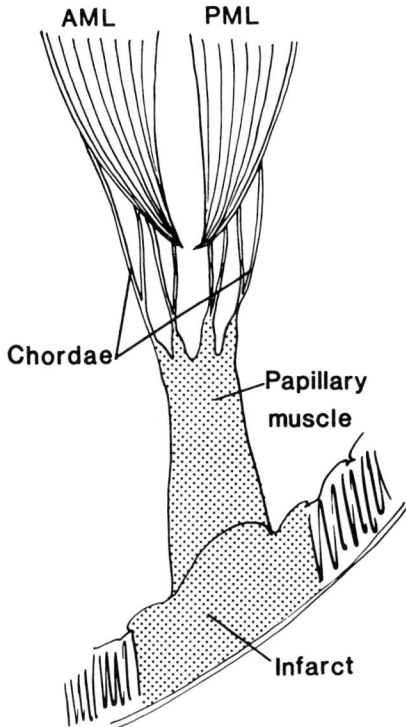

Fig. 4. Acute infarction involving the papillary muscle and adjacent myocardium. Although the papillary muscle remains intact, mitral regurgitation may still occur secondary to papillary muscle dysfunction (AML; anterior mitral leaflet, PML; posterior mitral leaflet).

artery and marginal branches of the circumflex artery. The posteromedial papillary muscle, on the other hand, usually has a single blood supply from the posterior descending artery. This single blood supply is thought to make the posteromedial papillary muscle more vulnerable to infarction and rupture *(30)*. In fact, studies have demonstrated that approximately 75% of postinfarction papillary muscle ruptures involve the posteromedial papillary muscle *(26,31,32)*.

The most common cause of mitral valve dysfunction as a result of coronary artery disease is ischemic papillary muscle dysfunction that produces intermittent episodes of mitral regurgitation and pulmonary edema. If the papillary muscle does not rupture but does not contract because of the infarction, it is termed papillary muscle dysfunction (Fig. 4). This can also result in severe mitral regurgitation and can often improve dramatically with coronary revascularization alone.

This chapter will focus on mitral regurgitation resulting from papillary muscle rupture. Papillary muscle rupture can involve the entire trunk of the muscle or, more commonly, partial rupture of one of the heads. Some studies indicate that approximately half of patients have complete muscle disruption *(33)*. Other studies have noted that the majority of ruptures are partial ruptures of either the main muscle trunk or one of the papillary muscle heads *(31,32,34)* (Fig. 5). This results in mitral regurgitation and hemodynamics that are often better tolerated than a complete papillary muscle rupture

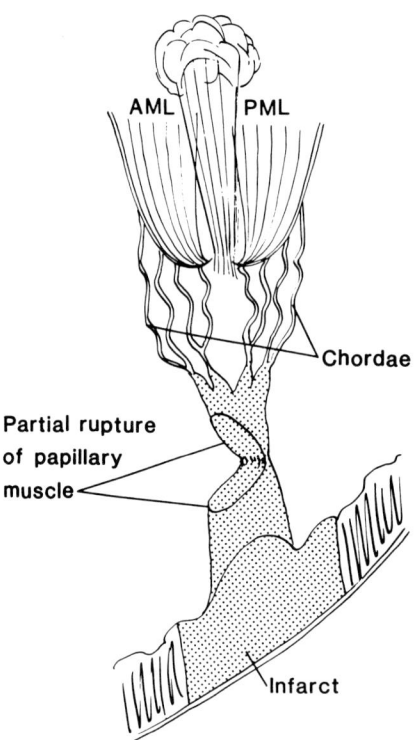

Fig. 5. A partial papillary muscle rupture resulting from myocardial infarction resulting in mitral valve regurgitation. Note the adjacent infarcted ventricular wall.

(30) (Fig. 6). However, a partial rupture may extend into a complete rupture, causing progressive deterioration in hemodynamics. The extent of the infarction can range from small (20% of the left ventricle) to large (50% of the left ventricle) *(26,31)*. The extent of coronary artery disease is often less severe than in patients with chronic ischemic mitral regurgitation, with single-vessel disease present in 25% *(35)*.

Medical treatment alone is unsuccessful. Sanders et al. *(36)* reported the dismal results of postinfarction papillary muscle rupture. One-third of the patients died immediately, with one-half not surviving the first 24 h. Only 6% survived beyond 2 mo. Given these poor results with medical therapy alone, urgent surgical intervention offers the best chance for survival.

Preoperative Strategy

The optimal timing of surgery has been a topic of controversy. In the past, delayed surgical intervention was preferred because it was felt that a successful operation was more likely if the infarcted tissue had healed and would be more likely to hold sutures. This approach, although associated with a lower surgical mortality, likely selected out patients with smaller infarcts who survived long enough to undergo operation *(12)*.

Nishimura and colleagues *(31)* reported the Mayo Clinic experience of 17 patients with postinfarction papillary muscle rupture. They looked at the medical and surgical groups and compared their outcomes based on the presentation of cardiogenic shock

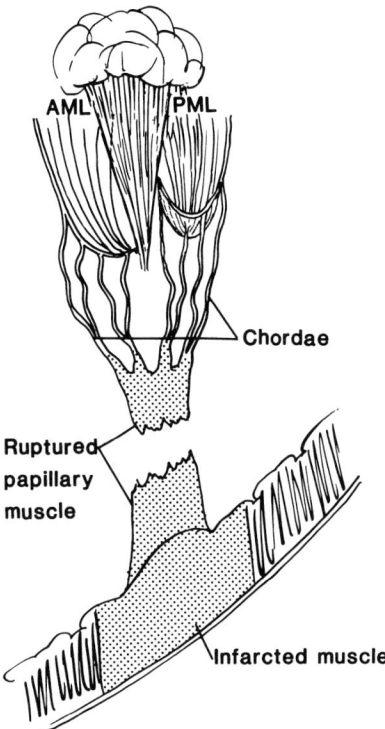

Fig. 6. A complete papillary muscle rupture resulting from myocardial infarction resulting in severe mitral valve regurgitation.

or congestive heart failure without shock. Among the patients with cardiogenic shock, four were treated medically and all four died. Two patients with cardiogenic shock were treated surgically; one of these patients survived. Of the patients who presented in congestive heart failure alone, the five patients treated medically all died. These deaths were characterized as sudden and unpredictable, occurring up to 60 d after papillary muscle rupture. There were six patients stabilized and taken to the operating room, and five of these patients survived. The authors concluded by recommending an early surgical approach in acute papillary muscle rupture to improve overall survival.

When a patient presents in cardiogenic shock as a result of acute papillary muscle rupture with pulmonary edema, initial treatment includes inotropic support to optimize cardiac output and stabilize hemodynamics. If possible, nitroprusside can be added to reduce afterload. IABP counterpulsation should be initiated to decrease left ventricular afterload and optimize cardiac output. One must recognize, however, that the hemodynamic improvement with IABP counterpulsation may be only temporary. Because the patient's clinical status may deteriorate rapidly, plans for surgical intervention should be promptly made once the diagnosis of papillary muscle rupture is confirmed by echocardiography *(12)*.

The role of preoperative coronary angiography is somewhat controversial. In the study by Nishimura et al. *(31)*, 13 of 17 patients had preoperative coronary angiograms. Approximately 50% of patients had only single-vessel disease. However, it has been shown that recurrent myocardial infarction and left ventricular dysfunction account for significant postoperative morbidity and mortality in patients with acute papillary muscle rupture *(12,31)*. Therefore, if hemodynamics are stable, we prefer an urgent coronary angiogram prior to transfer to the operating room.

Surgical Technique

Surgical options include mitral valve replacement or mitral valve repair. In general, valve replacement is most often performed for complete truncal papillary muscle rupture. Valve repair is sometimes performed when there is partial rupture (and occasionally with complete rupture) depending on the experience of the surgeon, the age and stability of the patient, and the anatomic findings at operation. It is important to note that the myocardial infarction rarely involves just the papillary muscle; there is typically an ecchymotic, friable lateral or inferior wall consistent with an acute infarct. This can often make valve repair more challenging. In addition, as the ventricle recovers and heals from the infarct, there is usually progressive apical displacement of the papillary muscles into the ventricle that can result in recurrent mitral regurgitation following a successful repair *(37)*.

The operation is approached through a median sternotomy. Intraoperative transesophageal echocardiography is used routinely. Standard cardiopulmonary bypass techniques with left heart venting and cardioplegic arrest are employed. We prefer bicaval cannulation to allow adequate mitral valve exposure given the typical small left atrium noted in these cases. If coronary artery bypass grafting is planned, it is generally performed first, followed by mitral valve replacement or repair.

In the majority of cases, exposure of the mitral valve is via a standard left atriotomy. In general, we recommend a mitral valve replacement as the procedure of choice for papillary muscle rupture. The choice of a mechanical or bioprosthesis is individualized and determined with the patient and family prior to surgery. We give careful consideration to valve repair in selected circumstances. In general, our approach is to attempt valve repair in younger patients in an effort to avoid a prosthesis, especially if the rupture is partial and the surrounding tissue is of satisfactory quality. Given that the majority of these patients arrive in the operating room in extremis, it is important for the surgeon to exercise conservative judgment about the feasibility of a successful and durable repair in an effort to avoid repeated attempts at repair with potentially multiple bypass runs.

If valve replacement is planned, our approach is to resect the flail papillary muscle and its respective chordae. We make an effort to maintain as much leaflet tissue and subvalvular apparatus intact as possible. If valve repair is planned, our technique is a transatrial or transeptal approach without a left ventriculotomy, as described by Rankin *(38)*. The papillary muscle head is reattached to its respective location on the left ventricular wall by placing a mattress suture reinforced with felt pledgets full thickness through the lateral or inferior left ventricular wall, as shown in Fig. 7. The repair is then reinforced with a flexible posterior annuloplasty ring (Figs. 8 and 9).

Cardiopulmonary bypass is discontinued with IABP counterpulsation and inotropic support initiated as needed. Transesophageal echocardiography is used to assess the repair or the function of the prosthesis. IABP counterpulsation is usually continued for 24–48 h or as needed depending on hemodynamics and left ventricular function.

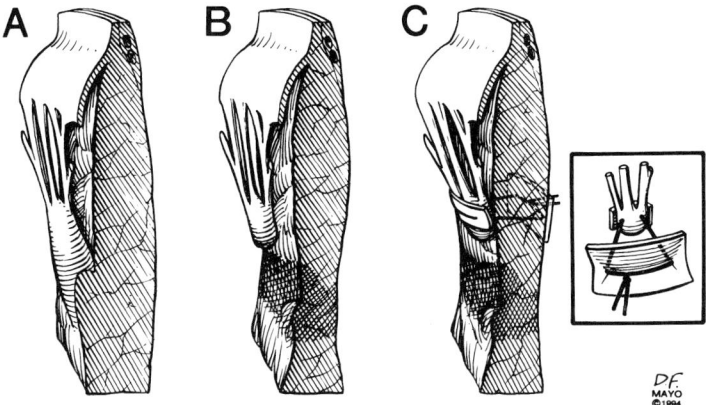

Fig. 7. A papillary muscle head is reattached to its proper location on the infarcted left ventricular wall utilizing a buttressed suture that is passed full thickness through the ventricular wall.

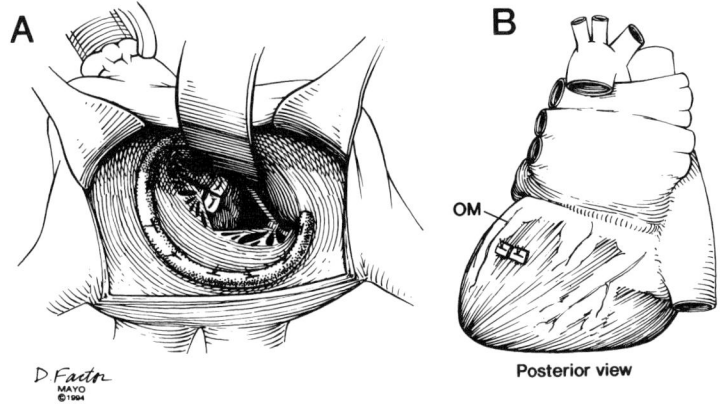

Fig. 8. The surgeon's view through the left atrium showing the completed repair of a ruptured *anterolateral* papillary muscle with a flexible posterior annuloplasty band.

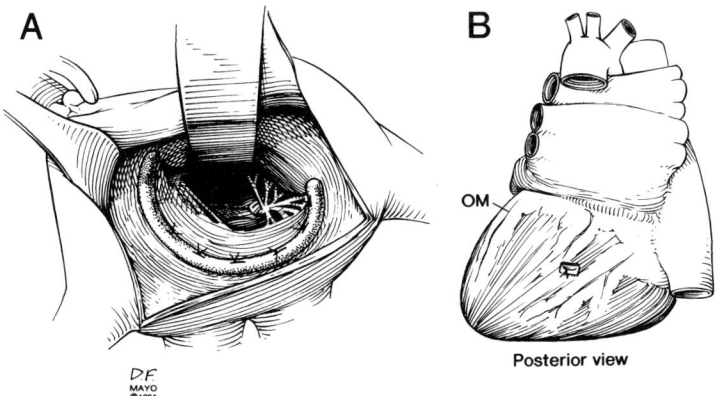

Fig. 9. The surgeon's view through the left atrium showing the completed repair of a ruptured *posteromedial* papillary muscle with a flexible posterior annuloplasty band.

Results

There are several series of acute papillary muscle rupture in the literature, with operative mortalities ranging from 17% to 40% *(33,39,40)*. Nishimura et al. *(12)* reported the Mayo Clinic experience on the surgical treatment of seven consecutive patients with postinfarction papillary muscle rupture. Five of the patients presented with cardiogenic shock and pulmonary edema, whereas two patients had just pulmonary edema. They all underwent "early" mitral valve replacement within 4 d of presentation. All of the patients survived the perioperative period. The authors concluded by recommending early surgical intervention in patients suffering a postinfarction papillary muscle rupture with acute mitral regurgitation.

VENTRICULAR FREE WALL RUPTURE

Rupture of the left ventricle free wall after myocardial infarction was first described by William Harvey in 1647 *(41)*. The first successful repair of a ventricular free wall rupture was performed by Cobbs and Hatcher in 1968 *(42)*. Postinfarction left ventricular free wall rupture accounts for up to 24% of fatal myocardial infarctions *(43)*. Most of these patients die before making it to emergency surgery.

Anatomy

Batts and colleagues *(44)* reported 100 consecutive autopsied cases of postinfarction rupture of the left ventricular free wall at the Mayo Clinic. All of the recent myocardial infarctions were transmural. One-half of the ruptures were classified as simple, through-and-through ruptures, whereas the other half were complex with a serpiginous route through the myocardium. Sixty-six of the ruptures occurred in the middle third of the ventricle rather than the apical or basal third. The rupture was most often in the lateral left ventricular wall (44%) as opposed to the anterior or inferior walls.

Critical coronary artery atherosclerotic lesions were noted in 98 of the 100 cases. Eighty-three of the patients had two or more vessel disease. Coronary artery thrombosis was present in 73 patients. This involved the left anterior descending artery in 23, left circumflex artery in 22, right coronary artery in 27, and left main artery in 1.

Pathophysiology

Clinically, ruptures can be classified as early (acute) or secondary (subacute) *(45)*. The early acute rupture, or "blowout," typically occurs immediately after the chest pain. This type of rupture quickly leads to cardiogenic shock and death from pericardial tamponade. These patients deteriorate rapidly prior to any surgical intervention.

Secondary or subacute ruptures are usually observed within the first 5 d after the myocardial infarction *(45)*. This type of rupture starts out as a small left ventricular tear that may not be actively bleeding *(5)*. Patients with subacute free wall ruptures can survive for days *(46)*. However, the nonbleeding small tear may progress to a larger tear, resulting in pericardial tamponade. It is these subacute ruptures that potentially provide the surgeon with a small window of opportunity for surgical intervention.

Preoperative Strategy

Once the diagnosis of postinfarction left ventricular free wall rupture has been established by echocardiography, no time is wasted in transferring the patient to the operating room. Often, the patient already has inotropic and IABP support that may have temporarily stabilized the patient. However, the immediate goal is surgical relief of the pericardial tamponade and closure of the rupture.

Controversy exists with regard to the necessity of a preoperative coronary angiogram. Most authors agree that given the high risk of mortality with a free wall rupture, no time should be wasted obtaining an angiogram (5,45,47–50). Zeebregts et al. (48) recommend consideration of coronary artery revascularization if significant stenoses were present on previously obtained coronary angiograms or if bypass grafting is necessary for successful discontinuation from cardiopulmonary bypass. In addition, if coronary angiography has not been performed, the coronary arteries should be palpated intraoperatively for proximal intraluminal plaques, and consideration should be given to bypass grafting.

Surgical Technique

Once in the operating room, the patient should be prepped and draped prior to anesthesia, as in any case of suspected pericardial tamponade. Further hypotension will result with anesthetic induction (5). Intraoperative transesophageal echocardiography is used routinely. A median sternotomy is performed and the tamponade is relieved. Often, there is no active bleeding at the site of rupture (5). In general, cardiopulmonary bypass with ascending aortic cannulation and bicaval or right atrial cannulation is employed. The left heart is vented via the right superior pulmonary vein. If coronary artery bypass grafting is planned, it is usually performed first. Saphenous vein conduits are generally used; consideration to internal mammary artery grafting is given for younger patients after cardiopulmonary bypass has been initiated.

A few techniques of repair should be mentioned (5). One way to repair the rupture is to perform an infarctectomy and close the defect with horizontal mattress sutures using felt strips to buttress the closure. An infarctectomy is not always necessary; sometimes, the rupture can be repaired directly with mattress sutures and felt. However, one must recognize that suture placement through necrotic muscle may risk further rupture (5). Thus, the decision about infarctectomy is made intraoperatively, depending on tissue quality. A modification was added by Nunez et al. (51), in which they covered the repair with a large Teflon patch and sutured it to the surrounding healthy myocardium. Padro et al. (47) reported a sutureless technique in which they glued a large felt patch to the heart to cover the rupture. They performed this technique successfully on 13 patients, with only 1 requiring the assistance of cardiopulmonary bypass.

After completion of the repair, cardiopulmonary bypass is discontinued and IABP counterpulsation and inotropic support are used as needed. The balloon pump is of critical importance following repair because it decreases left ventricular wall tension and thus decreases the stress on the suture lines. We generally continue the IABP for a minimum of 24–48 h, depending on the stability of the patient.

Results

Few series exist in the literature concerning the outcome of surgical repair of left ventricular free wall rupture. Padro et al. (47) reported on 13 patients undergoing their technique of gluing a felt patch over the infarct. There was 100% survival at a mean follow-up of 26 mo. Zeebregts and colleagues (48) reported 100% survival (mean follow-up, 36 mo) with five patients employing a combination of the aforementioned surgical techniques. Other small series report operative survival ranging from 40% to 100% *(45,49,52)*.

CONCLUSION

In summary, the diagnosis of a postinfarction mechanical complication is a surgical emergency. The diagnosis is established with echocardiography. For ventricular septal and papillary muscle ruptures, a preoperative coronary angiogram is preferable if possible. Inotropes and intra-aortic balloon counterpulsation are helpful in providing temporary hemodynamic stabilization while the patient is being prepared for transfer to the operating room. Intraoperative transesophageal echocardiography should be used routinely. IABP counterpulsation is an important adjunct in the early postoperative period to decrease left ventricular wall tension and thus decrease stress on the repair.

REFERENCES

1. Vlodaver Z, Edwards JE. Rupture of ventricular septum or papillary muscle complicating myocardial infarction. Circulation 1977;55:815–822.
2. Wei JY, Hutchins GM, Bulkley BH. Papillary muscle rupture in fatal acute myocardial infarction: A potentially treatable form of cardiogenic shock. Ann Intern Med 1979;90:149–152.
3. Lundberg S, Sodestrom J. Perforation of interventricular septum in myocardial infarction: a study based on autopsy material. Acta Med Scand 1962;172:413–422.
4. Cooley DA, Belmonte BA, Zeis LB, et al. Surgical repair of ruptured interventricular septum following acute myocardial infarction. Surgery 1957;41:930–937.
5. Madsen JC, Daggett WM Jr. Postinfarction VSD and free wall rupture. In: Edmunds LH Jr, ed. Cardiac Surgery in the Adult. McGraw-Hill, New York, 1997, pp. 629–655.
6. Edwards BS, Edwards WD, Edwards JE. Ventricular septal rupture complicating acute myocardial infarction: identification of simple and complex types in 53 autopsied hearts. Am J Cardiol 1984;54:1201–1205.
7. Deville C, Fontan F, Chevalier JM, Madonna F, Ebner A, Besse P. Surgery of post-infarction ventricular defect: risk factors for hospital death and long-term results. Eur J Cardiothorac Surg 1991;5:167–175.
8. Fananapazir L, Bray CL, Dark JF. Right ventricular dysfunction and surgical outcome in postinfarction ventricular septal defect. Eur Heart J 1983;4:155–167.
9. David TE, Dale L, Sun Z. Postinfarction ventricular septal rupture: repair by endocardial patch with infarct exclusion. J Thorac Cardiovasc Surg 1995;110:1315–1322.
10. Giuliani ER, Danielson GK, Pluth JR, et al. Postinfarction ventricular septal rupture: surgical considerations and results. Circulation 1974;49:455–459.
11. Daggett WM, Guyton RA, Mundth ED, et al. Surgery for post-myocardial infarct VSD. Ann Surg 1977;186:260–270.
12. Nishimura RA, Schaff HV, Gersh BJ, et al. Early repair of mechanical complications after acute myocardial infarction. JAMA 1986;256:47–50.
13. Daggett WM, Buckley MJ, Akins CW, et al. Improved results of surgical management of postinfarction ventricular septal rupture. Ann Surg 1982;196:269–277.
14. Montoya A, McKeever L, Scanlon P, et al. Early repair of ventricular septal rupture after infarction. Am J Cardiol 1980;45:345–348.
15. Madsen JC, Daggett Jr. WM. Repair of postinfarction VSDs. Semin Thorac Cardiovasc Surg 1998;10:117–127.
16. Pretre R, Ye Q, Grunenfelder J, et al. Role of myocardial revascularization in postinfarction ventricular septal rupture. Ann Thorac Surg 2000;69:51–55.
17. Muehrcke DD, Daggett WM, Buckley MJ. Postinfarction VSD repair: effect of coronary artery bypass grafting. Ann Thorac Surg 1992;54:876–883.
18. Skillington PD, Davies RH, Luff AL. et al. Surgical treatment for infarct-related VSDs. J Thorac Cardiovasc Surg 1990;99:798–808.
19. David TE. Operative management of postinfarction VSD. Semin Thorac Cardiovasc Surg 1995;7:208–213.

20. David TE, Armstrong S. Surgical repair of postinfarction VSD by infarct exclusion. Semin Thorac Cardiovasc Surg 1998;10:105–110.

21. Daggett WM, Burwell LR, Lawson DW. Resection of acute ventricular aneurysm and ruptured interventricular septum after myocardial infarction. N Engl J Med 1970;283:1507–1514.

22. Shumaker H. Suggestions concerning operative management of postinfarction VSDs. J Thorac Cardiovasc Surg 1972;64:452–457.

23. Heitmiller R, Jacobs ML, Daggett WM. Surgical management of postinfarction ventricular septal rupture. Ann Thorac Surg 1986;41:683–691.

24. Hill JD, Lary D, Kerth WJ, et al. Acquired VSDs. J Thorac Cardiovasc Surg 1975;70:440–450.

25. Deja MA, Svostek J, Widenka K. Post infarction VSD—can we do better? Eur J Cardiothorac Surg 2000;18:194–201.

26. Wei JY, Hutchins GM, Bulkley BH. Papillary muscle rupture in fatal acute myocardial infarction: A potentially treatable form of cardiogenic shock. Ann Intern Med 1979;90:149–152.

27. Stevenson RR, Turner WJ. Rupture of a papillary muscle in the heart as a cause of sudden death. Bull Johns Hopkins Hosp 1935;57:235.

28. Davidson S. Spontaneous rupture of a papillary muscle of the heart: a report of three cases and a review of the literature. Mt Sinai J Med 1948;14:941.

29. Austen WG, Sanders CA, Averill JH, et al. Ruptured papillary muscle: Report of a case with successful mitral valve replacement. Circulation 1965;32:597–601.

30. Nishimura RA, Gersh BJ, Schaff HV. The case for an aggressive surgical approach to papillary muscle rupture following myocardial infarction: "From paradise lost to paradise regained." Heart 2000;83:611–613.

31. Nishimura RA, Schaff HV, Shub C, et al. Papillary muscle rupture complicating acute myocardial infarction: Analysis of 17 patients. Am J Cardiology 1983;51:373–377.

32. Barbour DJ, Roberts WC. Rupture of a left ventricular papillary muscle during acute myocardial infarction: analysis of 22 necropsy patients. J Am Coll Cardiol 1986;8:558–565.

33. Kirklin JW, Barratt-Boyes BG. Mitral incompetence from ischemic heart disease. In: Kirklin JW, Barratt-Boyes BG, eds. Cardiac Surgery. 2nd ed. Churchhill Livingstone, New York, 1993, pp. 415–422.

34. Buckley MJ, Mundth ED, Daggett WM, Gold HK, Leinbach RC, Austen WG. Surgical management of ventricular septal defects and mitral regurgitation complicating acute myocardial infarction. Ann Thorac Surg 1973;16:598–609.

35. Becker AE. Anatomy of the coronary arteries with respect to chronic ischemic mitral regurgitation. In: Vetter HO, Hetzer R, Schmutzler H, eds. Ischemic Mitral Incompetence. Springer-Verlag, New York, 1991, p. 17.

36. Sanders RJ, Neubuerger KT, Ravin A. Rupture of papillary muscles: occurrence of rupture of the posterior muscle in posterior myocardial infarction. Dis Chest 1957;31:316–323.

37. David TE. Techniques and results of mitral valve repair for ischemic mitral regurgitation. J Cardiac Surg 1994;9(2 Suppl):274–277.

38. Rankin JS, Hickey MS, Smith LR, et al. Current management of mitral valve incompetence associated with coronary artery disease. J Cardiac Surg 1989;4:25–42.

39. Tepe NA, Edmunds LH. Operation for acute postinfarction mitral insufficiency and cardiogenic shock. J Thorac Cardiovasc Surg 1985;89:525–530.

40. Killen DA, Reed WA, Wathanacharoen S, Beauchamp G, Rutherford B. Surgical treatment of papillary muscle rupture. Ann Thorac Surg 1983;35:243–248.

41. Harvey W. Complete Works (1647). Willis R (transl.). Sydenham Society, London, p. 127.

42. Cobbs BW, Hatcher CR, Robinson PH. Cardiac rupture. Three operations with two long-term survivals. JAMA 1973;223:532–535.

43. Spiekerman RE, Brandenburg JT, Achor RWP, et al. The spectrum of coronary heart disease in a community of 30,000: A clinicopathologic study. Circulation 1962;25:57–65.

44. Batts KP, Ackermann DM, Edwards WD. Postinfarction rupture of the left ventricular free wall: Clinicopathologic correlates in 100 consecutive autopsy cases. Hum Pathol 1990;21:530–535.

45. Kretz JG, Eisenmann B, Bareiss P, Bauer MC, Desroche P, Kieny R. Acute postinfarction left ventricle rupture. Five operations with three long-term survivals. J Cardiovasc Surg 1985;26:244–247.

46. O'Rourke MF. Subacute heart rupture following myocardial infarction. Clinical features of a correctable condition. Lancet 1973;22:124–126.

47. Padro JM, Mesa JM, Silveste J, et al. Subacute cardiac rupture: repair with a sutureless technique. Ann Thorac Surg 1993;55:20–24.

48. Zeebregts CJ, Noyez L, Hensens AG, Skotnicki SH, Lacquet LK. Surgical repair of subacute left ventricular free wall rupture. J Card Surg 1997;12:416–419.
49. Coletti G, Torracca M, Zogno M, et al. Surgical management of left ventricular free wall rupture after acute myocardial infarction. Cardiovasc Surg 1995;3:181–186.
50. Feneley MP, Chang VP, O'Rourke MF. Myocardial rupture after acute myocardial infarction. Br Heart J 1983;49:550–556.
51. Nunez L, de la Llana R, Sendon L, et al. Diagnosis and treatment of subacute free wall ventricular rupture after infarction. Ann Thorac Surg 1982;35:525–529.
52. Pifarre R, Sullivan HJ, Grieco J, et al. Management of left ventricular rupture complicating myocardial infarction. J Thorac Cardiovasc Surg 1983;86:441–443.

V CARDIOGENIC SHOCK RELATED TO VALVULAR HEART DISEASE

11 Cardiogenic Shock Related to Valvular Heart Disease

Alex Sagie, MD, and Yaron Shapira, MD

CONTENTS

INTRODUCTION

Acute or chronic dysfunction of native or prosthetic valves may cause cardiogenic shock and should be considered in its differential diagnosis (Tables 1 and 2). In the SHOCK trial registry *(1)*, of 1190 patients with cardiogenic shock, 8% suffered from a pre-existing severe valvular disease, which caused or worsened their hemodynamic status.

A rapid diagnosis of a valvular etiology in a patient with cardiogenic shock is very important, because emergent interventions such as intensive medical therapy, percutaneous balloon valvuloplasty, or native valve replacement can be effective, and, at times, life-saving. Clinical clues (from the patient's history, symptoms, and signs) suggesting valvular etiology of cardiogenic shock are presented in Table 3.

In this chapter, we will discuss the clinical presentation, diagnosis, and treatment of patients presenting with cardiogenic shock related to valvular dysfunction. In the first section, we focus on native valvular disease, and in the second section, we focus on prosthetic valvular disease.

CARDIOGENIC SHOCK RELATED TO NATIVE VALVE DISEASE

Mitral Stenosis

The most common cause of cardiogenic shock caused by obstruction of left ventricular filling is critical mitral stenosis (MS). Other conditions that may cause obstruction

From: *Contemporary Cardiology: Cardiogenic Shock: Diagnosis and Treatment*
Edited by: David Hasdai et al. © Humana Press Inc., Totowa, NJ

Table 1
Cardiogenic Shock Caused by Native Valves Lesions

	Etiology
Mitral valve	
Critical stenosis	Postinflammatory (postrheumatic scarring)
Valve obstruction	Large thrombus
	Obstructive vegetation as a result of infective endocarditis (IE)
	Obstructive tumor (e.g., myxoma)
Acute mitral regurgitation	Ischemic (e.g., papillary muscle rupture)
	Valve leaflet perforation as a result of IE
	Spontaneus chordal rupture in myxomatous valve disease
	Blunt chest trauma
	Iatrogenic — complicating surgical or catheter-based valvuloplasty
Aortic valve	
Critical stenosis	Postinflammatory, degenerative, congenital deformity
Valve obstruction	Obstructive vegetation resulting from IE
	Familial hypercholesterolemia
	Ochronosis
Acute aortic regurgitation	Leaflet perforation resulting from IE
	Dissection of the ascending aorta
	Traumatic disruption of the valve
	Spontaneous rupture or prolapse secondary to degenerative disease
	Iatrogenic — surgical or catheter-based valvuloplasty
Tricuspid valve	
Valve obstruction	Obstructive tumor (e.g., myxoma)
	Obstructive vegetation resulting from IE
	Obstructive thrombus
Acute tricuspid regurgitation	Acute right ventricular infarction
	Blunt chest trauma
	Leaflet perforation resulting from IE
	Spontaneous chordal rupture
	Traumatic disruption of the valve or chordae after right ventricular biopsy

Table 2
Cardiogenic Shock Associated with Prosthetic Valve Malfunction

	Etiology
Prosthetic valve obstruction	Obstructive thrombosis
	Obstructive vegetation
	Obstruction resulting from valve remnants or ball variance
Prosthetic valve regurgitation	
Intravalvular	Disruption of tissue leaflets
	Valve sticking in open position
	Strut fracture and occluder escape
	Ball wear
	Ball variance
Paravalvular	Dehiscence

Table 3
Clinical Clues Suggesting Valvular Etiology of Cardiogenic Shock

Patient's history
    Pre-existing significant valvular disease
        Native
        Prosthetic
    A history of rheumatic heart disease
    Recent fever without obvious cause (possible endocarditis)
    Recent/current embolic phenomena
    Poor anticoagulation in a patient with mechanical prosthetic valve
    Syndromes associated with valvular pathology (e.g., Marfan syndrome)
Symptoms and signs
    Heart murmur: new or pre-existing.
    Evidence of predominant right-heart failure
    Signs of pulmonary hypertension
    Peripheral signs of infective endocarditis
    Peripheral signs of emboli
    Muffled/absent valve clicks of a prosthetic mechanical valve

of left ventricular filling, such as obstructive vegetations or tumor masses, are very rare (Table 1). The incidence of cardiogenic shock in patients with MS is unknown but is probably very low in developed countries, given that interventions to relieve mitral valve obstruction are usually performed before severe heart failure or shock develops. A rapid diagnosis of this condition is very important because emergency interventions such as valve replacement or percutaneous balloon mitral valvuloplasty (PBMV) are very effective and readily available. There have been few reports of cardiogenic shock resulting from critical MS *(2–7)*; a total of 63 critically ill patients have been reported in these studies examining the effectiveness of PBMV for the treatment of cardiogenic shock secondary to MS.

PATHOPHYSIOLOGY

The primary pathophysiologic abnormality in patients with MS is impairment of left ventricular filling at the mitral valve level. The mitral obstruction causes an increase in diastolic pressure gradients between the left atrium and left ventricle. Consequently, the elevated left atrial (LA) pressure results in a passive rise in pulmonary venous and arterial pressure. If the obstruction is not relieved, most patients develop significant pulmonary hypertension that is higher than expected for the degree of elevation of LA pressure. These phenomena result from reactive arterial vasoconstriction and morphologic changes in the pulmonary vasculature. Later, severe pulmonary hypertension causes right-heart abnormalities to develop, including right ventricular (RV) hypertrophy, RV dilatation, functional tricuspid regurgitation, an additional decrease in cardiac output, and, eventually, right-heart failure *(8–10)*.

Cardiogenic shock can be the final manifestation of these processes, but it is an uncommon presentation of MS. It occurs mainly in patients who remain untreated until the MS is very advanced. Several conditions such as sepsis, severe anemia, pregnancy, rapid atrial fibrillation, and associated valvular and myocardial disease may serve as triggers of cardiogenic shock in a stable patient with critical MS.

CLINICAL PRESENTATION

The clinical presentation of cardiogenic shock resulting from mitral stenosis may include pulmonary edema, hypotension with cold extremities, right-heart failure, and signs of multiple-organ failure. These are not specific for cardiogenic shock secondary to MS. Prominent pulmonary hypertension, right ventricular failure, and signs of tricuspid regurgitation (prominent jugular venous V-waves and pulsatile liver) may also lead the physician to suspect a valvular lesion as the primary cause of the shock, but these signs are not specific.

DIAGNOSIS

The classical auscultatory findings of MS include an opening snap, a diastolic murmur, and an accentuated first heart sound. These may be very difficult to appreciate in a critically ill patient on a mechanical ventilator with very low cardiac output. The low-pitched diastolic murmur, for example, is often of low intensity because of low transmitral gradients secondary to reduced cardiac output. The opening snap is not always audible in patients with severe valvular calcification.

The classical electrocardiographic abnormalities, which include LA enlargement, right axis deviation, and RV hypertrophy, are not specific.

A chest X-ray may be helpful in revealing interstitial and alveolar edema, a pulmonary hypertension pattern, right-heart dilatation, and associated pulmonary infection.

Echocardiography is an excellent tool for the initial diagnosis of cardiogenic shock secondary to mitral stenosis and for ruling out other causes of shock. Critical mitral stenosis can be easily diagnosed with transthoracic two-dimensional and Doppler echocardiography (11). Because of its superior resolution, transesophageal echocardiography (TEE) should be considered in cases of poor imaging quality. An echocardiographic examination can determine the severity of the stenosis and the morphology of the valve, evaluate coexisting aortic and tricuspid valve disease (12), and estimate the pulmonary pressure. It can also evaluate left and right ventricular function and size. Mitral valve morphology and the presence of mitral regurgitation or left atrial thrombus (13) (as assessed by TEE) are important variables when PBMV is considered.

TREATMENT

Medical treatment to stabilize these patients includes optimal ventilatory and inotropic support; catecholamines should be used with caution because of their positive chronotrophic effect. Excessive tachycardia in these patients shortens diastole and causes an undesired increase in pressure gradients across the mitral valve. Efforts should be made to identify and treat precipitating factors such as anemia, infection, and arrhythmias. Mechanical relief of MS is the treatment of choice and should be done as soon as possible.

Surgical treatment: Emergency commissurotomy or mitral valve replacement for relief of MS are associated with a high mortality rate mainly because of the precipitating events. Barlow (8) reported a 25% mortality rate for emergency closed mitral valvulotomy. Emergency surgery, therefore, should be restricted to patients who are not suitable for PBMV.

Percutaneous balloon mitral valvuloplasty (PBMV), if feasible, is an acceptable alternative to surgery for these patients, almost all of whom die without mechanical relief. There are several reports (2–5) about emergency PBMV in critically ill patients

Table 4
Reports on PBMV in Critically Ill Patients with Cardiogenic Shock
and/or Intractable Pulmonary Edema Secondary to Severe Mitral Stenosis

Authors (ref.)	No. of patients	Uneventful recovery	Complicated by significant MR	Required MVR	Mortality
Lokhandwala et al. (2)	40	24 (60%)	6 (15%)	6 (15%)	14 (35%)
Patel et al. (3)	12	12 (100%)	0	0	0
Wu et al. (4)	10	6 (60%)	2 (20%)	2 (20%)	2 (20%)
Goldman et al. (5)	1	1 (100%)	0	0	0
Total	63	43 (68%)	8 (13%)	8 (13%)	16 (25%)

Abbreviations: PBMV = percutaneous balloon mitral valvuloplasty; MR = mitral regurgitation; MVR = mitral valve replacement.

secondary to severe MS. A summary of the clinical presentation, complications, and outcome of these studies is presented in Table 4.

A summary of 63 critically ill patients with severe MS reveals a mortality rate of 25%, with significant mitral regurgitation (MR) in 13% (eight patients) and the need for mitral valve replacement (MVR) in 13% (eight patients). Most of the remaining patients, including pregnant women, had continuing clinical improvement. The outcome of these patients with mitral stenosis appeared to be better than that of patients with cardiogenic shock from other causes. (See Chapter 12 for a more detailed review of PBMV in critically ill patients with MS.)

Aortic Stenosis

PATHOPHYSIOLOGY

In adults with chronic aortic stenosis (AS), left ventricular function, and cardiac output can be well maintained by the development of left ventricular hypertrophy, which may sustain a large pressure gradient across the aortic valve for many years without a reduction in cardiac output, dilatation of the left ventricle, or the development of symptoms. The development of left ventricular hypertrophy is one of the principal mechanisms by which the heart adapts to chronic pressure overload caused by left ventricular outflow tract obstruction. The increase in wall thickness counterbalances the increased pressure, so that the peak systolic wall tension returns to normal or remains stable as long as the obstruction develops slowly (14,15).

Over time, some patients will develop left ventricular dysfunction as a result of increased wall stress, secondary to inadequate wall thickening, resulting in "afterload mismatch" (16,17). In others, the ejection fraction deteriorates secondary to decreased myocardial contractility. In some patients, massive left ventricular hypertrophy is associated with degenerative changes, including disruption of sarcomeres and interstitial fibrosis. Thus, increased afterload, altered contractility, or their combination are important determinants of left ventricular performance in patients with severe AS.

Cardiogenic shock as the final manifestation of these processes is an uncommon presentation of AS. It usually occurs in patients who remain untreated until reaching a very advanced stage. Conditions such as myocardial ischemia, sepsis, dehydration, excessive diuretic and vasodilator consumption, severe anemia, rapid atrial fibrillation, and associated valvular and myocardial diseases may trigger cardiogenic shock in the patient with severe AS. When left ventricular systolic dysfunction is caused by increased afterload (i.e., "afterload mismatch") with normal myocardial contractility, systolic function is expected to improve after relief of outflow obstruction. Even with superimposed myocardial dysfunction, ventricular performance may improve, although to a lesser extent, after relief of outflow obstruction.

INCIDENCE

The incidence of cardiogenic shock in patients with AS is unknown but is probably low in the current era because interventions to relieve aortic valvular obstruction (before severe progressive heart failure or shock develops) are performed at an earlier stage. In the NHLBI registry of percutaneous balloon aortic valvuloplasty (PBAV) for aortic valve stenosis, 39 (6%) of 674 patients were in cardiogenic shock *(18)*. A rapid diagnosis of this situation is very important, because emergency interventions such as valve replacement or PBAV can be lifesaving and are the only alternatives for these critical high-risk patients. Most information regarding cardiogenic shock resulting from critical AS is derived from several reports on the presentation and outcome of emergency PBAV *(19–27)*.

CLINICAL PRESENTATION

The classic symptoms of severe AS include angina, a gradual decrease in exercise tolerance as a consequence of exertional dyspnea or fatigue, and syncope. Some patients present with sudden onset of heart failure, including pulmonary edema and cardiogenic shock. These manifestations are often related to an acute infection, acute myocardial ischemia or infarction, anemia, or other causes of hemodynamic stress that lead to acute decompensation in a previously asymptomatic patient. Other symptoms such as anasarca, pedal edema, marked fatigability, debilitation, peripheral cyanosis, and other manifestation of low cardiac output are rare and represent late manifestations of untreated severe AS.

PHYSICAL EXAMINATION

The classical auscultatory findings of AS are difficult to appreciate in a critically ill patient with cardiogenic shock. When the left ventricle fails and cardiac output falls, the murmur becomes softer or disappears altogether. The clinical picture changes to that of severe left ventricular failure with low cardiac output. Thus, critical AS may be occult and should be ruled out by echocardiography in every patient presenting with intractable heart failure or cardiogenic shock.

DIAGNOSIS

Two-dimensional and Doppler echocardiography are the best noninvasive tests for revealing the various pathological and pathophysiological aspects of aortic stenosis as well as for assessing the severity of the disease. This is especially true in patients presenting in cardiogenic shock when the classical physical signs and hemodynamic features of severe AS are not specific and sometime occult. Two-dimensional echocardiography provides information about the underlying causes of aortic stenosis such as bicuspid aortic valve, degenerative calcific stenosis, or changes related to previous rheumatic fever. Doppler echocardiography provides information regarding transvalvular gradients and aortic valve area (using the continuity equation).

In the subset of patients who present in cardiogenic shock with left ventricular dysfunction and low cardiac output, the transvalvular gradient does not truly reflect the severity of the stenosis. In these patients, resting transvalvular gradients are usually modestly elevated because of the low transaortic flow rate. Therefore, calculation of the aortic valve area is mandatory.

In cases of a technically difficult transthoracic study, valve area planimetry by TEE can be helpful (28). This relatively new method for measuring valve area is still controversial, however, and some authors question its validity in patients with heavily calcified valves (29).

An evaluation of the change in valve area with a change in flow rate, by using pharmacological stress echocardiography, may be helpful in a subgroup of patients with aortic stenosis and coexisting significant left ventricular dysfunction. It is sometimes difficult to separate patients with true, anatomically severe AS from those with a reduced aortic opening owing to poor left ventricular function in the setting of only mild to moderate aortic valve obstruction (i.e., "functional aortic stenosis"). If the transaortic flow rate increases during dobutamine stress echocardiography, the resultant increase in flow rate increases the degree of aortic valve opening when the primary process is left ventricular dysfunction. In contrast, when severe valvular obstruction is present, the aortic valve area remains unchanged with increased transaortic velocity and pressure gradient. When there is no increase in flow rate, it remains unclear whether the failure to increase flow rate results from an unresponsive myocardium or a stiff aortic valve restricting an increase in ventricular outflow (30).

A patient with severe AS and poor left ventricular function may benefit from PBAV or aortic valve replacement, whereas a patient with primary left ventricular dysfunction and associated mild or moderate valvular disease may not (31,32). Although dobutamine stress is not always applicable in patients in cardiogenic shock, it may be useful in patients who are already on a regimen of catecholamines. In patients who recover from cardiogenic shock, dobutamine stress testing is very useful for selecting those who might benefit from surgery or PBAV.

TREATMENT

Medical therapy for patients with critical AS and cardiogenic shock should include optimal ventilatory and inotropic support. Occasionally, an intra-aortic balloon pump is required, providing there is no concomitant moderate or severe aortic regurgitation. Every effort should be made to identify and treat the precipitating factors such as anemia, infection, arrhythmias, and an acute coronary event. It is not, however, recommended that medical stabilization be the ultimate goal of treatment; these patients should have urgent or emergency interventional therapy (PBAV or aortic valve replacement) as soon as possible.

Surgical therapy: The experience with emergency or urgent aortic valve replacement (AVR) in patients with cardiogenic shock from critical aortic stenosis is limited. Aortic valve replacement in these patients is associated with high mortality and morbidity (33,34). Although AVR provides definitive and long-lasting relief of AS in some critically ill patients, surgeons consider most patients presenting with cardiogenic shock and multiorgan failure to be too risky for cardiac surgery; thus, the only alternative for these patients is PBAV.

Percutaneous balloon aortic valvuloplasty was reported in elderly patients with critical aortic stenosis and relative contraindications to surgery in several studies in the late

Table 5
Reports on PBAV in Critically Ill Patients with Cardiogenic Shock
or Intractable Pulmonary Edema and Critical Aortic Stenosis

Authors (ref.)	No. of patients	Developed significant AR	AVR at follow-up	Mortality (30 d)
Moreno et al. (21)	21	1 (5%)	4 (19%)	9 (43%)
NHLBI (18)	39	NA	NA	19 (49%)
Cribier et al. (23)	10	0	6 (60%)	2 (20%)
Smedira et al. (24)	5	0	5 (100%)	0
Total	75			30 (40%)

Abbreviations: AR= aortic regurgitation; PBAV = percutaneous balloon aortic valvuloplasty; AVR= aortic valve replacement; NA= not available.

1980s and early 1990s. The short-term results were acceptable, but there was rapid (i.e., within 4–9 mo) and frequent (42–83% of patients) restenosis of the aortic valve. The NHLBI registry reported the 3-yr outcome of 674 patients: 1-, 2-, and 3-yr mortality rates were 45%, 65%, and 77%, respectively (32,35,36).

There have been four moderate-sized studies (19,21,23,24) (Table 5) and several case reports (22,27,37) of PBAV in critically ill patients with critical aortic stenosis and cardiogenic shock (most of them at presentation). A summary of these studies reveals an in-hospital survival rate of 63%. Most of the patients eventually underwent AVR, and a significant number were in functional class I–II at mid-term follow-up. Thus, PBAV can be lifesaving in patients with AS and cardiogenic shock, and an improvement in functional class is expected in some patients.

The risk of developing severe aortic regurgitation with this procedure is not high, occurring in 4 (0.8%) out of 492 patients in the Mansfield scientific aortic valvuloplasty registry (36). Because the increase in the aortic valve area is small and many of these patients suffer from severe coronary disease that is not addressed during PBAV, many of them are at high risk for early postprocedural death. Therefore, PBAV should be considered as a bridge to AVR and myocardial revascularization if necessary in most, if not all, patients. Because AVR prolongs the life of symptomatic patients with severe aortic stenosis (35), the decision not to perform subsequent AVR because of comorbid conditions or for any other reason should be individualized on a risk/benefit basis. (See Chapter 12, on percutaneous valvuloplasty in cardiogenic shock for a more detailed review of PBAV in critically patients with aortic stenosis.)

Acute Aortic Regurgitation

Although rare, some patients with acute aortic regurgitation (AR) present with the clinical picture of cardiogenic shock. The most common causes of acute AR that can cause cardiogenic shock are infective endocarditis, dissection of the ascending aorta, trauma, or spontaneous rupture of a myxomatous valve (Table 1).

PATHOPHYSIOLOGY

Acute severe AR is defined as hemodynamically significant AR of sudden onset in a patient with a previously normal or mildly diseased valve, usually with a nondilated left ventricle not previously subject to volume overload. In these patients, eccentric hypertrophy and dilatation of the left ventricle are usually absent. Therefore, the compliance of the ventricle is normal and remains so despite the sudden volume overload resulting from a large regurgitant volume pouring into the ventricle (38,39). This volume overload is poorly tolerated by the left ventricle resulting in a sharp increase of end-diastolic pressure, almost approaching aortic diastolic pressure. The rise in left ventricular end-diastolic pressure can lead to elevated left atrial and pulmonary capillary pressures of sufficient magnitude to cause pulmonary edema. In addition, the rise in left ventricular end-diastolic pressure causes a decrease in coronary perfusion related to a decrease in diastolic coronary perfusion pressure (40,41). The noncompliant left ventricle cannot acutely increase its end-diastolic volume sufficiently to maintain forward stroke volume in this setting. Cardiac output usually declines and systemic arterial blood pressure is maintained by a reflex increase in peripheral vascular resistance. With time, the reduced cardiac output leads to impaired perfusion to vital organs. With extreme reduction of tissue perfusion, cardiogenic shock may develop.

CLINICAL PRESENTATION AND PHYSICAL EXAMINATION

The patient with acute AR presents with progressive symptoms related to pulmonary congestion (resulting from a sudden rise in left atrial pressure), which include exertional dyspnea, orthopnea, paroxysmal nocturnal dyspnea, and pulmonary edema. The symptoms reflecting the reduction of cardiac output are not prominent in the early stages and are often overshadowed by those resulting from pulmonary congestion. If left untreated, prominent signs of low cardiac output and decreased tissue perfusion dominate the picture, and cardiogenic shock eventually develops.

The classical physical signs of chronic severe AR include a collapsing pulse, a widened arterial pulse pressure, laterally displaced apical impulse, marked parasternal retraction (reflecting left ventricular volume overload), and a long high-pitched diastolic murmur. These signs are usually absent in patients with acute severe AR. The peripheral arterial palpatory and auscultatory signs reflecting volume overload and high output are absent, the precordium is usually quiescent, the first heart sound is soft or absent, the third heart sound is common, and the diastolic murmur is short. When the patient is already in cardiogenic shock, these signs are even less prominent.

The diagnosis of severe AR can be easily overlooked, and signs related to low cardiac output and reduced tissue perfusion predominate. There are, however, specific symptoms and physical signs that can help the physician in making the correct diagnosis. Abrupt onset of severe chest and back pain are characteristic of aortic dissection. Fever, chills, a recent history of dental treatment, gastrointestinal or genito-urinary surgery or instrumentation, and evidence of peripheral embolism suggest the diagnosis of infective endocarditis. A history of recent chest trauma raises the likelihood of traumatic disruption of the aortic valve. A difference in the intensity of the left and right brachial pulses suggests aortic dissection. When the patient is tall, thin, and has a long arm span and hyperextensible joints, one should consider the possibility of acute AR and aortic dissection complicating Marfan syndrome.

DIAGNOSIS

Echocardiography. Echocardiographic study provides information concerning the etiology of AR (e.g., bicuspid valve, endocarditis, dissection), the severity of AR, involvement of other valves, the size and function of the left ventricle, and the presence of other cardiac abnormalities. The echocardiographic manifestations of severe AR that are acute (rather than chronic) include early mitral valve closure (best assessed by M-mode), occasionally diastolic mitral regurgitation (resulting from extremely high end-diastolic pressure), and diastolic fluttering of the mitral valve, usually with normal LV function and size *(42,43)*. Color flow Doppler mapping is highly accurate in estimating regurgitation severity by measuring the width and area of the jet at its origin, as well as its extension to the left ventricle. A rapid deceleration slope of the regurgitant jet as assessed by continuous-wave Doppler is also a useful sign of acute severe AR; diastolic reversal of flow in the ascending aorta is another important sign *(44)*.

Transesophageal echocardiography is necessary only when a good quality transthoracic echocardiographic (TTE) study cannot be obtained or when the question of aortic dissection or endocarditis is raised. In many instances, where high-quality echocardiographic studies are obtained and interpreted by experienced cardiologists, cardiac catheterization is not required to confirm the diagnosis of acute severe AR.

Cardiac catheterization is needed if the echocardiographic diagnosis is uncertain or when coronary artery disease is suspected. The decision whether to catheterize the patient depends on a careful assessment of the clinical condition. For example, in a young patient presenting with cardiogenic shock without previously diagnosed cardiac disease, urgent AVR without prior cardiac catheterization may be lifesaving. In contrast, in the elderly patient in a relatively stable condition and with suspected coronary artery disease, cardiac catheterization should be favorably considered *(45)*.

During left ventricular catheterization, the most striking hemodynamic findings are equilibration of left ventricular and aortic pressure at end diastole and the marked elevation of left ventricular end-diastolic pressure that may exceed left atrial pressure at end diastole *(46)*. The risk of cardiac catheterization in a critically ill patient is related to the additional hemodynamic stress imposed by the procedure and the administration of contrast agents. In addition, there is risk of arterial embolization secondary to catheter-induced traumatic disruption of one or more friable aortic valve vegetations *(47)*. In a patient with aortic dissection, there is the risk of injection of contrast into the false lumen.

TREATMENT

When a patient with acute AR presents in cardiogenic shock, it is essential to have bedside hemodynamic assessment to monitor administration of appropriate vasopressors, diuretics, and vasodilators.

Vasodilators decrease regurgitant volume per beat by reducing afterload and preload, improve forward cardiac output, and lower left ventricular end-diastolic volume. Nitroprusside infusion with careful titration may produce a significant increase in cardiac output and decline in pulmonary artery wedge pressure with only a modest reduction in blood pressure. In patients with severe hypotension, sympathomimetic agents such as dobutamine should be added. Such agents ($\beta 1$ myocardial stimulant) can augment myocardial contractility and raise cardiac output with little or no increase in heart rate. Dobutamine, unlike dopamine, lacks intrinsic α-adrenergic agonist activity. Therefore, dobutamine elevates neither arterial resistance (increase afterload) nor venous tone (increase preload). Dobutamine should be given to maintain systolic blood pressure in excess of 90 mm Hg *(45)*. Intra-aortic balloon pump (IABP) counter pulsation is contraindicated in patients with acute or chronic severe AR because the augmented diastolic blood pressure that results from the IABP increases the volume of aortic regurgitation.

Patients with acute AR who require inotropic and vasodilator therapy to reverse cardiogenic shock require prompt AVR. Patients with acute AR related to infective endocarditis suffer from a mortality rate as high as 50–90% without surgical intervention. It is desirable to perform AVR in these patients after a few days of antibiotic therapy, if possible, with an acceptable low risk of reinfection. However, when the patient presents with cardiogenic shock, AVR should be undertaken immediately. The increased operative mortality risk consequent to delaying surgery exceeds the potential benefit of completing a full course or even a few days of antibiotic therapy before AVR *(48,49)*.

Acute Mitral Regurgitation

Cardiogenic shock secondary to acute mitral regurgitation (MR) is most commonly related to acute papillary muscle rupture in the setting of acute myocardial infarction. (See Chapter 10 for a detailed discussion of the diagnosis and surgical treatment of this complication.) Several additional causes of acute MR can cause cardiogenic shock (Table 1). These include valve leaflet perforation or ruptured chordae tendinae resulting from infective endocarditis, spontaneous chordal rupture in myxomatous valve disease, and blunt chest trauma. Iatrogenic trauma to the mitral apparatus can complicate cardiac surgery or percutaneous balloon valvuloplasty. Although uncommon, it is very important to recognize this complication because a rapid diagnosis and appropriate therapy can be lifesaving.

PATHOPHYSIOLOGY

In acute severe MR, the regurgitant valve imposes a sudden volume and pressure overload on an unprepared, nondilated, and nonhypertrophied left atrium and ventricle. Because the atrium is poorly compliant, the massive systolic regurgitant flow results in a large pressure peak in systole, manifested by a giant "V"-wave in the left atrial pressure tracing. The sudden increase in left atrial pressure is transmitted retrogradely, resulting in increased pulmonary venous pressure and, often, increased pulmonary artery pressure as well. If pulmonary venous pressure exceeds plasma oncotic pressure, interstitial pulmonary edema will occur. If the rate at which fluid accumulates exceeds the ability to remove it, alveolar pulmonary edema will result. Despite the increased left ventricular preload and contractility and decreased afterload, overall left ventricular pump function declines. The total left ventricular stroke volume is usually increased, but a large amount of this flow is directed into the left atrium rather than to the aorta *(50)*. Forward cardiac output declines and, occasionally, cardiogenic shock may ensue, especially in cases where there is pre-existing LV dysfunction or if LV dysfunction develops from acute myocardial ischemia or other factors.

Clinical Presentation and Physical Examination

The clinical presentation of acute severe MR is usually that of acute pulmonary edema. The patient generally complains of a sudden onset of severe dyspnea, orthopnea, paroxysmal nocturnal dyspnea, and cough. The patient appears ill, often in respiratory distress, and sinus tachycardia is common. In severe cases, systemic hypotension and full-blown cardiogenic shock occur. Systemic venous pressure can be elevated as a result of elevated right ventricular end-diastolic pressure from the acute onset of pulmonary hypertension.

In a patient with acute MR, there is no apical displacement or left ventricular heave. Because the "V"-wave is markedly elevated, the pressure gradient between the left ventricle and atrium declines at the end of systole and the murmur may be decrescendo rather than holosystolic, but ending well before the second heart sound. It is usually lower pitched and softer than the murmur of chronic MR. Jets directed posteriorly into the left atrial cavity are more difficult to detect during precordial auscultation. On the other hand, with a flail posterior leaflet and an anteriorly directed jet, the precordial basal murmur may be mistaken for an aortic murmur. When the patient is already in cardiogenic shock, the murmur may not be heard at all (i.e., "silent MR") *(51)*. Both left-sided S4 and S3 are frequently present. Pulmonary hypertension, which is common in acute MR, may be associated with an increased intensity of P2, and murmurs of pulmonary and tricuspid regurgitation and a right-sided S4 may also develop. Other physical findings may provide clues to the etiology of the regurgitation. For example, a patient with infective endocarditis may have signs of vasculitis, septic emboli, fever, or other systemic features of this disease.

DIAGNOSIS

Electrocardiogram. Patients with acute MR demonstrate neither left atrial enlargement nor left ventricular hypertrophy on the ECG. The ECG changes can be related to the etiology of MR such as myocardial infarction with associated papillary muscle rupture or nonspecific ST-T changes typically found in patients with mitral valve prolapse.

Echocardiography. Two-dimensional and Doppler echocardiography are very useful tools for achieving the following three goals in patients with acute MR: define the pathology responsible for the mitral regurgitation; assess the severity of the lesion; and seek associated cardiac pathologies, such as LV dysfunction, aortic and tricuspid valve disease, and pericardial effusion. By establishing the etiology and severity of the lesion, a decision can be made about the appropriate medical or surgical therapy. TEE is frequently indicated in these patients, especially if the image quality by TTE is limited. TEE is especially important for assessing the severity of the lesion in cases of suspected endocarditis and for determining the suitability of surgery for mitral valve repair.

There are many methods of estimating the severity of MR based on the characteristics of regurgitant jet using color flow Doppler *(52)*. These include left atrial regurgitant jet area, or jet area relative to the left atrial size, jet width at the vena contracta, proximal isovelocity surface area, and other quantitative methods based on the calculation of total and forward cardiac output and calculation of regurgitation fractions. These methods are especially important in patients presenting with acute MR, in whom other clues to lesion severity such as left atrial and ventricular enlargement are unlikely. In addition, Doppler interrogation of pulmonary vein flow can be very useful for assessing regurgitation severity. Typically, reversal of the systolic flow is detected.

Cardiac catheterization. When echocardiography cannot assess the severity of regurgitation with certainty, bedside right-heart catheterization can be performed to further assess the hemodynamic significance of the lesion *(53)*. An increase in left atrial pressure during systole (a large "V"-wave) supports the diagnosis but is not specific; other mechanisms for a large "V"-wave include severe acute congestive heart failure and acute ventricular septal rupture. Semiquantitative assessment of the amount of radiopaque contrast delivered into the left atrium during left ventriculography has many of the drawbacks of color flow Doppler interrogation. Quantitative calculation of regurgitation fraction based on the left ventricular volumes and total and forward cardiac output is technically challenging and adds little to the quantification of MR.

TREATMENT

Acute MR presenting in cardiogenic shock is a medical and surgical emergency. The patient should be stabilized by intravenous afterload reduction therapy such as nitroprusside as long as the systolic blood pressure is not too low. In most cases, an intra-aortic balloon pump is necessary to further reduce afterload and improve coronary perfusion *(54–57)*.

Surgical intervention is usually needed as soon as the patient is stabilized to correct the underline lesion causing the acute severe MR. Whenever possible, the mitral valve apparatus and continuity between the leaflets and papillary muscle should be preserved. Thus, either mitral valve repair or replacement with chordal preservation is the preferred procedure in order to minimize left ventricular damage. (See Chapter 10 for a fuller discussion of operative issues surrounding mitral valve repair or replacement.)

Tricuspid Valve Trauma

Traumatic tricuspid regurgitation is very rare; fewer than 100 cases have been reported in the literature *(58)*. An early autopsy study revealed tricuspid valve injury in only 1.5% of patients with blunt chest trauma, always with cardiac rupture or other cardiac injuries *(59)*. Later studies revealed that acute tricuspid regurgitation is rather well tolerated and may be underdiagnosed *(60)*. In one series, patients were eventually operated after a median delay of 17 yr (range 1 mo to 37 yr) *(61)*. A rare cause of tricuspid valve injury may be iatrogenic damage to the valve during cardiac catheterization (e.g., by trying to pull back an open atrial septal defect occluder).

The commonest mechanisms underlying traumatic tricuspid regurgitation are ruptured anterior papillary muscle, a tear in the anterior leaflet, or, rarely, a tear of the septal leaflet. The physical diagnosis may be misleading. A systolic tricuspid murmur may not always be heard because of the low systolic gradient over the tricuspid valve. Elevated jugular venous pressure (JVP) may be detected but may be attributed to positive-pressure ventilation or associated lung injury. Extreme cases may be associated with hypotension and signs of right-heart failure. Occasionally, cyanosis may be noted, a result of a right-to-left shunt caused by an elevated right atrial pressure and a pre-existing patent foramen ovale.

The diagnosis of traumatic tricuspid regurgitation may be suggested first by enlargement of the cardiac silhouette or by an echocardiogram done routinely or for other reasons. If left untreated, traumatic tricuspid regurgitation will eventually lead to right-heart failure and should therefore be corrected. Shock has rarely been reported in acute tricuspid regurgitation *(62,63)*.

If the pulmonary pressure is normal and there is no previous right ventricular dysfunction, patients can tolerate complete absence of the tricuspid valve for years, as is the case in drug addicts with right-sided endocarditis who have their tricuspid valve excised *(64)*. In a patient with shock and proven traumatic tricuspid regurgitation, additional lesions (cardiac and extracardiac) should be sought systematically.

SHOCK ASSOCIATED WITH PROSTHETIC HEART VALVES

General Approach

Shock may be attributed to numerous factors in a patient with a prosthetic heart valve (Table 2). It may be associated with structural or nonstructural valve dysfunction, which may interfere with the opening of the valve and/or with its occluder mechanism. Shock may also develop in a patient with a prosthetic heart valve despite preserved integrity of the valve mechanism. Examples include acute myocardial infarction, progression of advanced pre-existing myocardial or valvular heart disease, septic shock (which may be associated with prosthetic or native valve endocarditis), hemorrhagic shock (possibly attributable to excessive anticoagulation), intermittent mitral obstruction as a result of left atrial ball thrombus, and so forth.

The responsibility of the cardiologist who encounters a patient with a prosthetic heart valve who presents with shock is to determine the etiology, explore valvular and myocardial functions, provide medical or mechanical supportive therapy, and identify pathologies amenable to either pharmacological therapy or surgical correction.

Patient History

The patient's history may provide clues to the underlying mechanism of shock. The abrupt occurrence of shock in a patient who was previously in a good functional class may indicate leaflet escape, acute blockage of a mechanical valve, or acute perforation of a bioprosthesis. A gradual decrease in functional capacity is less helpful from a diagnostic point of view, although it usually rules out a sudden loss of valve competence. A history of systemic embolic phenomena, inappropriately low levels of anticoagulation, or a recent transient cessation of oral anticoagulants as a result of bleeding or a scheduled noncardiac surgery makes the diagnosis of valve thrombosis more likely. It is advisable to ask the patient about valve clicks: If the patient could previously hear them but is currently unable to hear them, a stuck valve should be considered. A sudden, intermittent electromechanical dissociation very soon after valve replacement raises the possibility of an extrinsic valve block (usually because of valve remnants). A history of fever and/or shaking chills may be indicative of infective endocarditis. Embolic phenomena usually imply the presence of either a thrombus or a vegetation, but valve components may embolize as well.

Knowing the valve model may be helpful, as certain valves are more susceptible to certain complications. Knowing the valve model can prevent a fruitless search for a missing second leaflet in a monoleaflet model, for example. The medical chart, the patient, or an identification card are possible sources of these data.

Additional information should be sought to identify causes of shock that are not directly valve related. These include a history of chest pain, gastrointestinal bleeding, recent trauma, and so forth. Therefore, the physician should take a thorough medical history not restricted to the valvular disease.

Physical Examination

The physical examination is of paramount importance. There are the general signs of shock (i.e., low blood pressure, tachycardia, apprehension, clammy skin appearance, obtundation, and low urinary output). Additional signs may be observed in patients with prosthetic valves who are in a shock state. These include auscultatory clues, such

Table 6
Comparison Among Diagnostic Modalities for the Diagnosis of Prosthetic Valve Complications

	Modality			
Quality	TTE	TEE	Cinefluoro-scopy	Plain X-ray
Bedside availability	+++	+++	–	+++ (portable)
Demonstration of leaflet motion abnormality	+/++[a]	+/++*	+++	–
Quantification of leaflet motion abnormality	+/–	+/++*	+++	–
Demonstration of intravalvular regurgitation	+/++[b]	+++	–	–
Demonstration of a thrombus	+/–	+++	–	–
Demonstration of absent occluder	++/+++ [a]	++/+++[a]	+++	++
Demonstration of embolized occluder	+/–	+/–	+++	+++
Data on left and right ventricular function	+++	+++	–	–
Data on associated valvular lesions	+++	+++	–	–

[a] Less efficient in aortic position.

[b] Less efficient in mitral position.

as muffled or absent valve clicks, the appearance of a diastolic murmur over an atrio-ventricular valve, a loud and prolonged systolic aortic murmur, or the appearance of a new regurgitant murmur. These auscultatory signs may, however, be barely detected in a noisy environment, which may be expected if the patient develops pulmonary edema or is mechanically ventilated. Sometimes, the auscultatory findings are intermittent. For example, this may happen when two cardiac cycles (and rarely more) are needed to develop sufficient pressure to open a stuck valve. Material (solid valve components or biologic material, such as a vegetation or a thrombus) may embolize anywhere in the arterial tree and produce signs according to the affected organ (paralysis/paresis in case of brain damage, limb ischemia, intestinal symptoms in case of an acute mesenteric vascular event, etc.).

Additional signs may indicate other reasons for shock. Pallor may indicate anemia, which may be attributed to internal blood loss or profound hemolysis, which often accompanies structural valve dysfunction. Fever may implicate an infectious etiology. Peripheral signs of infective endocarditis should be sought (e.g., Janeway lesions, Osler's nodes).

Imaging Modalities

The main imaging modalities for the diagnosis of prosthetic valve malfunction are echocardiography (transthoracic and transesophageal), cinefluoroscopy, and, occasionally, plain X-ray. Table 6 compares these modalities with regard to the diagnosis of valve malfunction. In general, fluoroscopy provides the best images of the radiopaque components, including the occluder part, whereas it provides no hemodynamic information or data about radiolucent materials. Echocardiography provides hemodynamic data and information about radiolucent materials (vegetations, thrombi, cloth, etc.) but is inferior to fluoroscopy in imaging the occluder part of the valve. TEE provides invaluable data with high resolution on both the valve anatomy and its physiology. It is especially useful for posterior structures and is, therefore, most suitable to assess prosthetic mitral valves, but it is helpful in other valves as well. It can be done at the bedside or in the operating theater. It is, however, a semi-invasive procedure and requires expertise.

The following section reviews the diagnosis and management of disorders specific to prosthetic heart valves that can be associated with shock: (1) stuck valve, which is sometimes amenable to medical (thrombolytic) therapy; (2) disk escape, which is the extreme case of loss of occluder mechanism and acute prosthetic valve insufficiency; (3) acute nonthrombotic valve block, which is at the other extreme of valve malfunction; and (4) degeneration of bioprosthetic valves. Cardiologists should be familiar with all other types of valve malfunction that may culminate in a state of shock (Table 2).

OBSTRUCTIVE VALVE THROMBOSIS (STUCK VALVE)

Thrombosis is by far the most common cause of valve immobilization. Although its yearly incidence varies among reports, it lies between 0% and 0.5% in the aortic position, between 0% and 2.6% in the mitral position, and up to 4% in the tricuspid position (65–67). This variability is multifactorial, depending on the valve model, flow rate across the valve, loss of atrial contraction (atrial fibrillation), irregular prosthetic valve surface, as well as a general prothrombotic tendency (cancer, chronic infections, use of oral contraceptive drugs, etc.).

The composition of the material that blocks the valve may be variable. In a pathological study of 112 explanted stuck valves, Deviri et al. found pure thrombosis in 77.7%, pure pannus in 10.7%, and a combination of the two in 11.6% (68). Vitale et al. studied the pathology of 87 stuck prosthetic valves and found pure thrombosis in only 24.1%, pure pannus in 31.0%, and their combination in 44.8% (69). The true incidence of valve thrombosis is probably closer to that found by Deviri et al., given the high response rate to thrombolysis (80–85%) in most stuck valve series, suggesting the presence of a predominantly thrombotic component.

Some findings may support the diagnosis of thrombus formation, as opposed to pure pannus formation. These clues include shorter symptom duration, a history of inadequate anticoagulation, shorter time interval from surgery, larger thrombi (extending beyond the ring in mitral prostheses), and softer echo densities (70). These clues have limited positive and negative predictive values. In the individual patient, one may not reach a conclusive answer on the composition of the obstructive material, even after thorough diagnostic efforts. However, shock is unlikely to occur in cases of pure tissue ingrowth, as a result of the gradual nature of its evolution.

There is also no linear relationship between the amount of accumulated thrombotic material and the severity of leaflet immobility. This is especially true for bileaflet valves, in which a small thrombus may entrap the hinge points and immobilize both leaflets (68,71,72).

The clinical presentation of obstructive valve thrombosis is variable (Table 7). The proportion of patients in shock is not always reported, and they might be included among patients reported to be in NYHA functional class IV. The proportion of patients in NYHA functional class IV varies from 25% to 75%, whereas the proportion of patients in shock is <20%. The discussion herein concerns only patients in hemodynamic compromise, but it should be remembered that patients with stuck valves may be only mildly symptomatic, especially when only one of two leaflets is trapped.

Table 7
Stuck Valves: Distribution of Functional Class at Presentation

Authors (ref)	No. of episodes	FC I–III	FC IV	Shock
Deviri et al. (68)	106	43 (40.6%)	63 (59.4%)	8 (7.5%)
Vitale et al. (69)	87	65 (74.7%)	22 (25.3%)	NA[a]
Shapira et al. (72)	17	11 (64.7%)	6 (35.3%)	0
Roudaut et al. (73)	74	46 (62.2%)	28 (37.8%)	11 (14.9%)
Reddy et al. (74)	44	11 (25%)	33 (75%)	8 (18.2%)
Vasan et al. (75)	16	8 (50%)	8 (50%)	NA
Manteiga et al. (76)	22	13 (59.1%)	9 (40.9%)	NA

[a] NA = not available.

Patient History

The time interval from valve implantation to its obstruction is quite variable. The mean interval in many series is 3–4 yr, but periods may vary from a few days to 16 yr. Symptoms of heart failure can also exist for variable periods of time, from a few days to more than a month. They usually follow a progressive course. Patients occasionally note muffled valve clicks, but this may be quite misleading: Patients may become unaware of the valve clicks over time, and newer generation valves are generally quiet. An important clue to the diagnosis of a stuck valve is a history of inadequate anticoagulation, which can be elicited in 60–70% of patients. This is usually evident from the first blood sample drawn at admission but may be tracked back to the blood tests performed in the preceding days or weeks.

Physical Examination

Aside from signs of shock and congestive heart failure, the physical examination of patients with a stuck valve may add useful information: (1) muffled or absent valve clicks, (2) a diastolic mitral murmur, which should not be generally heard, and (3) a regurgitant murmur (aortic or mitral) in case the leaflet is stuck in an open position. All of these signs may be difficult to note in an unstable patient, in full-blown pulmonary edema, with the noise of the respirators, and so forth, but when noted, they are very useful.

Diagnostic Considerations

The questions to be asked when stuck valve is suspected are as follows: (1) Is the excursion of the valve leaflet(s) limited? (2) What is the extent of leaflet motion abnormality? (3) Is there a high-risk left-sided thrombus that may embolize? (4) What are the hemodynamic consequences of leaflet immobilization? (5) Are there markers of high operative risk?

The diagnostic modalities to answer these questions are transthoracic echocardiography (TTE), TEE, and fluoroscopy, each of which has advantages and disadvantages (77–79). Table 6 compares the various modalities as to their ability to answer the above-posed questions.

TTE is usually the most valuable diagnostic tool to begin with because it can be done bedside, needs no patient preparation, and provides most of the data needed to confirm the diagnosis of stuck valve. It has, however, several drawbacks. First, it cannot usually provide accurate data regarding the amount of thrombotic material, which may influence the therapeutic considerations. Second, it is largely based on the demonstration of markedly increased transvalvular gradients. A patient in a state of shock may display deceptively low or normal gradients, because cardiac output is an important determinant of transvalvular gradients. Third, the visualization of valve leaflets using TTE is limited. In the mitral position, the ability to image both leaflets of a bileaflet prosthetic valve is quite satisfactory (>80%), whereas aortic valve leaflets are imaged in only 25% *(80)*. Quantification of leaflet motion abnormality is quite unreliable with TTE.

Transesophageal echocardiography offers the most valuable data on the soft-tissue structures, especially on thrombus burden. It has been suggested that a thrombus size of <5 mm is associated with favorable results when thrombolysis is applied *(81)*. The safety of this approach was recently validated in patients with thrombosed bileaflet mitral valves *(72)*. TEE may provide data on a thrombus attached to the affected valve or elsewhere in the heart, especially in the left atrium. The ability of TEE to demonstrate leaflet motion is better than that of TTE, although it is inferior to that of cinefluoroscopy, especially when the aortic valve is involved.

Fluoroscopy is the most powerful tool for identifying leaflet motion abnormality, both for older-generation valves *(82,83)* and for bileaflet valves *(84,85)*.

In the noncritically ill patient, the diagnosis is usually raised by the clinical presentation and supported by TTE. Validation of leaflet motion abnormality can then be achieved by either fluoroscopy or TEE. If thrombolysis is planned, TEE is highly recommended to rule out large left-sided thrombi. TTE should then be performed serially to identify a change in the pressure gradient and gross changes in leaflet motion. Fluoroscopy should be the main tool for verifying therapeutic success *(71)*. When the patient is in shock, the need for a quick diagnosis may prompt the performance of TEE as an initial strategy. Fluoroscopy should be performed only if it does not cause an undue delay in therapy.

Therapy

In general, there are three therapeutic modalities for obstructive valve thrombosis: intensified anticoagulation, thrombolysis, and surgical (valve re-replacement or, rarely, thrombectomy) *(86,87)*.

An intensified antithrombotic option is irrelevant in a patient in shock because of the slow rate of thrombus dissolution using this method. This leaves the choices of thrombolysis and surgery. These modalities have never been compared head to head in a randomized fashion in thrombosed valves, in general, or in critically ill patients, in particular. Thus, any comparison is subject to flaws such as selection bias, therapeutic regimens, and so forth.

Two studies included detailed information about patients with thrombosed prosthetic heart valves in shock who were given thrombolytic therapy (Table 8). The total number of patients analyzed was small (19 patients) and the success rate was about 50%. In both studies, there were no details about the thrombotic burden, so that the embolic risk could not be predicted.

Table 8
Thrombolytic Therapy in Patients with Thrombosed Prosthetic
Heart Valves Who Were in Shock

Author (ref).	Valve position		Valve model		Success	Complication	Mortality
	M	A	ML	BL			
Roudaut et al. (73)	9	2	8	3	6 (54.5%)	3 (27.3%)	2 (18.2%)
Reddy et al. (74)	7	1	0	8	4 (50%)	0	4 (50%)

Abbreviations: A = aortic; BL = bileaflet; M = mitral; ML = monoleaflet.

The American College of Cardiology/American Heart Association (ACC/AHA) Task Force on Valvular Heart Disease recommends surgery for patients with stuck valves who are in NYHA functional class III–IV but are not at high surgical risk (87). The rationale behind these recommendations is not detailed in these guidelines. There are insufficient data to point out the operative risk of patients in shock because of stuck valves. Deviri et al. reported an operative mortality of 17.5% in patients with stuck valves who were in NYHA functional class III–IV, compared with 4.7% in patient who were in NYHA I–II (68). No mortality data were given on eight patients who were already in shock at admission. Husebye et al. reported the results of reoperation in patients with prosthetic valves. The operative mortality in emergency procedures in this study was 38% for aortic valves and 55% for mitral valves (88). Bortolotti et al. reported 57% mortality in emergency reoperative valve surgery, as compared with 11% in nonemergency surgery (89).

Given that the operative risk in emergency valve reoperation is similar to that of thrombolysis in the same setting, additional factors must be taken into account. For example, if the operating room with a skillful team is unavailable for several hours, thrombolysis should be attempted. It may result in complete success, which may obviate the need for surgery or bring about partial resolution of the leaflet abnormality. If surgery is still indicated in such a case, it can be performed in a more favorable hemodynamic state. If thrombolysis fails, concern is raised regarding heart surgery soon after thrombolytic therapy. Emergency coronary artery bypass graft (CABG) surgery soon after streptokinase (SK) administration is associated with significant difficulties in bleeding control and increased blood consumption (90,91). Tissue-type plasominogen activator (tPA) is more fibrin-specific and was associated with less postoperative blood requirement in patients undergoing CABG within 24 h of tPA infusion (92,93). Thus, if thrombolysis fails and the patient needs an emergency operation, bleeding control may be achieved more effectively after tPA than after SK.

The coexistence of additional significant valvular lesions or myocardial dysfunction further increases the surgical risk, although it is unclear whether medically treated patients fare better.

The obstructive thrombus size is strongly associated with embolic phenomena. Thrombolysis is quite safe when the thrombus size is <5 mm (72). Larger thrombi can put the patient at increased thromboembolic risk and argue against thrombolytic therapy if the surgical option is readily available.

Obstructive thrombosis of a mechanical tricuspid valve usually follows an insidious course, with fatigue and signs of increased systemic pressure with volume retention

(94). Shock is unlikely to occur in patients with bileaflet mechanical tricuspid valves. There have, however, been fatal cases associated with valve thrombosis in older models *(95)*. Unlike the debate about left-sided valves, there is a wide acceptance of thrombolysis as the modality of choice in stuck tricuspid prostheses. There are no comparative data on thrombolysis versus a surgical approach in patients who are in shock.

DISK ESCAPE

Disk escape is an ominous complication of mechanical valves that results from abrupt failure of the occluder mechanism. This catastrophic complication has been reported with the Björk–Shiley convexo-concave prosthesis, primarily with large (≥29 mm) valves, mitral position, an opening angle of 70°, age <50 yr at implantation, male gender, certain welding groups, and welding dates between January 1981 and June 1982 *(96–100)*.

By the end of 1994, Shiley Inc. received reports on 564 cases of complete strut fracture. The incidence of this event is highly variable and may be as high as >0.6% per year in high-risk patients and <0.1% in low-risk patients. This risk can be formulated according to the above-mentioned risk factors, and prophylactic valve re-replacement may be judiciously considered if the risk of disk escape is considerably higher than the reoperative risk.

Although the majority of complete strut fractures reported to Shiley Inc. were fatal, there were reports of successful emergency reoperation in patients with disk escape from mitral prostheses. In a literature review from 1989, 13 (59%) of 22 patients died, and 9 survived, 5 of whom underwent disk removal during the same operation *(101)*. The Dutch experience revealed a similar mortality rate (24/42, 57%), which was better in patients with mitral prostheses (18/35, 51%) than in aortic prostheses (6/7, 86%) *(98)*. The mean time from onset of symptoms to death was 2.3±0.9 h in the aortic position and 12±12 h in the mitral position *(98)*. The patients who survived to surgery had better outcomes: 17/22 survived in the Dutch study (77%), and 9/16 (56%) in the other study *(98,101)*.

The underlying mechanism for the disk escape is fracture of the outlet strut. Occasionally, a single leg separation of the outlet strut, which may lead to complete fracture, may be identified by X-ray imaging *(102)*. Indeed, this is now an accepted indication for prophylactic replacement of the valve.

Disk escape is extremely rare in other valve models, but there have been a few reports of its occurrence in the following models: Beall *(103)*, Harken *(104)*, St. Jude Medical *(105)*, Edwards-Duromedics *(106,107)*, Edwards TENKA *(108)*, and Omnicarbon *(109)*.

The clinical presentation of an embolized valve disk is usually catastrophic, as expected from sudden free regurgitation into a cardiac chamber. Full-blown pulmonary edema and cardiogenic shock are the rule. Additional symptoms (e.g., neurologic deficits, extremity or mesenteric ischemia, etc.) may be attributed to the organ affected by the dislodged disk. The valve clicks are no longer heard. Regurgitant murmurs are less likely to be heard and, if they are, they are brief related to rapid pressure equalization with the receiving cardiac chamber.

Because the clinical course quickly deteriorates, the physician should choose the most readily available diagnostic modality (Table 6), as well as the one with which the staff is most experienced. Once the diagnosis is confirmed, the patient should be taken

Table 9
Etiology of Nonthrombotic Extrinsic Interruption
of Disk Movement

Valve position	Mitral	Aortic
Chordal remnants	+	–
Leaflet remnants	+	+
Too long knots	+	+
Left ventricular wall	+	–
Aortic commissure remnants	–	+

without delay to the operating room for valve re-replacement. If echocardiography was not previously performed, it is prudent to perform intraoperative TEE. While the patient is prepared for emergency surgery, supportive measures should be taken. An intra-aortic balloon should be inserted in patients with mitral disk escape, but it is strictly contraindicated in patients with aortic disk escape, because it worsens the regurgitation. Other measures include intravenous inotropic support, careful use of vasodilators, and mechanical ventilatory support, as needed.

The management of the embolized disk is important. The disk usually embolizes to the abdominal aorta, although, rarely, it can remain in the heart chambers or the thoracic aorta *(101)*. It can be seen using overpenetrated chest X-ray and abdominal films, which should be ordered as a part of the initial evaluation, provided they can be performed promptly. Embolized disks have usually been retrieved during the valve operation in order to avoid distal ischemia. There are, however, reports of delayed retrieval, up to 1 mo after the cardiac operation *(110)*.

NONTHROMBOTIC VALVE BLOCK

There are a few reports of patents with cardiogenic shock related to extrinsic interruption of leaflet motion *(111–118)*. Some of the underlying causes are depicted in Table 9.

This complication is generally limited to tilting disk valves, and its reported incidence was 0.24% for mitral prostheses and 0.33% for aortic prostheses *(117)*. The clinical presentation is quite typical. It occurs in the very early postoperative period, usually within the first 48 h and, occasionally, shortly after weaning from cardiopulmonary bypass. The longest reported postoperative delay has been 10 wk *(118)*. This complication is characterized by sudden, unexpected, intermittent electromechanical dissociation. Echocardiography demonstrates intermittent blockage of the valve opening, as detected by M-mode imaging or pulsed-Doppler interrogation of the valve. Sometimes, a long observation period is needed because of the intermittent character of the blockage, and a TEE probe may left *in situ* for this purpose.

A blocked mitral valve calls for emergency redo surgery during which the excess tissue blocking the valve should be removed. The valve may be left *in situ,* replaced, or reoriented. Blocked aortic valves may undergo spontaneous release, as the left ventricular pressure may overcome the blockage. There are reports about such valves that were left unattached, with a favorable outcome *(117)*. Currently, implanted mechanical valves, mostly bileaflet, are vary rarely subject to this complication.

Table 10
Factors Associated with Structural
Dysfunction of Prosthetic Biological Valves

Young age at implantation
Long postoperative period
Mitral position
Chronic renal failure
Hypercalcemia

COMPLICATIONS ASSOCIATED WITH PROSTHETIC
BIOLOGICAL VALVES

Biological valves can undergo structural dysfunction over time. The rate of degeneration depends on several factors (Table 10). About 30% of bioprosthetic valves will degenerate within 10 yr. By 15 yr, the actuarial freedom from bioprosthetic primary tissue failure ranges from 30% to 60% *(119,120)*.

The pathological finding in the degenerated valves include cuspal tears, fibrin deposition, disruption of the fibrocollagenous structure, perforation, fibrosis, and calcification.

The most common indication for reoperation in patients with a degenerated prosthetic valve is valvular regurgitation *(121,122)*. The clinical presentation of prosthetic valve regurgitation may range from an asymptomatic finding to dramatic hemodynamic derangement. In most cases, the valve does not fail suddenly, leaving sufficient time to schedule elective reoperation. Caution should be taken to differentiate between central jets, indicative of structural dysfunction, and perivalvular leak. If intravalvular regurgitation seems significant or progressive, elective valve replacement is desirable. The reoperative risk in most series is 10–15% *(89,123–126)* in a wide range of ages and clinical settings.

Despite the relatively indolent nature of structural dysfunction of biological valves, patients may suddenly become severely ill, especially following an acute tear of a cusp *(127,128)*. This can occur, for example, in a porcine bioprosthesis, which can undergo commissural dehiscence of the aortic wall, whereas the other two leaflets remain relatively uninvolved *(127,128)*.

When a patient with a bioprosthesis is admitted in a state of shock, structural dysfunction should be sought. The odds are higher if the patient is in a high-risk category (Table 10) or when previous evaluation revealed significant intravalvular regurgitation. In case of a tear, a loud regurgitant murmur is often heard, and the patient can appreciate an audible "honking noise" coming from the chest *(129)*. A patient may point out the precise moment of leaflet rupture, noting a sudden vibrating sensation in the chest *(130)*. Echocardiography may detect intravalvular regurgitation of variable degrees. The audio signal of the valvular regurgitation may be honking *(131)*. The precordium may be hyperkinetic.

TTE is usually the first diagnostic step to be taken and it may be all that is needed to make a solid diagnosis. TEE may be required if TTE does not provide the requested information. TEE is better than TTE in estimating bioprosthetic mitral valves, differentiating intravalvular from perivalvular regurgitation, and demonstrating thickened valves resulting from degeneration *(132)*. Fluoroscopy is usually useless in the case of biological valve. It may show valve calcification, but not its hemodynamic consequences. It may also show significant rocking of the base of the valve in cases of dehiscence, but color-Doppler will provide much more comprehensive data.

Patients with cardiogenic shock attributable to structural dysfunction of a biological prosthetic valve should undergo emergency surgery. Until then, they should be given supportive therapy. In a series of 400 patients who required reoperation for degenerated bioprostheses, 153 (38%) were nonelective, including 4 (1%) urgent operations *(121)*. Using multivariable analysis, a nonelective surgery was a strong predictor of hospital death and prolonged postoperative hospital stay.

Bioprosthetic valves may sometimes require replacement because of progressive valve stenosis rather than regurgitation. The progression to stenosis is obviously slower than regurgitation, which may occur or progress suddenly. The likelihood of presenting in cardiogenic shock resulting from stenosed bioprosthetic valve is low. Therapy is usually surgical. There are some reports on balloon valvuloplasty of stenosed bioprostheses *(133–138)*, but the results are less favorable than in native mitral valve valvuloplasty. Ex vivo and intraoperative studies showed that there is a high frequency of dislodgment of friable fragments of calcific deposits and thrombi during inflation, dislodgment of calcific deposits during insertion and withdrawal of the balloon, fracture and dislodgment of portions of stiffened cusps *(138)*, and high rate of severe valvular regurgitation *(137)*. The long-term results of a successful procedure are unknown.

In situ thrombosis may occur on top of a degenerated bioprosthetic valve. The occurrence is low: In the series of Oliver et al., it was 10/161 (6.2%) among patients with prosthetic valve malfunction *(139)*. Two of these patients were operated, but eight received anticoagulants and seven of them achieved long-term clinical and hemodynamic improvement.

REFERENCES

1. Hochman JS, Buller CE, Sleeper LA, et al. Cardiogenic shock complicatiog acute myocardial infarction-etiologies, management and outcome: a report from the SHOCK trial registry. Should we emergently revascularize occluded coronaries for cardiogenic shock. J Am Coll Cardiol 2000;36:1063–1070.
2. Lokhandwala YY, Banker D, Vora AM, et al. Emergent balloon mitral valvotomy in patients presenting with cardiac arrest, cardiogenic shock or refractory pulmonary edema. J Am Coll Cardiol 1998;32:154–158.
3. Patel JJ, Munclinger MJ, Mitha AS, Patel N. Percutaneous balloon dilatation of the mitral valve in critically ill young patients with intractable heart failure. Br Heart J 1995;73:555–558.
4. Wu JJ, Chern MS, Yeh KH, Chen YC, Fu M, Hung JS. Urgent/emergent percutaneous transvenous mitral commissurotomy. Cathet Cardiovasc Diagn 1994;31:18–22.
5. Goldman JH, Slade A, Clague J. Cardiogenic shock secondary to MS treated by balloon mitral valvuloplasty. Cathet Cardiovasc Diagn 1998;43:195–197.
6. Chow WH, Chow TC. Percutaneous balloon mitral valvotomy as a bridge to elective mitral valve replacement. Cathet Cardiovasc Diagn 1998;45:102.
7. Strick S, Seggewiss H, Fassbender D, et al. Emergent percutaneous mitral valve repair with Inoue balloon-catheter in severe MS and cardiogenic shock. Dtsch Med Wochenschr 1994 19;119:1110–1114.
8. Barlow JB: Perspective of the Mitral Valve. FA Davis, Philadelphia, 1987, pp. 247–250.
9. Otto CM. Valvular Heart Disease. WB Saunders, Philadelphia, 1999, p. 218.
10. Sagie A, Freitas N, Padial LR, et al. Doppler echocardiographic assessment of long-term progression of mitral stenosis in 103 patients: valve area and right heart disease. J Am Coll Cardiol 1996;28:472–479.
11. Reid CL. Echocardiography in patients undergoing catheter balloon mitral commissurotomy. In Otto CM, ed. The Practice of Clinical Echocardiography. WB Saunders, Philadelphia, 1997, pp. 373–388.

12. Sagie A, Freitas N, Chen MH, Marshall JE, Weyman AE, Levine RA. Echocardiographic assessment of mitral stenosis and its associated valvular lesions in 205 patients and lack of association with mitral valve prolapse. J Am Soc Echocardiol 1997;10:141–148.

13. Aschenberg NK, Schluter M. Kremer P, et al. Transesophageal-two-dimensional echocardiography for the detection of left atrial appendage thrombus. J Am Coll Cardiol 1986;7:163–168.

14. Donner R, Carabello BA, Black I, Spain JF. Left ventricular wall stress in compensated aortic stenosis in children. Am J Cardiol 1983;51:946.

15. Spann JF, Bove AA, Natarajan G, Kreulens T. Ventricular performance, pump function, and compensatory mechanism in patients with aortic stenosis. Circulation 1980;62:576–582.

16. Ross J Jr. Afterload mismatch and preload reserve: a conceptual framework for the analysis of ventricular function. Prog Cardiovasc Dis 1976;18:255–264.

17. Gunter S, Grossman W. Determinant of ventricular function in pressure overload hypertrophy in man. Circulation 1979;59:679.

18. NHLBI Balloon Valvuloplasty Registry Participants. Percutaneous balloon aortic valvuloplasty. Acute and 30-day follow-up results in 674 patients from the NHLBI Balloon Valvuloplasty Registry. Acute and 30-day follow-up. Circulation 1991;84:2383–2397.

19. Otto CM, Mickel MC, Kennedy JW, et al. Three years outcome after balloon aortic valvuloplasty: insights into prognosis of valvular aortic stenosis. Circulation 1994;89:642–650.

20. Christ G, Zehetgruber M, Mundigler G, et al. Emergency aortic valve replacement for critical aortic stenosis. A lifesaving treatment for patients with cardiogenic shock and multiple organ failure. Intensive Care Med 1997;23:297–300.

21. Moreno PR, Jang IK, Newell JB, Block PC, Palacios IF. The role of percutaneous aortic balloon valvuloplasty in patients with cardiogenic shock and critical aortic stenosis. J Am Coll Cardiol 1994;23:1071–1075.

22. Bhatia A, Kumar A, Seth A, Bhatia ML, Trehan N. Successful aortic balloon valvuloplasty in critical aortic stenosis with shock. Cathet Cardiovasc Diagn 1993;29:296–297.

23. Cribier A, Remadi F, Koning R, Rath P, Stix G, Letac B. Emergency balloon valvuloplasty as initial treatment of patients with aortic stenosis and cardiogenic shock. N Engl J Med 1992;27:646.

24. Smedira NG, Ports TA, Merrick SH, Rankin JS. Balloon aortic valvuloplasty as a bridge to aortic valve replacement in critically ill patients. Ann Thorac Surg 1993;55:914–916.

25. Sprigings DC, Jackson G, Chambers JB, Monaghan MJ, Thomas SD, Meany TB, et al. Balloon dilatation of the aortic valve for inoperable aortic stenosis. Br Med J 1988 22;297:1007–1011.

26. Jackson G, Thomas S, Monaghan M, Forsyth A, Jewitt D. Inoperable aortic stenosis in the elderly: benefit from percutaneous transluminal valvuloplasty. Br Med J 1987;294:83–86.

27. Vaitkus PT, Manicini D, Herrmann HC. Percutaneous balloon aortic valvuloplasty as a bridge to heart transplantation. Transplant 1993;12:1062–1064.

28. Kim KS, Maxted W, Nanda NC, et al. Comparison of multiplane and biplane transesophageal echocardiography in the assessment of aortic stenosis. Am J Cardiol 1997;79:436–441.

29. Bernard Y, Meneveau N, Vuillemenot A, et al. Is planimetry of aortic valve area using multiplane transesophageal echocardiography a reliable method in assessing severity of aortic stenosis? Heart 1997;78:68–73.

30. Otto CM. Valvular Heart Disease. WB Saunders, Philadelphia, 1999, p. 193.

31. Fremes SF, Goldman BS, Ivanov J, Weisl RD, David TE, Salerno T. Valvular surgery in the elderly. Circulation 1989:80(Suppl I):I-177–I-190.

32. Otto CM, Mickel MC, Kennedy JW, et al. Three year outcome after aortic balloon valvuloplasty: insights into prognosis of valvular aortic stenosis. Circulation 1994;89:642–650.

33. Hutter A Jr, De Sanctis R, Nathan M, et al. Aortic valve surgery as an emergency procedure. Circulation 1970;51:623–627.

34. Kirklin JW. Aortic valve disease. In: Kirklin JW, Barrat-Boys B, eds. Cardiac Surgery: Morphology, Diagnostic Criteria, Natural History, Techniques, Results and Indications: Churchill Livingstone, New York, 1993, p. 528.

35. Rahimtoola SH. Catheter balloon valvuloplasty for severe calcific aortic stenosis: a limited role. J Am Coll Cardiol 1994;89:642–650.

36. Isner JM. Acute catastrophic complications of balloon aortic valvuloplasty. The Mansfield Scientific Aortic Valvuloplasty Registry Investigators. J Am Coll Cardiol 1991;17:1436–1444.

37. Whisenant B, Sweeney J, Ports TA. Combined PTCA and aortic valvuloplasty for acute myocardial infarction complicated by severe aortic stenosis and cardiogenic shock. Cathet Cardiovasc Diagn 1997;42:283–285.

38. Welch GH, Braunwald E, Sarnoff SJ. Hemodynamic effects of quantitavely varied experimental aortic regurgitation. Circ Res 1957;5:546.

39. Miller GA, Kiklin JW, Swan JH. Myocardial function and left ventricular volumes in acquired valvular insufficiency. Circulation 1965;31:374.

40. Nakao S, Nagatomo T, Kiyonaga K, et al. Influence of localized aortic valve damage on coronary artery blood flow in acute aortic regurgitation. An experimental study. Circulation 1987;59:1144–1148.

41. Ardehali A, Segal J, Cheitilin MD. Coronary blood flow reserve in acute aortic regurgitation. J Am Coll Cardiol 1995;25:1387–1392.

42. Mann T, McLaurin L, Grossman W, et al. Assessing the hemodynamic severity of acute aortic regurgitation due to infective endocarditis. N Engl J Med 1975;293:108–113.

43. Sareli P, Klein HO, Schamroth CL, et al. Contribution of echocardiography and immediate surgery to the management of severe aortic regurgitation from active infective endocarditis. Am J Cardiol 1986;57:413–418.

44. Otto CM, Perlman AS. Textbook of Clinical Echocardiography, WB Saunders, Philadelphia, 1995.

45. Alpert JS, Dalen JE, Rahimtoola SH. Valvlar Heart Disease. 3rd ed. Lippincott Williams and Wilkins, Baltimore, MD, 2000, Chap. 9.

46. Morganroth J, Perloff JK, Zeldis SM, et al. Acute severe aortic regurgitation. Ann Intern Med 1977;87:223.

47. Welton DE, Young JB, Raizner AE, et al. Value and safety of cardiac catheterization during active endocarditis. Am J Cardiol 1978;44:1306–1310.

48. Wilson WR, Danielson GK, Giulian ER, et al. Cardiac valve replacement in congestive heart failure due to infective endocarditis. Mayo Clin Proc 1979;54:223–232.

49. Labalestier RI, Kinchala NM, Aranki SF, et al. Acute bacterial endocarditis — optimizing surgical results. Circulation 1992;86(Suppl II):II-68–II-74.

50. Carabello BA. Mitral regurgitation. Part I. Basic pathophysiologic principles. Mod Concepts Cardiovasc Dis 1988;57:53.

51. Sutton GC, Craige E. Clinical signs of severe acute mitral regurgitation. Am J Cardiol 1967;20:141–144.

52. Alpert JS, Dalen JE, Rahimtoola SH. Valvar Heart Disease. 3rd ed. Lippincott Williams and Wilkins, Baltimore, MD, 2000, Chap. 5.

53. Slater J, Gindea AJ, Freedberg RS. Comparison of cardiac catheterization and Doppler echocardiography in the decision to operate in aortic and mitral valve disease. J An Coll Cardiol 1991;17:1037–1038.

54. Chatterjee K, Parmley WW, Swan HJ, Berman G, Forrester J, Marcus HS. Beneficial effects of vasodilator agents in severe mitral regurgitation due to dysfunction of subvalvar apparatus. Circulation 1973;48:684–690.

55. Harshaw CW, Grossman W, Munro AB, McLaurin LP. Reduced systemic vascular resistance as therapy for severe mitral regurgitation of valvular origin. Ann Intern Med 1975;83:312–316.

56. Greenberg BH, Massie BM, Brundage BH, Botvinick EH, Parmley WW, Chatterjee K. Beneficial effects of hydralazine in severe mitral regurgitation. Circulation. 1978;58:273–279.

57. Horstkotte D, Schulte HD, Niehues R, Klein RM, Piper C, Strauer BE. Diagnostic and therapeutic considerations in acute, severe mitral regurgitation: experience in 42 consecutive patients entering the intensive care unit with pulmonary edema. J Heart Valve Dis 1993;2:512–522.

58. Maisano F, Lorusso R, Sandrelli L, et al. Valve repair for traumatic tricuspid regurgitation. Eur J Cardiothorac Surg 1996;10:867–873.

59. Parmley LF, Manion WC, Mattingly TW. Nonpenetrating traumatic injury of the heart. Circulation 1958;18:371.

60. Gayet C, Pierre B, Delahaeye JP, Champsaur G, Andre-Fouet X, Roueff P. Traumatic tricuspid insufficiency: an underdiagnosed disease. Chest 1987;92:429–432.

61. Van Son JAM, Danielson JK, Schaff HV, Miller FA. Traumatic tricuspid valve insufficiency. Experience in thirteen patients. J Thorac Cardiovasc Surg 1994;108:893–898.

62. Bolinger BS, Winslow TM. Transesophageal echocardiographic diagnosis of a ruptured tricuspid valve chordae tendineae as the etiology for cardiogenic shock. Chest 1994;105:1286–1288.

63. Chares M, Lamm P, Leischik R, Lenz G, Steinmann EH, Polonius MJ. Highly acute course of ruptured papillary muscle of the tricuspid valve in a case of blunt chest trauma. Thorac Cardiovasc Surg 1993;41:325–327.

64. Arbulu A, Holmes RJ, Asfaw I. Tricuspid valvulectomy without replacement: twenty years' experience. J Thorac Cardiovasc Surg 1991;102:917–922.

65. Horstkotte D, Burckhardt D. Prosthetic valve thrombosis. J Heart Valve Dis 1995;4:141–153.

66. Thorburn CW, Morgan JJ, Shanahan MX, Chang VP. Long-term results of tricuspid valve replacement and the problem of prosthetic valve thrombosis. Am J Cardiol 1983;51:1128–1132.

67. Cannegieter SC, Rosendaal FR, Briet E. Thromboembolic and bleeding complications in patients with mechanical heart valve prostheses. Circulation 1994;89:635–641.

68. Deviri E, Sareli P, Visenbaugh T, Cronje SL. Obstruction of mechanical heart valve prostheses: clinical aspects and surgical management. J Am Coll Cardiol 1991;17:646–650.

69. Vitale N, Renzulli A, Agozzino L, et al. Obstruction of mechanical mitral prostheses: analysis of pathologic findings. Ann Thorac Surg 1997;63:1101–1106.

70. Barbetseas J, Zoghbi WA. Evaluation of prosthetic valve function and associated complications. Cardiol Clin 1998;16:505–530.

71. Silber H, Khan S, Matloff JM, et al. The St. Jude valve: thrombolysis as the first line of therapy for cardiac valve thrombosis. Circulation 1993;87:30–37.

72. Shapira Y, Herz I, Vaturi M, et al. Thrombolysis is an effective and safe therapy in stuck bileaflet mitral valves in the absence of high-risk thrombi. J Am Coll Cardiol 2000;35:1874–1880.

73. Roudaut R, Labbe T, Lorient-Roudat M, et al. Mechanical cardiac valve thrombosis: is fibrinolysis justified? Circulation 1992;86(Suppl II):II-8–II-15.

74. Reddy N, Padmanabhan T, Singh S, et al. Thrombolysis in left-sided prosthetic valve occlusion: immediate and follow-up results. Ann Thorac Surg 1994;58:462–471.

75. Vasan RS, Kaul U, Sanghvi S, et al. Thrombolytic therapy for prosthetic valve thrombosis: a study based on serial Doppler echocardiographic evaluation. Am Heart J 1992;123:1575–1580.

76. Manteiga R, Souto JC, Ites A, et al. Short-course thrombolysis as the first line of therapy for cardiac valve thrombosis. J Thorac Cardiovasc Surg 1998;115:780–784.

77. Shapira Y, Herz I, Sagie A. Fluoroscopy of prosthetic heart valves: does it have a place in the echocardiography era? J Heart Valve Dis 2000;9:594–599.

78. Montorsi P, De Bernardi F, Muratori M, Cavoretto D, Peppi M. Role of cine-fluoroscopy, transthoracic and transesophageal echocardiography in patients with suspected prosthetic heart valve thrombosis. Am J Cardiol 2000;85:58–64.

79. Nottestad SY, Zabalgoitia M. Echocardiographic recognition and quantitation of prosthetic valve dysfunction. In: Otto CM, ed. The Practice of Clinical Echocardiography. WB Saunders, Philadelphia, 1997; p. 809.

80. Panidis IP, Ren J-F, Kotler MN, et al. Clinical and echocardiographic evaluation of the St. Jude cardiac valve prosthesis: follow-up of 126 patients. J Am Coll Cardiol 1984;4:454–462.

81. Hurrell DG, Schaff HV, Tajik JA. Thrombolytic therapy for obstruction of mechanical prosthetic valves. Mayo Clin Proc 1996;71:605–613.

82. Vogel W, Stoll HP, Bay W, Frohlig G, Schieffer H. Cineradiography for determination of normal and abnormal function in mechanical heart valves. Am J Cardiol 1993;71:225–232.

83. Montorsi P, Repossini A, Bartorelli AL. Cinefluoroscopic identification of Bjork–Shiley prosthetic heart valves. Eur Heart J 1993;14:1514–1518.

84. Montorsi P, Cavoretto D, Repossini A, Bartorelli AL, Guazzi MD. Valve design characteristics and cine-fluoroscopic appearance of five currently available bileaflet prosthetic heart valves. Am J Cardiac Imag 1996;10:29–44.

85. Montorsi P, Arena V, Muratori M, et al. Fluoroscopic functional evaluation of bileaflet prostheses: effect of different intraoperative valve orientation. Am J Cardiac Imag 1996;10:101–107.

86. Lengyel M, Fuster V, Ketlai M, et al. Guidelines for management of left-sided prosthetic valve thrombosis: a role for thrombolytic therapy. Consensus conference on prosthetic valve thrombosis. J Am Coll Cardiol 1997;30:1521–1526.

87. Bonow RW, Carabello B, De Leon AC Jr, et al. ACC/AHA guidelines for the management of patients with valvular heart disease. J Am Coll Cardiol 1998;32:1486–1588.

88. Husebye DG, Pluth JR, Piehler JM, et al. Reoperation on prosthetic heart valves: an analysis of 552 patients. J Thorac Cardiovasc Surg 1983;4:543–552.

89. Bortolotti U, Milano A, Mossuto E, Mazzaro E, Thiene G, Casarotto D. Early and late outcome after reoperation for prosthetic valve dysfunction: analysis of 549 patients during a 26-year period. J Heart Valve Dis 1994;3:81–87.

90. Skinner JR, Phillips SJ, Zeff RH, Kongtahworn C. Immediate coronary bypass following failed streptokinase infusion in evolving myocardial infarction. J Thorac Cardiovasc Surg 1984;87:567–570.

91. Lee KF, Mandell J, Raskin JS, et al. Immediate versus delayed coronary grafting after streptokinase treatment. Postoperative blood loss and clinical results. J Thorac Cardiovasc Surg 1988;95:216–222.

92. Kereiakes DJ, Topol EJ, George BS, et al. Emergency coronary artery bypass surgery preserves global and regional left ventricular function after intravenous tissue plasminogen activator therapy for acute myocardial infarction. J Am Coll Cardiol 1988;11:899–907.

93. Gersh BJ, Chesebro JH, Braunwald E, et al. Coronary artery bypass surgery after thrombolytic therapy in the Thrombolysis in Myocardial Infarction Trial, Phase II (TIMI II). J Am Coll Cardiol 1995;25:395–402.

94. Shapira Y, Sagie A, Jortner R, Adler Y, Hirsch R. Thrombosis of bileaflet tricuspid valve prosthesis — clinical spectrum and the role of nonsurgical treatment. Am Heart J 1999;137:721–725.

95. Van Nooten GJ, Caes F, Taeymans Y, et al. Tricuspid valve replacement: postoperative and long-term results. J Thorac Cardiovasc Surg 1995;110:672–679.

96. Schondube FA, Althoff W, Dorge HC, et al. Prophylactic reoperation for strut fractures of the Björk–Shiley convexo-concave heart valve. J Heart Valve Dis 1994;3:247–253.

97. Van der Meulen JH, Steyerberg EW, van der Graaf Y, et al. Age thresholds for prophylactic replacement of Björk–Shiley convexo-concave heart valves: a clinical and economic evaluation. Circulation 1993;88:156–164.

98. Van der Craaf Y, de Waard P, van Herwerden LA, Defauw JJ. Risk of strut fracture of Björk–Shiley valves. Lancet 1992;339:257–261.

99. Ericsson A, Lindblom D, Semb C, et al. Strut fracture with Björk–Shiley 70 degrees convexo-concave valve: an international multi-institutional follow-up study. Eur J Cardiothorac Surg 1992;6:339–346.

100. Smith JK, for the Supervisory Panel Bowling–Pfizer Settlement. Important updated information for physicians about patients with Björk–Shiley convexo-concave heart valves. Proposed by the Bowling-Pfizer Supervisory Panel and adopted on March 8, 2000 by the U.S. District Court, Southern District, Western Division, Cincinnati, Ohio.

101. Hendel PN. Björk–Shiley strut fracture and disc escape: literature review and method of disc retrieval. Ann Thorac Surg 1989;47:436–440.

102. O'Neill WW, Chandler JG, Gordon RE, et al. Radiographic detection of strut separations in Björk–Shiley convexo-concave mitral valves. N Engl J Med 1995;333:414–419.

103. Chauve A, Alfieri O. Escape of the disc occluder from a Beall model 104 mitral prosthesis. Thorac Cardiovasc Surg 1982;30:53–55.

104. Federico J, Masters RG, Walley VM, Keon WJ. Retrograde dislodgement of a Harken mitral valve disc occluder. Can J Cardiol 1994;10:377–379.

105. Hjelms E. Escape of a leaflet from a St. Jude Medical prosthesis in a mitral position. Thorac Cardiovasc Surg 1983;31:310–312.

106. Tsui BC, Kinley CE, Miller RM. Optimal imaging techniques for locating leaflets after escape from prosthetic heart valves. Can Assoc Radiol J 1994;45:93–96.

107. Moritz A, Klepetko W, Rodler S, Foger A, Schreiner W, Grabenwoger F, et al. Six-year follow-up after heart valve replacement with the Edwards Duromedics bileaflet prosthesis. Eur J Cardiothorac Surg 1993;7:84–90.

108. Hemmer WB, Doss M, Hannekum A, Kalper X. Leaflet escape in a TENKA and an original duromedics bileaflet valve. Ann Thorac Surg 2000;69:942–944.

109. Kornberg A, Wildhirt SM, Schulze C, Kreuzer E. Leaflet escape in Omnicarbon monoleaflet valve. Eur J Cardiothorac Surg 1999;15:867–869.

110. Larrieu AJ, Puglia E, Allen P. Strut fracture and disc embolization of a Bjork–Shiley mitral valve prosthesis: localization of embolized disc by computerized axial tomography. Ann Thorac Surg 1982;34:192–195.

111. Jones AA, Otis JB, Fletcher GF, Roberts WC. A hitherto undescribed cause of prosthetic mitral valve obstruction. J Thorac Cardiovasc Surg 1977;74:116–117.

112. Blasko EC, Plzak LF, Shon M, Manion WL. Acute, complete, extrinsic obstruction of the Björk–Shiley valve in the immediate postoperative period. J Thorac Cardiovasc Surg 1983;86:630–631.

113. Trites PN, Kiser JC, Johnson G, Tycast FJ, Gobel FL. Occlusion of Medtronic–Hall mitral prosthesis by ruptured papillary muscle and chordac tendineae. J Thorac Cardiovasc Surg 1984;88:301–302.

114. Pai G, Ellison RG, Rubin JW, Moore HY, Kamath MV. Disc immobilization of Björk Shiley and Medtronic–Hall valves during and immediately after valve replacement. Ann Thorac Surg 1987;44:73–76.

115. Masters RG, Keon WG. Extrinsic obstruction of the Medtronic–Hall disc valve in the mitral position. Ann Thorac Surg 1988;45:210–212.

116. Borowski A, Reib N, Klaer R. Intermittent obstruction of the Omnicarbon-valve prosthesis in the mitral position due to interference by papillary muscle. Diagnostic and surgical consideration. J Cardiovasc Surg (Torino) 1992;33:305–307.

117. Santé P, Renzulli A, Festa M, et al. Acute post-operative block of mechanical prostheses: incidence and treatment. Cardiovasc Surg 1994;2:403–406.

118. Greenwood GP, Nolan J, Mackintosh AF. Late, intermittent obstruction of a mitral prosthesis by chordal remnants. Eur J Cardiothorac Surg 1997;12:804–806.

119. Grunkemeier GL, Bodnar E. Comparison of structural valve failure among different "models" of homograft valves. J Heart Valve Dis 1994;3:556–560.

120. Grunkemeier GL, Jamieson WR, Miller DC, Starr A. Actuarial versus actual risk of porcine structural valve deterioration. J Thorac Cardiovasc Surg 1994;108:709–718.

121. Akins CW, Buckley MJ, Daggett WM, et al. Risk of reoperative valve replacement for failed mitral and aortic bioprostheses. Ann Thorac Surg 1998;65:1545–1552.

122. Jones EL, Weintraub WS, Craver JM, et al. Ten-year experience with the porcine bioprosthetic valve: Interrelationship of valve survival and patient survival in 1,050 valve replacements. Ann Thorac Surg 1990;49:370–383.

123. Lytle BW, Corsgrove DM, Taylor PC, et al. Reoperation for valve surgery: perioperative mortality and determinants of risk for 1000 patients. Ann Thorac Surg 1986;42:632–643.

124. Cohn LA, Aranki SF, Rizzo RJ, et al. Decrease in operative risk of reoperative valve surgery. Ann Thorac Surg 1993;56:15–21.

125. Mazzuco A, Milano A, Mazzaro E, Bortolotti U. Reoperation in patients with a bioprosthesis in the mitral position: indications and early results. J Heart Valve Dis 1993;2:646–648.

126. Tyres GFO, Jamieson WRE, Munro AI, et al. Reoperation in biological and mechanical valve populations: fate of the reoperative patient. Ann Thorac Surg 1995;60:S464–S469.

127. Naqvi TZ, Siegel RJ, Buchbinder NA, Fishbein MC. Clinical, echocardiographic and pathologic features of aortic wall dehiscence of porcine bioprosthetic valves: a cause of rapidly progressive mitral regurgitation and heart failure after bioprosthetic mitral valve replacement. J Am Soc Echocardiogr 1998;11:720–728.

128. Ha JW, Chang BC, Chung N, Cho SH. Acute severe mitral regurgitation due to unusual detachment of bioprosthetic valve leaflet. Clin Cardiol 1998;23:213–215.

129. Errington M, Bloomfield P, Starkey IR, Shaw TR. Patients' observations of bioprosthetic valve failure: "my heart is honking, doctor." Br Heart J 1990;64:393–394.

130. Voyce SJ, Gore GM, Murphy KR, VanderSalm TJ, Dalen JE. Accurate patient diagnosis of acute porcine valve failure. Arch Int Med 1987;147:585–586.

131. Alam M, Rosman HS, Lakier JB, et al. Doppler and echocardiographic features of normal and dysfunctioning bioprosthetic valves. J Am Coll Cardiol 1987;10:851–858.

132. Alam M, Serwin JB, Rosman HS, Polanco GA, Sun I, Silverman NA. Transesophageal echocardiographic features of normal and dysfunctioning bioprosthetic valves. Am Heart J 1991;121:1149–1155.

133. Calvo OL, Sobrino N, Gamallo O, Olover J, Dominguez F, Iglesias A. Balloon percutaneous valvuloplasty for stenotic bioprosthetic valves in the mitral position. Am J Cardiol 1987;60:736–737.

134. Cox DA, Friedman PL, Selwyn AP, Lee RT, Bittl JA. Improved quality of life after successful valvuloplasty of a stenosed mitral bioprosthesis. Am Heart J 1989;118:839–841.

135. Babic UU, Grujicic S, Vucinic M. Balloon valvuloplasty of mitral prosthesis. Int J Cardiol 1991;30:230–232.

136. Ludman P, Pitt MP. Inoue balloon dilatation of a mitral bioprosthesis. Heart 2000;81:320.

137. Lin PJ, Chang JP, Chu JJ, Chang CH, Hung JS. Balloon valvuloplasty is contraindicated in stenotic mitral bioprostheses. Am Heart J 1994;127:724–726.

138. Waller BF, McKay C, VanTassel J, Allen M. Catheter balloon valvuloplasty of stenotic porcine bioprosthetic valves. Part II: Mechanisms, complications, and recommendations for clinical use. Clin Cardiol 1991;14:764–772.

139. Oliver JM, Gallego P, Gonzalez A, Dominguez FJ, Gamello C, Mesa JM. Bioprosthetic mitral valve thrombosis: clinical profile, transesophageal echocardiographic features, and follow-up after anticoagulant therapy. J Am Soc Echocardiogr 1996;9:691–699.

12

Percutaneous Valvuloplasty in Cardiogenic Shock

Alec Vahanian, MD, Bernard Iung, MD, and Olivier Nallet, MD

CONTENTS

INTRODUCTION

Cardiogenic shock is far less frequently caused by valvular disease than by coronary disease or cardiomyopathies. For two main reasons, however, assessment of the treatment of cardiogenic shock in patients with valvular disease is of interest. First, the frequency of valvular disease remains high in both developing and industrialized countries even though the etiologies are different *(1)*. Second, until the early 1980s, surgery was the only possible treatment, but the introduction of percutaneous techniques has reoriented the treatment of valvular stenoses *(2,3)*. This led to an expectation that the minimally invasive nature of percutaneous techniques would make them more suited to patients with cardiogenic shock than surgery, which carries a very high risk as a result of the advanced stage of the disease and the urgent nature of the interventions.

Fifteen years of experience in tens of thousands of patients has shown that percutaneous mitral commissurotomy (PMC) is an effective treatment for a wide range of patients with mitral stenosis. The risk is low when performed by experienced teams, and follow-up at 10 yrs shows good durability. These encouraging results has led to the increased use of this technique, which now has an important place in interventional cardiology *(4–7)*.

Conversely, after great initial enthusiasm, percutaneous aortic valvuloplasty (PAV) for degenerative aortic stenosis has largely lost favor owing to the high procedural risk and lack of midterm benefit *(3,8)*.

The aim of this chapter is to review current experience with these procedures when performed in emergency circumstances in patients with cardiogenic shock. The chapter will encompass percutaneous valvuloplasty in both mitral stenosis and aortic stenosis

From: *Contemporary Cardiology: Cardiogenic Shock: Diagnosis and Treatment*
Edited by: David Hasdai et al. © Humana Press Inc., Totowa, NJ

and will consider the clinical presentation of patients with cardiogenic shock, the results of percutaneous intervention, and the practical implications.

MITRAL STENOSIS

Rheumatic mitral stenosis continues to be endemic in developing countries where it is the most frequent valve disease. Although the prevalence of rheumatic fever has greatly decreased in Western countries, it continues to represent an important clinical entity resulting from recurrent mitral stenosis after surgical commissurotomy and, even more so, because of emigration from developing countries (1,9).

Clinical Presentation of Patients with Cardiogenic Shock

In the vast majority of cases of mitral stenosis, symptoms may be controlled by medical therapy so that PMC rarely becomes a matter of urgency in patients in shock. This may, however, occur in two main clinical settings:

1. In developing countries, where rheumatic disease has an accelerated course and where there are socioeconomic constraints, it is not uncommon for young patients to present with an advanced stage of the disease with pulmonary edema, low cardiac output, and cardiogenic shock (10–13).
2. In the Western world, despite the fact that the degree of valvular obstruction may be similar, clinical and anatomic features are different. Patients with refractory heart failure are often at an advanced age and in poor general condition with frequent comorbidities. They may be at the end stage of the disease and present with large cardiomegaly, atrial fibrillation, and a high degree of valve deformity and calcification. Left ventricular function may be more severely depressed, and coexistent coronary disease is frequent (14–17).

In both situations, there is often a precipitating event such as respiratory infection, anemia, atrial fibrillation, or, more specifically, pregnancy in developing countries and myocardial infarction in the West. Acute pulmonary edema leading to shock has been described during the procedure of PMC using retrograde transarterial nontransseptal techniques, which have now been abandoned (18). Finally, in some cases, mitral stenosis may go undiagnosed and only be discovered by an echocardiographic examination performed to elucidate the cause of shock or a cardiac arrest.

Results of Percutaneous Mitral Commissurotomy

The precise evaluation of the results of PMC in patients with mitral stenosis and cardiogenic shock is difficult because, despite the large number of publications on PMC, we have only a limited number of series available and a small number of patients. In addition, the definition of shock is often imprecise, and in the published reports, patients with definite shock are often grouped among others with intractable heart failure or critical conditions that do not strictly fulfill the definition of shock.

Overall, it is not possible to analyze separately the results of PMC in elderly patients with mitral stenosis and shock because older age is merged in publications with other high-risk variables such as low ejection fraction or respiratory insufficiency (14–17).

The publications on PMC in patients with cardiogenic shock come mostly from developing countries and report on relatively young patients (Table 1). The largest series is that of Lokhandwala et al. (12), which includes 40 patients who had cardiogenic shock (65%),

Table 1
Percutaneous Mitral Commissurotomy

Authors (ref.)	n	Mean age (yr)	Unfavorable anatomy[a] (%)	Mortality (%)	Secondary MVR (%)	Follow-up (mo)	Late results
Lokhandwala et al. (12)	40 (26)[b]	40	40	35	12.5	8	2 Late MVR, 19/20 NYHA CL I/III, 4 unknown
Patel et al. (11)	12 (3)[b]	29	60	0	0	10	1 sudden death, 1 MVR, 10 NYHA CL I/II
Wu et al. (10)	10 (4)[b]	38	30	20	20	26	6 NYHA CL I/II
Chow and Chow (13)	(1)[b]	59	100	0	0	6	NYHA CL II
Goldman et al. (19)	(1)[b]	49	0	0	0	—	—

Abbreviation: MVR = mitral valve replacement.

[a] Unfavorable anatomy = echo score >8 or valve calcification.

[b] Proven cardiogenic shock.

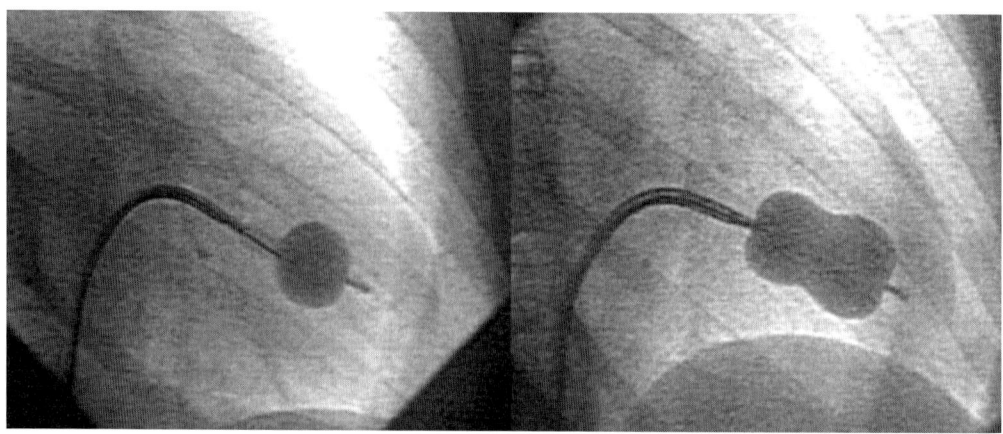

Fig. 1. Percutaneous mitral commissurotomy using an Inoue balloon.

cardiac arrest (28%), or pulmonary edema refractory to medical treatment (7%) and underwent emergency PMC. The second largest is by Patel et al. *(11)* and deals with 12 younger patients with intractable heart failure, among whom three required mechanical ventilatory support. Finally, Wu et al. *(10)* discussed 10 patients with severe pulmonary edema; 1 was moribund and 4 required a mechanical respirator. The other series are case reports *(13,19)*. Notably, five cases concern pregnant patients *(10,11)*.

Taking into account the limitations previously mentioned, these preliminary reports suggest the following:

1. Emergency PMC is feasible, even though its success rate is somewhat lower than in scheduled cases. The performance of the procedure in patients with cardiogenic shock has a number of specific features.
   • Before the procedure, transesophageal echocardiography is recommended in order to exclude the presence of left atrial thrombosis because these patients are at high risk of embolism.
   • Performance of PMC is often a technical challenge at each step. The transseptal puncture is more difficult because of the large dilatation of the left and right atria as well as thoracic deformities. In patients with severe orthopnea, it may be necessary to make the puncture with the patient in a semirecumbent position *(10)*. Crossing the valve and stabilizing the balloon are more challenging as a result of the distorted valve and subvalvular anatomy. Inflation of the balloon may be poorly tolerated in patients with poor hemodynamic condition and possible associated coronary or carotid disease.
   • For successful performance of emergency PMC, the following measures are recommended to make this difficult procedure safe, effective, and quick. The procedure should only be performed by experienced interventionists and should be shortened by using mainly echocardiographic monitoring and by excluding full right-heart catheterization, cardiac output measurements, and left ventriculography. The Inoue balloon (Fig. 1), which has a short inflation–deflation time and makes the procedure simpler and safer, is the device of choice over the double-balloon technique (Fig. 2) or new, still unevaluated devices such as the multitrack balloon *(20)* or the metallic commis-

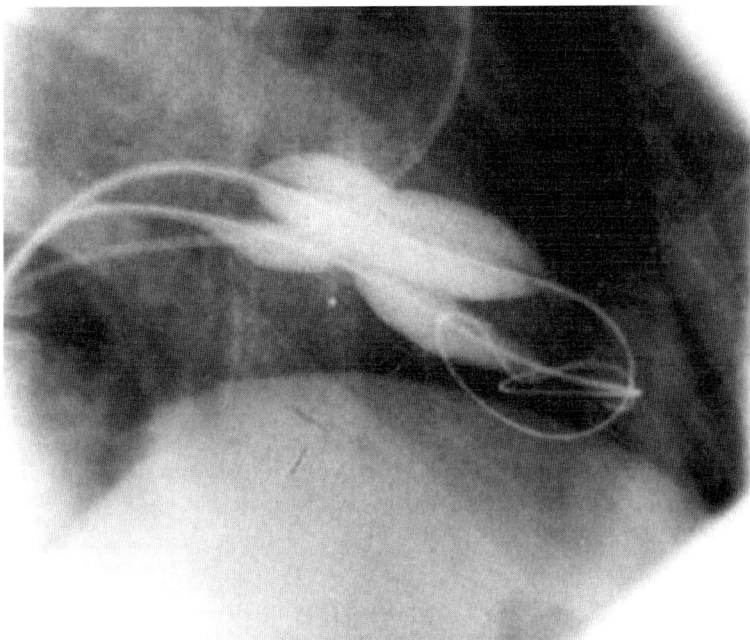

Fig. 2. Percutaneous mitral commissurotomy using a double balloon.

surotome *(21)*. Finally, the goal of the procedure should be to significantly improve valve function and not to aim for a perfect result because of the inherent risk of traumatic mitral regurgitation with catastrophic consequences.

- After the procedure, management of these patients may remain difficult as a result of cardiac cachexia, severe pulmonary hypertension, respiratory infections, and impaired renal and cerebral function. The problems are magnified in cases where PMC fails or if a complication occurs.

2. Percutaneous mitral commissurotomy carries an acceptable risk. No fatalities occurred in the series from Patel et al. *(11)*, but mortality rose to 35% in that of Lokhandwala et al. *(12)*, which included somewhat older patients at a more advanced stage of the disease. In the latter report, as in the NHLBI cooperative study *(22)*, unfavorable anatomy, high pulmonary pressures, and lower cardiac output were predictors of immediate death. Half of the deaths in the Lokhandwala et al. study were related to unsatisfactory results or complications such as mitral regurgitation. Other deaths occurred despite a satisfactory improvement in valve function, reflecting the advanced stage of the disease. Finally, the outcome of the pregnant patients was good, and PMC allowed uneventful delivery *(10,11)*.

3. Percutaneous mitral commissurotomy provides moderate to significant improvement in valve function (Table 2). Modest improvement may be the result of unfavorable anatomy and of a deliberate decision to prioritize safety over efficacy.

4. After the procedure, the majority of patients improved functionally. In the young population of Patel et al. *(11)*, even a modest increase in the valve area resulted in a midterm clinical improvement and a decrease in pulmonary hypertension. In the other cases, either secondary surgery was necessary because of complications or unsatisfactory results, or incapacity remained because of associated disease or because hemodynamic improvement was limited by extensive valve deformity and calcification.

Table 2
Valve Area Before and After PMC

Authors (ref.)	n	Before PMC (cm²)	After PMC (cm²)
Lohandwala et al. (12)	40	0.7	1.5
Patel et al. (11)	12	0.7	1.4
Wu et al. (10)	10	0.8	2
Chow and Chow (13)	1	0.5	1.1
Goldman et al. (19)	1	0.8	1.5

Overall, the analysis of these results must take into account unfavorable characteristics of patients and the alternative risk of surgery. The patients in question combine several of the factors identified as predictors of poor immediate and long term results after PMC: atrial fibrillation, history of previous commissurotomy, high functional class, unfavorable anatomy, small valve area, severe tricuspid regurgitation, high pulmonary pressures, and less than optimal immediate results (6,7).

On the other hand, these patients were also at very high risk for surgery; surgery was denied by anesthesiologists and surgeons in most of the cases reported. The parameters previously mentioned, as well as pulmonary hypertension, low ejection fraction, or associated coronary disease are most strongly associated with an adverse outcome after surgery (23,24). Depending on the presenting characteristics, the mortality of mitral valve replacement in the elderly ranges from 17% to 54%. In addition, the emergency nature of the intervention further increases the operative risk: In a recent survey, the operative mortality for mitral valve replacement was 4% for elective surgery, rising to 43% in salvage operations (25). Similarly, the operative mortality for closed surgical commissurotomy in this group may be as high as 25% (26).

Practical Implications

The limited available data and the absence of randomized studies make it difficult to evaluate the results with certainty and establish indications. With these limitations in mind, we can make the following comments on the indications for PMC.

The first step is to exclude contraindications. Here, where surgery is contraindicated or very high risk, the contraindications for the procedure are more limited than usual. The most important is the presence of a thrombus in the left atrium (4,5). A contraindication is self-evident if the thrombus is floating, localized in the left atrial cavity or on the interatrial septum. In the setting of shock, we consider performing PMC if the thrombus is located in the left atrial appendage and not protruding and when using an Inoue balloon. PMC can be performed in cases with moderate mitral regurgitation if the stenosis is tight and the overall anatomy satisfactory, but a severe regurgitation should be considered a contraindication. Massive valvular calcification is a relative contraindication. In such cases, PMC can be attempted as a tentative bridge to surgery if other characteristics allow for it.

Percutaneous mitral commissurotomy is a viable option in young patients because good immediate and midterm results can be obtained, despite a high immediate risk.

This is of particular interest during pregnancy. In such cases, even if the initial results are suboptimal, PMC can be a useful life-saving procedure and serves as a bridge to lower-risk secondary surgery. In the elderly population, the decision is much more difficult because data are lacking *(27)*. Some offer PMC despite the high risk because unexpected good results may be obtained and individual results remain largely unpredictable *(16)*. The objective here is to obtain, at best, a modest improvement in life expectancy. We favor an individualized approach, taking into account the multifactorial nature of the prediction of the results of PMC. The procedure should not be performed in elderly patients at the end stage of the disease, where all the predictors of poor results *(6,7)*, both anatomic and clinical, are present. Here, the procedure is highly likely to be unsuccessful, the risk is very high, and secondary surgery cannot be considered. In contrast, PMC seems to be a useful, even if palliative treatment, as a bridge to surgery in patients with unfavorable anatomy if all other characteristics are favorable *(28)*.

AORTIC STENOSIS

Severe aortic stenosis is the most frequent valve disease in Western countries. It is now mostly degenerative in origin and affects elderly patients. The occurrence of cardiogenic shock in aortic stenosis is rare but associated with catastrophic consequences *(29)*.

Clinical Presentation of Cardiogenic Shock

In patients with severe aortic stenosis, cardiogenic shock may occur at the end stage of the disease. The condition may deteriorate continuously or be precipitated by a complication that may be cardiac, such as atrial fibrillation or acute myocardial infarction, noncardiac (e.g., a respiratory infection), or a complication of an invasive examination *(30)*. Aortic stenosis can result in cardiogenic shock based on other causative factors, such as left ventricular failure resulting from excessively high wall stress and afterload mismatch or more severe left ventricular failure despite less severe aortic stenosis *(31)*, associated coronary artery disease leading to acute myocardial infarction *(32)*, or ischemic cardiomyopathy. Furthermore, hypotension and/or coronary disease could initiate a vicious circle of myocardial ischemia, leading to an exacerbation of left ventricular dysfunction, which could further reduce myocardial perfusion and increase myocardial ischemia. As an illustration, 52% of the patients in the largest series of PAV for cardiogenic shock had non-Q myocardial infarction at admission *(33)*. Finally, aortic stenosis may be discovered only at the onset of shock or after cardiac arrest, the diagnosis being made by echocardiography or suggested by the presence of valvular calcification.

Results of Percutaneous Aortic Valvuloplasty

Aortic stenosis complicated by cardiogenic shock is a rare clinical situation. In large series of PAV *(33,34)*, patients with shock account for only 6% of cases. The results in this specific subgroup have been described only in short series *(33–37)* and a few case reports *(38–41)* (Table 3). The largest series included 21 patients with strict criteria for shock *(33)*, whereas that by Cribier in which the criteria for shock were less precisely defined *(37)*, included 10 patients. Contrary to mitral stenosis, the patients included in these series were almost exclusively elderly with severe comorbidities.

Table 3
Percutaneous Aortic Valvuloplasty

Authors (ref.)	n	Mean age (yr)	Comorbidity (%)	Hospital mortality (%)	Secondary AVR (%)	Follow-up (mo)	Late results
Moreno et al. (33)	21	74	100	43	33	6–18	Survival 38±11%
Cribier et al. (37)	10	69	70	20	75	27	No late death
Smedira et al. (39)	5	29–88[a]	1 Acute MI	0	100	—	5 Good postop outcomes
Losordo et al. (30)	3	—[a]	1 Cancer	—	33	11	1 Death (1 wk), 2 NYHA Class II
Desnoyer et al. (38)	2	75–84	—	—	—	5.8	2 NYHA Class II
Whisenant et al. (32)	1	87	Acute MI	0	—	6	Death
Friedman et al. (40)	1	70	—	0	—	3	NYHA Class II
Bhatia et al. (41)	1	42	—	0	100	6	NYHA Class II

Abbreviation: AVR = aortic valve replacement.

[a] Unkown.

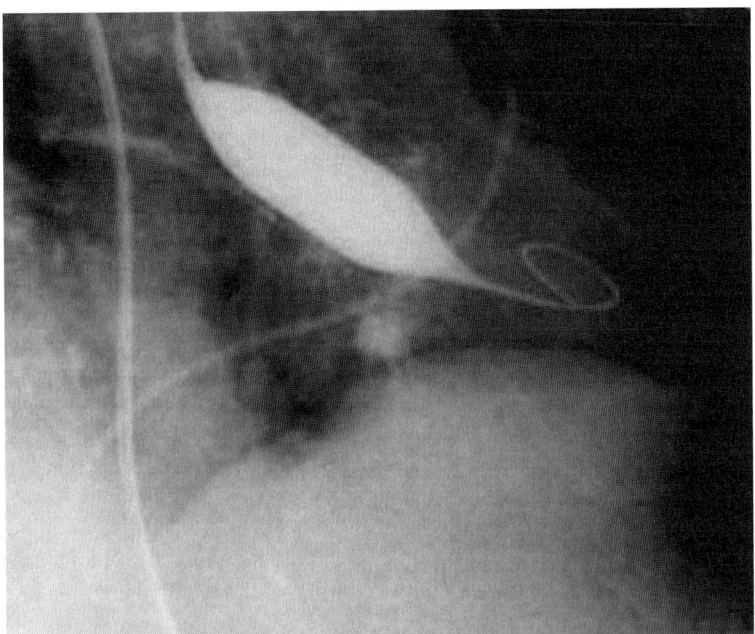

Fig. 3. Percutaneous aortic valvuloplasty.

The results of the available studies suggest the following:

1. Percutaneous aortic valvuloplasty is feasible in critically ill patients. The following points can be made regarding the technical aspects (Fig. 3):
   - An intra-aortic balloon pump is useful for stabilizing patients with left ventricular failure and frequent concomitant coronary disease.
   - In patients with shock, the procedure should follow the same principles of speed and safety as PMC. This may be technically challenging owing to many interventionists' lack of experience in the following: (1) Crossing the severely stenotic aortic valve, which is now seldom necessary during degenerative calcific stenosis, because of the accuracy of echocardiography. This is the most difficult technical part of the procedure because elderly patients frequently have tortuous iliac arteries and aorta and a tight and distorted aortic orifice. (2) Lack of experience in performing PAV, which has been abandoned in most centers and is very seldom used in others. The difficulty is further increased by the emergency nature of the intervention. Therefore, because the reported results came from experienced centers at a time when PAV was more popular, they might not be applicable in real-world current practice.
2. As is usually the case with PAV, the procedure results in a modest improvement in valve function (Table 4). This may, however, improve clinical condition: Cribier's series shows that shock signs disappeared in all patients after several hours *(37)*. In cases reported by Moreno, 90% of survivors after dilatation were weaned off inotropic agents within 1–24 h *(33)*.
3. Immediate mortality remains high. Deaths are related to cardiac causes and to major comorbid conditions. Mortality figures were two times higher in Moreno's series and in the NHLBI registry than in Cribier's series. These somewhat conflicting results may be

Table 4
Valve Area Before and After PAV

Authors (ref.)	n	Before PAV (cm^2)	After PAV (cm^2)
Moreno et al. (33)	21	0.5	0.8
Cribier et al. (37)	10	0.5	0.9
Smedira et al. (39)	5	0.6	0.9
Losordo et al. (30)	3	0.4	0.7
Desnoyers et al. (38)	2	0.2	0.6
Friedman et al. (40)	1	0.4	0.8

explained by the younger age and lower incidence of comorbidities in the latter. Morbidity was also high, mainly related to severe vascular complications and stroke.

4. At midterm follow-up, the overall outcome was poor because in the largest series, survival was 38% at 27 mo (33). Two-thirds of the deaths were cardiac in origin, whereas the others were due to comorbidities. However, in selected survivors, PAV may allow for a secondary surgery with satisfactory results: No operative deaths occurred in a total of 17 patients operated on from 6 d to 18 mo after PAV, and 15 of them (88%) survived in good functional condition at midterm (33,37,39,41).

5. Finally, there have been three reported cases of shock complicating catheterization in patients who were previously in a stable condition. PAV improved the patients' condition in all and enabled successful valve replacement in two; the last patient died from extra-cardiac causes several days later (30).

On the whole, these results are worse than the overall findings after PAV. However, as was the case for PMC, the patients presented with several high-risk characteristics that significantly worsen the immediate and short-term outcome of PAV: advanced age, low output, low ejection fraction, and concomitant coronary artery disease (34–36).

Aortic valve replacement may be performed with a low mortality rate, good palliation of symptoms, and satisfactory survival in selected patients after PAV (42). The preliminary results observed with valve replacement following "bridging PAV" in patients with shock are encouraging, but confirmatory larger series are needed that include patients with a precise assessment of the risk of surgery and with strict criteria for shock.

Generally speaking, surgery is the most appropriate treatment for aortic stenosis. The operative risk is low; after the operative period, results are good; and most of the survivors are in a good functional state (43–45). In addition, surgery enables the correction of severe associated coronary disease.

In patients with cardiogenic shock, there are limited data (mostly old) that consistently show that aortic valve replacement carries a very high risk with a perioperative mortality ranging from 29% to 50% (43–47). This high mortality rate results from the high-risk characteristics of the patients and the salvage or emergency nature of the operation, which further increases the operative risk. However, with the most recent improvements in surgical and postoperative care, better results were recently achieved involving younger patients who had few comorbidities (48).

At the present time, it remains difficult to compare the results of surgery with those of PAV because most patients who underwent PAV generally had a worse cardiac condition and were refused surgery because of comorbidities. This difficulty is particularly the case for cardiogenic shock where data are limited and lack precision.

Practical Conclusions

The question today is whether or not there is still a place for PAV *(49,50)*. Most groups have abandoned the technique, whereas for others, it would appear that there is a limited role for PAV in some circumstances, one of which is cardiogenic shock.

Percutaneous aortic valvuloplasty alone could not be considered as a satisfactory option because of its limited efficacy on valve function and the fact that it does not cure associated coronary disease. The recent ACC/AHA guidelines for the management of patients with valvular heart disease state that "PAV can be proposed as a 'bridge' to surgery in hemodynamically unstable patients who are at high risk for valve replacement" *(51)*. This recommendation has a grade IIa and is supported by only a few data. To provide a definite answer, PAV followed by surgery should be evaluated in a randomized way as an alternative to immediate surgery in patients with strict criteria of shock and a quantitative assessment of the surgical risk *(52)*. Unfortunately, such a study is unlikely to be conducted.

In our opinion, "bridging PAV" has a limited role, even more so because of the general disaffection for the technique. Its indication can only be decided after close consultation among cardiologists, surgeons, interventionists, and, whenever possible, the patient or the relatives. "Bridging PAV" could be proposed if all of the following criteria are met: institutions have experience in PAV; life expectancy is otherwise acceptable or, at a minimum, uncertain; temporary contraindication for surgery exists resulting from an acute decompensation; and patients have progressive renal, hepatic, or respiratory failure. If the procedure is to be successful, aortic valve surgery with or without bypass grafting should be performed early.

On the other hand, medical treatment is probably the best option in definitively inoperable patients (e.g., frail octogenarians or those with malignant disease, severe respiratory insufficiency, or severe left ventricular dysfunction resulting from a large myocardial scar from myocardial infarction). In other patients, surgery should be considered whenever possible.

The limited experience in the combined use of PAV and coronary angioplasty, in general, and in cardiogenic shock patients, in particular, does not allow us to draw many conclusions. These conclusions are limited to a primarily elderly population with calcific aortic stenosis. However, PAV might be a useful option for younger patients with rheumatic disease, especially if surgery is not immediately available.

CONCLUSIONS

The available data on percutaneous valvuloplasty in patients with valve stenosis and cardiogenic shock are very limited. The few interventions performed show that percutaneous interventions are feasible, but they are insufficient to evaluate the results accurately and establish indications.

Valvuloplasty appears to have a place, if limited, in the emergent treatment of mitral and aortic stenosis. The different indications for PMC and PAV reflect current opinion regarding their applicability. The need for PMC is infrequent, but, when required, could represent an effective lifesaving treatment, mostly in young patients. On the other hand, the future of PAV even in patients with shock is more uncertain; at a maximum, it could serve as a bridge to surgery in selected patients.

REFERENCES

1. Soler-Soler J, Galve E. Worldwide perspective of valve disease. Heart 2000;83:721–725.
2. Inoue K, Owaki T, Nakamura T, et al. Clinical application of transvenous mitral commissurotomy by a new balloon catheter. J Thorac Cardiovasc Surg 1985;87:394–402.
3. Cribier A, Savin T, Saoudi N, et al. Percutaneous transluminal valvuloplasty of acquired aortic stenosis in elderly patients: an alternative to valve replacement? Lancet 1986;11:63–7.
4. Vahanian A. Balloon valvuloplasty. Heart 2001;85:223–228.
5. Inoue K, Hung JS. Percutaneous transvenous mitral commissurotomy: the Far East experience. In: Topol EJ, ed. Textbook of Interventional Cardiology. WB Saunders, Philadelphia, 1994; pp. 1226–1243.
6. Iung B, Cormier B, Ducimetiere P, et al. Immediate results of percutaneous mitral commissurotomy. Circulation 1996;94:2124–2130.
7. Iung B, Garbarz E, Michaud P, et al. Late results of percutaneous mitral commissurotomy in a series of 1024 patients: Analysis of late clinical deterioration: frequency, anatomic findings, and predictive factors. Circulation 1999;99:3272–3278.
8. Rahimtoola SH. Catheter balloon valvuloplasty for severe calcific aortic stenosis: a limited role. J Am Coll Cardiol 1994;203:1076–1078.
9. Carroll JD, Feldman T. Percutaneous mitral balloon valvotomy and the new demographics of mitral stenosis. JAMA 1993;270:1731–1736.
10. Wu JJ, Chern MS, Yeh KH, et al. Urgent/emergent percutaneous transvenous mitral commissurotomy. Cathet Cardiovasc Diagn 1994;31:18–22.
11. Patel JJ, Munclinger MJ, Mitha AS, et al. Percutaneous balloon dilatation of the mitral valve in critically ill young patients with intractable heart failure. Br Heart J 1995;73:555–558.
12. Lokhandwala YL, Banker D, Vora AM, et al. Emergent balloon mitral valvotomy in patients presenting with cardiac arrest, cardigenic shock or refractory pulmonary edema. J Am Coll Cardiol 1998;32:154–158.
13. Chow WH, Chow TC. Percutaneous balloon mitral valvotomy as a bridge to elective mitral valve replacement. Cathet Cardiovasc Diagn 1998;45:102.
14. Iung B, Cormier B, Farah B, et al. Percutaneous mitral commissurotomy in the elderly. Eur Heart J 1995;16:1092–1099.
15. Lefèvre T, Bonan R, Serra A, et al. Percutaneous mitral valvuloplasty in surgical high risk patients. J Am Coll Cardiol 1991;17:348–354.
16. Sutaria N, Elder AT, Shaw TRD. Long term outcome of percutaneous mitral balloon valvotomy in patients aged 70 and over. Heart 2000;83:433–438.
17. Shaw TRD, McAreavey D, Essop AR, et al. Percutaneous balloon dilatation of the mitral valve in patients who were unsuitable for surgical treatment. Br Heart J 1992;67:454–459.
18. Romero M, Melina F, Suarez de Lezo J, et al. Transarterial mitral valvuloplasty in conditions of acute pulmonary oedema. Am Heart J 1990;119:1416–1419.
19. Goldman JH, Slade A, Clague J. Cardiogenic shock to mitral stenosis treated by balloon mitral valvuloplasty. Cathet Cardiovasc Diagn 1998;43:195–197.
20. Bonhoeffer P, Piechaud JF, Sidi D, et al. Mitral dilatation with the multi-track system: an alternative approach. Cathet Cardiovasc Diagn 1995;36:189–193.
21. Cribier A, Eltchaninoff H, Koning R, et al. Percutaneous mechanical mitral commissurotomy with a newly designed metallic valvotome: immediate results of the initial experience in 153 patients. Circulation 1999;99:793–799.
22. NHLBI Balloon valvuloplasty registry report on immediate and 30-day follow-up results. Multicentre experience with balloon mitral commissurotomy. Circulation 1992;85:448–461.
23. Christakis GT, Kormos RL, Weisel RD, et al. Morbidity and mortality in mitral valve surgery. Circulation 1985;72(Suppl II):I-I120–I-I128.
24. Jamieson WRE, Burr LH, Munro AI, et al. Cardiac valve replacement in the elderly: clinical performance of biological prostheses. Ann Thorac Surg 1989;48:173–185.
25. Edwards FH, Peterson ED, Coombs LP, et al. Prediction of operative mortality after valve replacement surgery. J Am Coll Cardiol 2001;37:885–892.
26. Barlow JB. Surgical aspects of mitral valve disease. In: Barlow JB, ed. Perspective on the Mitral Valve. FA Davis, Philadelphia, 1987, pp. 247–250.

27. Hildick-Smith DJ, Shapiro, LM. Balloon mitral valvuloplasty in the elderly. Heart 2000;83:374–375.
28. Iung B, Garbarz G, Doutrelant L, et al. Late results of PMC for calcific mitral stenosis. Am J Cardiol 2000;85:1308–1314.
29. Turina J, Hess O, Krayenbuehl F, et al. Spontaneous course of aortic valve disease. Eur Heart J 1987;8:471–483.
30. Losordo DW, Ramaswamy K, Rosenfeld K, et al. Use of emergency balloon dilation to reverse acute hemodynamic decompensation developing during diagnostic catheterisation for aortic stenosis (bail-out valvuloplasty). Am J Cardiol 1989;63:388–389.
31. Carabello BA, Green LH, Grossman W, et al. Hemodynamic determinants of prognosis of aortic valve replacement in critical aortic stenosis and advanced congestive heart failure. Circulation 1980;62:42–48.
32. Whisenant B, Sweeney J, Ports TA. Combined PTCA and aortic valvuloplasty for acute myocardial infarction complicated by severe aortic stenosis and cardiogenic shock. Cathet Cardiovasc Diagn 1997;42:283–285.
33. Moreno PR, Jang I-K, Newell JB, et al. The role of percutaneous aortic balloon valvuloplasty in patients with cardiogenic shock and critical aortic stenosis. J Am Coll Cardiol 1994;5:1071–1075.
34. Percutaneous balloon aortic valvuloplasty. Acute and 30-day follow-up results in 674 patients from the NHLBI balloon valvuloplasty registry. Circulation 1991;84:2383–2397.
35. McKay KG. The Mansfield Scientific Aortic Valvuloplasty Registry: overview of acute hemodynamic results and procedural complications. J Am Coll Cardiol 1991;2:485–491.
36. O'Neill WW. Predictors of long-term survival after percutaneous aortic valvuloplasty: report of the Mansfield Scientific Balloon Aortic Valvuloplasty Registry. J Am Coll Cardiol 1991;1:193–198.
37. Cribier A, Remadi F, Koning R, et al. Emergency balloon valvuloplasty as initial treatment of patients with aortic stenosis and cardiogenic shock. N Engl J Med 1992;326–646.
38. Desnoyers MR, Salem DN, Rosenfeld K, et al. Treatment of cardiogenic shock by emergency aortic balloon valvuloplasty. Ann Intern Med 1998;108:833–835.
39. Smedira NG, Ports TA, Merrick SH, et al. Balloon aortic valvuloplasty as a bridge to aortic valve replacement in critically ill patients. Ann Thorac Surg 1993;55:914–916.
40. Friedman HZ, Cragg DR, O'Neill WW. Cardiac resuscitation using emergency aortic balloon valvulo-plasty. Am J Cardiol 1989;63:387.
41. Bhatia A, Kumar A, Seth A, et al. Successful aortic balloon valvuloplasty in critical aortic stenosis with shock. Cathet Cardiovasc Diagn 1993;29:296–297.
42. Lieberman EB, Wilson JS, Harrison K, et al. Aortic valve replacement in adults after balloon aortic valvuloplasty. Circulation 1994;90(Suppl II):II-205–II-208.
43. Kirklin JW. Aortic valve disease. In: Kirklin JW, Barrat-Boyes B, eds. Cardiac Surgery: Morphology, Diagnostic Criteria, Natural History, Techniques, Results and Indications. Churchill Livingstone, New York, 1993, p. 528.
44. Logeais Y, Langanay T, Roussin R, et al. Surgery for aortic stenosis in elderly patients: as study of surgical risk and predictive factors. Circulation 1994;90:2891–2898.
45. Culliford A, Galloway A, Colvin S, et al. Aortic valve replacement for aortic stenosis in persons aged 80 years and over. Am J Cardiol 1991;67:1256–1260.
46. Scott WC, Miller DC, Haverich A, et al. Determinants of operative mortality in patients undergoing aortic valve replacement. Discriminate analysis of 1470 operations. J Thorac Cardiovasc Surg 1985;89:400–413.
47. Hutter A Jr, De Sanctis R, Nathan M, et al. Aortic valve surgery as an emergency procedure. Circulation 1970;51:623–627.
48. Christ G, Zehetgruber M, Mundigler G, et al. Emergency aortic valve replacement for critical aortic stenosis. A lifesaving treatment for patients with cardiogenic shock and multiple organ failure. Intensive Care Med 1997;23:297–300.
49. Vahanian A. Valvuloplasty. In: Topol EJ, ed. Comprehensive Cardiovascular Medicine. Lippincott–Raven, Philadelphia, 1988.
50. Wang A, Harrison K, Bashore T. Balloon aortic valvuloplasty. Prog Cardiovasc Dis 1997;40:27–36.
51. Bonow RO, Carabello B, de Leon AC Jr, et al. ACC/AHA guidelines for the management of patients with valvular heart disase: executive summary. A report of the American College of Cardiology/American Heart Association Task Force on Practice Guidelines. Circulation 1998;98:1949–1984.
52. Roques F, Nashef SAM, Michel P, et al. Risk factors and outcome in European cardiac surgery: analysis of the EuroSCORE multinational database of 19030 patients. Eur J Cardiothorac Surg 1999;15:816–823.

13

Operative Management
of Nonischemic Cardiogenic Shock

David G. Cable, MD,
and Joseph A. Dearani, MD

CONTENTS

INTRODUCTION

The spectrum of presentations for cardiogenic shock resulting from nonischemic etiologies can range from extremis, where there is little time for preparation or thought before intervening surgically, to cardiogenic failure that can be temporized with measures such as inotropic support or assist devices, allowing more preparation and planning before surgery. These diverse etiologies range from traumatic to iatrogenic and include infectious, ischemic, and degenerative causes. (For a detailed discussion of ischemic valvular disease, see Chapter 11.) This chapter will review penetrating and blunt cardiac trauma, iatrogenic cardiac injuries, and obstructive and infectious valvular heart disease. Various operative techniques required by each entity will be reviewed.

TRAUMATIC HEART DISEASE

Operative intervention for an individual patient in cardiogenic shock mandates expedient investigation of all contributing pathologic processes, prompt transport to the operative suite, and the appropriate delivery of available surgical techniques in a timely manner. Conceptualization of these logistical restraints is highlighted when a patient has sustained multiple trauma. Although this volume focuses on the cardiac pathophysiology, one must be cognizant of concomitant injuries, in particular those of the central nervous system, as they may dramatically alter the therapeutic plan.

From: *Contemporary Cardiology: Cardiogenic Shock: Diagnosis and Treatment*
Edited by: David Hasdai et al. © Humana Press Inc., Totowa, NJ

Traumatic injury to the heart can be classified according to the mechanism of injury, *penetrating* or *blunt* trauma. The incidence of both has increased in recent decades, continued crime and violence and rapid emergency medical transport systems have contributed to the increase in patients with penetrating cardiac injury who reach the hospital, whereas high-speed motor vehicle accidents have contributed to the increasing frequency of blunt trauma. Each has a different clinical presentation and may require dramatically different operative approaches; thus, each will be discussed separately. In addition, each injury associated with blunt cardiac trauma will be reviewed separately because most also involve additional medical personnel (general surgery, orthopedic surgery, neurosurgery, etc.) and require thoughtful planning of intervention.

Penetrating Cardiac Injury

The mechanism of a penetrating cardiac injury dictates the location of affected heart chambers. It is not surprising that the right ventricle, secondary to its anterior position, is the most commonly involved cardiac chamber. In a collective review of 1802 patients, Karrell et al. identified right ventricular injury in 43%, left ventricular injury in 33%, and atrial injury in 21% collectively *(1)*. The remainder had had injury to the great vessels. In another review of 109 patients, Attar et al. identified right ventricular injury in 47%, left ventricular in 28%, and atrial in 14% of patients *(2)*. Fully 12% of patients had mutliple chambers injured.

Penetrating injury to the heart will typically present in one of two manners; tamponade or hemorrhage. In stab wounds, pericardial tamponade predominates, with 80–90% of cases in most series presenting with signs of tamponade *(1,3,4)*. The prevailing opinion is that adjacent pericardial fat and clot formation seal the pericardial tear, localizing the extent of hemorrhage. However, this is dependent on the location of injury. Demetriades and Vander Veen noted that whereas 93% of right ventricular wounds presented with tamponade, only 43% of left ventricular wounds presented in a like fashion *(5)*. In contrast, gunshot wounds will present with tamponade in only 20% *(6,7)*, with the predominant hemorrhage varying from clinically overt to clinically ambiguous.

The importance of presentation is underscored by the rapidity at which surgery must be performed. As in all traumatized patients, the Advanced Trauma Life Support Management Protocols formulated by the American College of Surgeons should be instituted *(8)*. Rapid deterioration of a patient with initial signs of life may mandate an emergency room thoracotomy, performed most expeditiously through a left anterolateral approach. The intercostal space (usually fourth) is opened sharply, a thoracotomy retractor is inserted, and the lung is retracted laterally. A longitudinal incision in the pericardium preserves the phrenic nerve posteriorly. Direct finger pressure may allow transport to the operative suite or, at times, direct suture repair of the cardiac wound is required in the emergency room. If injuries to the right atrium or posterior mediastinum are identified, the incision can be extended across the sternum. It is our practice to clamp the aorta to facilitate volume resuscitation and improve blood flow to the coronary and cerebral circulations.

The diagnosis of cardiac injury should be suspected in any patient with penetrating injury to the chest, neck, back, or abdomen. Injuries to the precordium, epigastrium, or superior mediastinum are in the "danger zone" and are most likely to involve the heart *(2,9)*. When vital signs are stable, transthoracic echocardiography has been used with increasing frequency to aid in the diagnosis of injury to the heart *(10–13)*. Although findings of pericardial tamponade or valvular or septal defects are often apparent, a normal echocardiogram does not exclude an intrapericardial injury *(10)*. If the diagnosis is in doubt or if any degree of pericardial fluid on echocardiography is associated with an unstable patient, then a subxiphoid pericardial window can detect the presence of blood within the pericardial space. A small, midline incision is made inferior to the xiphoid, the rectus sheath is entered, and dissection is carried cephalad. Meticulous hemostatis is required so that, upon opening the pericardium, return of hemorrhagic fluid correctly identifies the cardiac injury. If cardiac damage is found, the incision can rapidly be converted to a midline sternotomy.

The operative approach for penetrating injuries is ideally through a median sternotomy. This allows full exposure with access to all cardiac chambers, especially the right atrium and right ventricle, the most commonly involved, as well as access for cardiopulmonary bypass. Cardiopulmonary bypass is used only when hemodynamics do not tolerate positioning of the heart or, rarely, when intracardiac valvular or septal injuries or major coronary arterial injuries are identified. The majority of distal coronary artery injuries in this predominantly young population can be ligated without significant detriment. Anterior descending coronary artery injuries occur most frequently and should be repaired, usually with bypass grafting. Fistulas may also occur. Management has typically involved ligation proximal and distal to the fistula and distal bypass grafting.

When lacerations to the right or left ventricle are present, attempts are made to preserve coronary perfusion when suture repairing these lacerations. Chamber lacerations are typically closed with pledgetted mattress sutures. If a coronary artery is near the laceration, the suture is passed deep to the arterial course, preserving truncal flow while ligating small perforators (Fig. 1).

Blunt Cardiac Injury

Because the heart is surrounded by the bony thorax and soft tissue and is suspended in the middle of the mediastinum, injury can occur by direct anterior compression of the sternum (or between the sternum and vertebral column) against the heart; a classic example is the "steering wheel injury." The heart and, more commonly, the great vessels arising from the heart are also at risk for "tears" from sudden deceleration injuries. Cardiac chamber rupture can also occur from blunt trauma. Atrial rupture may occur from compressive forces to the heart at the end of ventricular systole when the atria are filled and the ventricles contracted. Vena caval and pulmonary vascular pressures may be significantly elevated from concomitant compressive forces to both the abdomen and chest *(14)*. The result is increased atrial pressure at the time of atrioventricular valve closure with rupture of the thin atrial wall. In contrast, ventricular rupture likely occurs from sudden compressive forces at the end of diastole when the ventricle is full *(15)*. Free wall rupture is more common than septal rupture (early and delayed) *(16)*.

The majority of blunt cardiac injury is the result of motor vehicle accidents. During a 3-yr period, 515 patients sustained blunt cardiac trauma out of 5378 admission to the Maryland Institute for Emergency Medical Services Systems, with motor vehicle accidents accounting for 71% of mechanisms and pedestrian accidents accounting for only 10% *(17)*. Fully 28% of patients were hypotensive on arrival and 6% had no pulse. In contrast to penetrating trauma, only 16% of the patients in this series of blunt cardiac trauma had sustained an isolated injury; in fact, 48% of patients had three or more organ systems traumatized, including the thoracic injury.

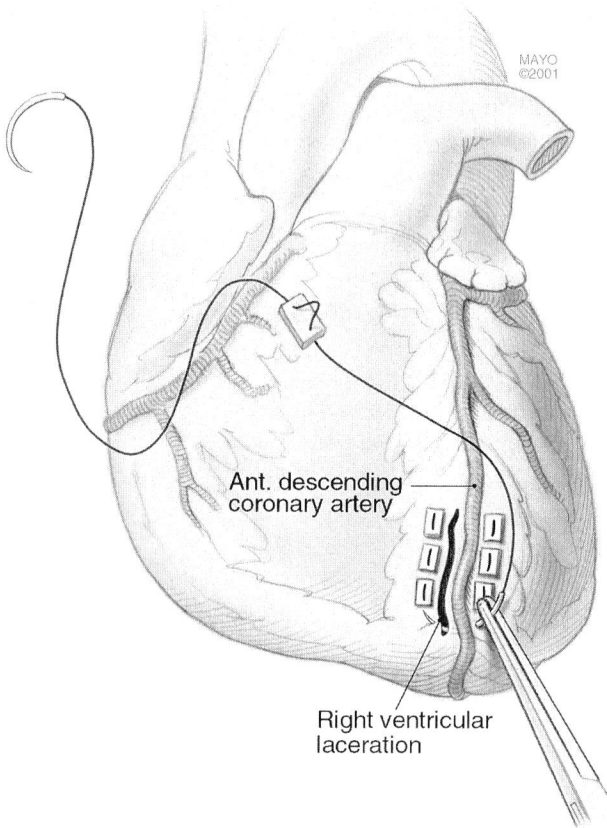

Fig. 1. Lacerations near an important coronary artery require passage of the suture deep to the arterial course to provide hemostatis. Although these maneuvers preserve truncal flow, small branches will be ligated. A resulting myocardial infarction is inevitable.

MYOCARDIAL CONTUSION

A diagnosis of contusion must be considered for any patient sustaining blunt cardiac trauma. For completeness, some points should be addressed, as contusions may coincide with other cardiac injuries. The most common adverse sequela of myocardial contusion is arrhythmia, and McLean et al. noted significant ventricular arrhythmias in 9% of 312 patients with myocardial contusions (18). Electrocardiography (19) and echocardiography (20) typically make the diagnosis. Creatinine kinase levels do not significantly correlate with myocardial contusion, likely the result of the polytraumatized state and associated skeletal muscle injury (21), but recent reports suggest troponin levels may be helpful in the diagnosis (22,23). The few patients who develop cardiac failure as a result of myocardial contusion typically respond to inotropic or intra-aortic balloon pump support.

SEPTAL DEFECTS

Despite the seemingly protected nature of the atrial and ventricular septums, they can sustain injury in blunt cardiac trauma with some frequency. In an animal study of

Table 1
Representative Traumatic Tricuspid Valve Injury Reported in the Literature

Author (ref.)	Age (yr)	Trauma mechanism	Operative interval	Valve pathology	Operative strategy
Halstead et al. (30)	19	MVA	Initial	Papillary rupture	Repair
Doty et al. (31)	27	Gunshot	4 yr	Leaflet perforation	Repair
Morelli et al. (32)	25	Stab wound	1 yr	N.A.	None
Trotter et al. (33)	15	MVA	Initial	Annulus rupture	Bioprosthesis
Pearson et al. (34)	5	Crush injury	2 mo	Annulus rupture	N.A.
Pearson et al. (34)	7	Pedestrian	7 yr	Chordal rupture	N.A.
Banning et al. (35)	19	MVA	Initial	Chordal rupture	Bioprosthesis
Stahl et al. (36)	30	MVA	Initial	Papillary rupture	Bioprosthesis
Chirillo et al. (37)	N.A.	Blunt chest	N.A.	N.A.	N.A.
Bolton et al. (38)	37	Stab wound	17 yr	Leaflet disruption	Repair

Abbreviations: MVA = motor vehicle accident; N.A. = not available.

Note: There are well over 100 cases of traumatic tricuspid valve injury cited in the literature since the first credited report by Williams in 1829.

blunt chest trauma, DeMuth et al. noted ventricular septal lacerations in 33% of canines, and 60% ventricular septums sustained contusions (24) despite a grossly uninjured appearance to the epicardium. In an autopsy series from the Armed Forces Institute of Pathology, traumatic atrial septal defects were noted in 4.5% of cases and traumatic ventricular septal defects were noted in 5.5% (25). Only 20% of these defects were isolated injuries, most commonly associated with valvular injury. Awareness of this prevalence is important when evaluating patients with blunt cardiac injury, as the prevailing valvular dysfunction may divert attention from the associated septal defect.

Operative intervention for traumatic septal defects requires cardiopulmonary bypass, and a midline sternotomy is preferred. Intraoperative transesophageal echocardiography is used routinely in our practice. Closure of traumatic ventricular septal defects have been described with both a direct suture approximation (26) and use of a patch (27,28). The choice of cardiac incisions, use of prosthetic material versus autologous pericardium, and timing of intervention will depend on the concomitant procedures performed, as well as surgeon preferences. As the majority of reported traumatic ventricular septal defects occur within the apical muscular septum, residual defects may remain; the literature contains at least one report of spontaneous closure of a small residual shunt (29).

ATRIOVENTRICULAR VALVE INJURY

The mechanism of atrioventricular valve injury is thought to be a sudden compressive force to the heart at the end of diastole, when the heart is full and the atrioventricular valves are closed. Diagnosis of atrioventricular valve abnormalities can be confirmed by transthoracic or transesophageal echocardiography.

Tricuspid Valve Injury: Tricuspid valve injury is predominantly confined to motor vehicle accidents in the developed countries, although deceleration falls and crush injuries have been reported (Table 1). Because of the anterior location of the right ventricle, traumatic injury to the tricuspid valve may occur with greater frequency than mitral injury. Over 100 cases had been reported in the literature up to 1992 *(39)*.

In a series of 13 patients reported by our institution, all but 1 case was secondary to motor vehicle accidents *(40)*. Chordal rupture was noted in nine patients, papillary rupture in another three patients, and leaflet tear in an additional patient. The mean interval from the trauma to operative intervention was 9.4 yr, ranging from 1 mo to 29 yr. A total of eight valves were replaced and repair was performed in five valves. Pertinent to the above discussion, two patients had concomitant septal defects closed at the time of operative intervention. This series is representative of the literature at large.

Traumatic tricuspid valve injury may be initially well tolerated in the relatively young patient population, delaying surgical intervention. FitzGibbon described a patient followed for 32 yr *(41)*. In contrast, Trotter et al. described a case requiring intervention within hours of presentation and noted that seven other presentations had been described within the literature by 1998 *(33)*. They attributed the acuity of presentation to rupture of the papillary muscle; however, our series contained one papillary muscle rupture that presented 10 mo later. Operative techniques have included valve replacements *(42)*, leaflet repair *(43)*, leaflet resuspension *(38)*, and papillary and chordal reattachment. In general, successful repair is more likely early after injury, in contrast to a delayed operation where the papillary muscles and the involved leaflet(s) are frequently found in a contracted and atrophic state making valvuloplasty more difficult *(16)*. Consequently, a shorter duration between trauma and operation may be advantageous in terms of feasibility of tricuspid valvuloplasty.

Mitral Valve Injury: Traumatic mitral valve injury occurs less frequently than tricuspid trauma. Although the Armed Forces autopsy series *(25)* found no isolated mitral valve lesions, injury to the mitral valve was associated with other cardiac injuries in 5% of fatal cases. During the same time period, McLaughlin et al. *(44)* reviewed 15 cases reported within the literature. In a 1996 review from our institution, 24 cases from the literature were analyzed *(45)*. Although less common than tricuspid injury, traumatic injury to the mitral valve apparatus is more commonly associated with dramatic hemodynamic compromise (Table 2). The majority of cases are operated within hours or days of injury, with the longest reported delay being 9 yr.

The majority of mitral valve injuries are the result of papillary muscle disruption or necrosis. Less frequently, chordae tendineae rupture has been described, and valve leaflet tears are rare. Prosthetic valve replacement, historically, has been used for complex valvular abnormalities *(47,49–53)*, with the increasing experience in reparative degenerative mitral valvular disease, however, traumatic lesions are increasingly being repaired. Whereas postinfarction rupture of the papillary muscle has traditionally required prosthetic replacement, traumatic rupture of the papillary muscle is often associated with less myocardial necrosis and diffuse injury *(54)*. As such, a papillary muscle can often be reinserted following trauma *(55)*. Repairs of papillary muscle avulsion are similar in technique to those used following myocardial infarction (see Chapter 10 for a full description of these procedures). Chordal injury and, on occasion, papillary muscle avulsion *(56)* may involve only a small portion of the subvalvular apparatus, lending itself to excision of the posterior flail leaflet, reapproximation of the triangular resection, and eccentric or ringed annuloplasty *(46)*. Additional techniques used for chordal rupture include reattachment or replacement with prosthetic material such as Gore-Tex® sutures; this is more common with unsupported segments of the anterior leaflet (Fig. 2). Various techniques have been

Table 2
Representative Traumatic Mitral Valve Injury Reported in the Literature

Author (ref.)	Age (yr)	Trauma mechanism	Operative interval	Valve pathology	Operative strategy
Halstead et al. (30)	29	MVA	Initial	Papillary rupture (posteromedial)	Repair
Grinberg et al. (46)	47	MVA	1 wk	Chordal rupture	Repair
Pearson et al. (34)	3	Fall	2 mo	Leaflet tear	N.A.
Wilke et al. (47)	68	Fall	Initial	Papillary rupture (anterolateral)	Mechanical prosthesis
Stahl et al. (36)	30	MVA	Initial	Papillary rupture	Bioprosthesis
Wilson et al. (48)	9	Stab wound	Initial	Leaflet tear	Repair
McDonald et al. (45)	42	Crush	Initial	Papillary rupture (anteriolateral)	Repair
Chirillo et al. (37)	N.A.	Blunt chest	N.A.	Anterior annular disruption	N.A.

Abbreviations: MVA = motor vehicle accident; N.A. = not available.

Note: There are approximately 31 cases of traumatic mitral valve injury cited in the literature since the first credited report by Glendy and White in 1936. The review by McDonald et al. in 1996 documents the findings in the remaining cases.

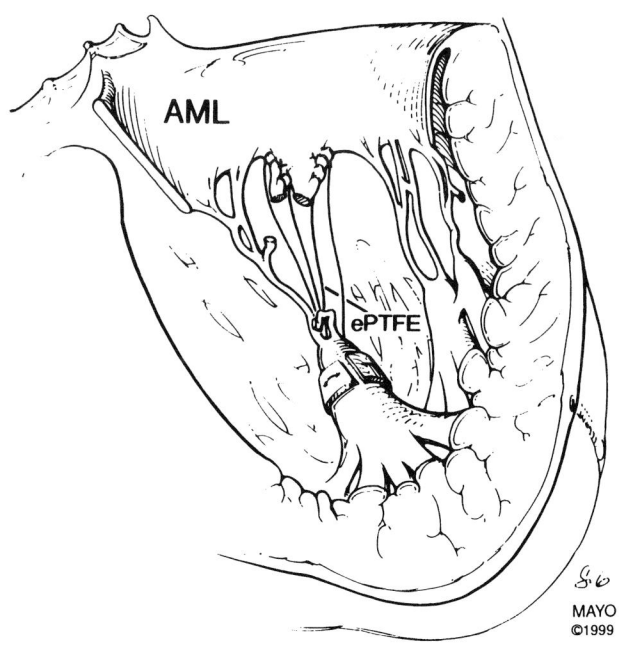

Fig. 2. Chordal rupture to the anterior mitral valve leaftlet can be repaired with prosthetic material to provide "neochordae." A pledgetted suture is placed in the anteromedial papillary muscle and attached to the unsupported segments of the anterior leaflet. Reproduced with permission from ref. *57.*

Table 3
Representative Traumatic Aortic Valve Injury Reported in the Literature

Author (ref.)	Age (yr)	Trauma mechanism	Operative diagnosis interval	Valve pathology	Operative strategy
Halstead et al. (30)	19	MVA	Initial	Cusp tear	Repair
Pearson et al. (34)	15	MVA	Initial	N.A.	None
Loeb et al. (60)	72	MVA	Initial (60 h)	Commissural tear	Repair
Miralles et al. (61)	65	Horse fall	6 mo	Intimal tear	Repair

Abbreviations: MVA = motor vehicle accident; N.A. = not available.

Note: There are few reports of traumatic aortic valve injury cited in the literature.

used in annular or leaflet disruption (58), dependent on the anatomical location of injury and the quality of the tissue (59).

Aortic Valve Injury: Injury to the aortic valve can occur in isolation or with concomitant aortic injury (Table 3). Because traumatic injury to the aortic valve is almost always associated with regurgitation (often severe), aortic valve injury must be separated from injury to the atrioventricular valves because mechanical support in the form of intraaortic balloon pump counterpulsation cannot be used to stabilize hemodynamic decompensation. Aortic valve abnormalities can be detected by two-dimensional echocardiography.

Traumatic aortic valve injury occurs less frequently than injury to the atrioventricular valves. Pretre and Faidutti noted only 37 cases described in the literature before 1993 (62). Of the 35 cases with complete descriptions of the valvular injury, 18 had avulsion of an aortic cusp from the annulus. Commissural avulsion was the next most common mode of injury, occurring in eight patients. Additionally, a patient with cuspal tear has been described after a motor vehicle accident (63). On occasion, reconstructive repairs may be feasible (64) (e.g., commissural disruption may require only resuspension of the valve). More commonly, however, the fragile, nonpathologic aortic valve cusp requires replacement (65). It is interesting to note that valve replacement occurred more frequently in recent years as reported in the review of Pretre and Faidutti (97); only six cases of primary repair have been reported since 1964.

IATROGENIC COMPLICATIONS

The advent and advances of invasive cardiac catheterization procedures enable both diagnostic and therapeutic interventions to be performed without the morbidity of an open, surgical approach. However, these percutaneously performed procedures are also associated with potential risks, and surgical intervention may be required to address such complications.

Endomyocardial Biopsy

Biopsy of the right ventricular myocardium is most commonly being used for rejection surveillance following cardiac allotransplantation, but it is also necessary for evaluating selected patients for restrictive cardiomyopathies and infiltrative processes such as hypereosinophilic syndrome. Several forms of intracardiac injury are unique to this procedure, some of which may require surgical intervention.

To reduce the incidence of ventricular perforation of the free wall, endomyocardial biopsies are often obtained from the interventricular septum. Mechanistically, it is understandable how a ventricular septal defect could arise, although it is uncommon. Katta et al. also described an atrioventricular septal defect allowing communication between the right atrium and left ventricle *(66);* spontaneous closure ensued. Although echocardiographic guidance of myocardial biopsies might reduce complications, particularly right ventricular free wall perforation, it is not used routinely. Despite this advancement, though, risks remain to the valvular and subvalvular apparatus.

Tricuspid regurgitation following endomyocardial biopsy may be well tolerated in the early postprocedure period, analogous to the natural history noted with traumatic tricuspid injury. This is usually the result of leaflet injury or disruption of the chordae or papillary muscle(s). Left ventricular biopsy is rarely required in the current era. When it is necessary, the complication rate can be higher, especially injury to the mitral valve or subvalvular apparatus. In addition, when mitral valve injury does occur, it is more likely to present with significant hemodynamic compromise requiring insertion of an intra-aortic balloon pump and urgent surgical intervention. When left ventricular biopsy is required, transesophageal echocardiographic guidance may be helpful in reducing potential complications.

Coronary artery fistulas following biopsy for cardiac allotransplantation can occur. Lazar and Uretsky evaluated the incidence and natural history of these fistulas in a group of 480 patients with transplanted hearts and serial coronary angiography *(67).* They demonstrated the incidence to be approximately 3.0%. Notably, however, angiographic follow-up demonstrated that approx 70% of fistulas resolved spontaneously within 3 yr. Although an indolent course follows the majority of these complications, one must always remain vigilant of possible coronary arterial complications of myocardial biopsies.

Balloon Valvuloplasty

Although mitral stenosis, usually the result of rheumatic valvular heart disease, is uncommon in North America, balloon valvuloplasty is occasionally indicated, depending on the specific anatomy. When it is deemed appropriate, percutaneous balloon valvuloplasty is preferred to open surgical valvotomy or replacement. Despite grading scales to reduce the incidence *(68,69),* severe mitral regurgitation still occurs in 2.5–12% of patients *(70–72).* Mortality related to the procedure occurs in 1% of patients *(72).* Herrmann et al. noted that not all patients with severe mitral regurgitation require urgent operative intervention; nearly 24% did not require surgery during 18-mo follow-up *(70).* Kannan and Jeyamalar reported a case of severe mitral regurgitation following balloon valvuloplasty that completely resolved on long-term follow-up *(73).* Although cases of resultant mitral regurgitation noted immediately following the procedure are sometimes observed, the majority of these patients will ultimately require surgery, usually valve replacement.

Leaflet rupture was noted in all the patients with severe mitral regurgitation in the series of Padial et al., occurring in the anterior leaflet in 60% and the posterior leaflet in 40% of the cases *(69).* In contrast, the North American Inoue Balloon Investigators noted that rupture of chordae tendineae was the most prevalent mechanism of severe regurgitation, occurring in 40% of cases *(70)*. Leaflet tearing was present in only 30%, whereas wide splitting of commissures resulting in a central jet occurred in 26% of cases. In a case series by Ramondo et al., leaflet tearing and shearing of the free leaflet edges was noted *(74)*.

Operative intervention for these traumatic injuries is, of course, dependent on the anatomic damage and severity of the regurgitation. As severe mitral stenosis prompted invasive therapeutic procedures initially, the vast majority will ultimately require valve replacement.

Percutaneous aortic valvuloplasty is also performed in certain centers and has been associated with the need for urgent cardiac surgery in 1% *(75)*. In the adult population in North America, the etiology of aortic stenosis is often calcific. Percutaneous treatment of this subgroup is generally reserved for those patients felt not to be operative candidates for valve replacement.

PROSTHETIC VALVE OBSTRUCTION

One of the most serious complications of the mechanical prosthetic valve is acute obstruction, with a reported incidence ranging from 0.2% to 4.5% per patient-year. Several risk factors have been identified, exclusive of inadequate levels of anticoagulation. Renqulli et al., in an analysis of 3231 prosthetic valves, identified the prosthetic model, large prostheses, atrial fibrillation, an enlarged left atrium, and an age between 40 and 50 yr to be significantly associated with prosthetic valve thrombosis *(76)*. Burckhardt has noted a seasonal increase in prosthetic valve thrombosis during the winter, coinciding with the known seasonal variation in fibrinogen levels *(77)*.

Although the development of symptoms, in retrospective analysis, was insidious and gradual, Buttard et al. noted that 90% of patients presented in congestive heart failure, among whom 38% were in cardiogenic shock *(78)*. Mortality was 40%, and 66% of deaths occurred before operative intervention could be contemplated. Deviri et al. noted that 63% of their patients were in NYHA class IV heart failure, 25% in a low cardiac output syndrome or cardiogenic shock, and an additional 3% presented with cardiac arrest *(79)*. Mortality strongly correlated with NYHA class, with a perioperative mortality of 18% for patients presenting in NYHA class IV.

The mainstay of treatment has been reoperation with valve re-replacement or mechanical thrombectomy. The administration of thrombolytic therapy has been reserved for high-risk surgical candidates with left-sided prosthetic valve thrombosis *(80)* because cerebral thromboembolism may occur in 12% of patients. Isolated reports have depicted alternative techniques. Jabbour et al. described a desperate case in which percutaneous catheter manipulation was used for a frozen bileaflet prosthesis after cardiac arrest *(81)*. Al-Halees described the use of a flexible fiberoptic choledochoscope for mechanical thrombectomy in two patients *(82)*.

At time of operative intervention, most thrombosed prosthetic valves are re-replaced rather than undergoing thrombectomy. In the series of Deviri et al., 76% patients underwent valve re-replacement and the remainder had thrombectomy *(79)*. All of the patients in the series of Buttard et al. underwent re-replacement *(78)*. In contrast, a small series from Taiwan described a series of 10 patients who all underwent thrombectomy *(83)*.

The reported incidence of prosthetic valve re-replacement in the setting of thrombosis is likely the result of the fact that most prosthetic valve obstruction is not from
thrombosis alone. Rizzoli et al. noted that pannus, or fibrous ingrowth, accounted for
62% of reoperations in their large series of prosthetic valve obstructions *(84)*. Pannus
was present in 12% of thrombotic occlusion in the series of Deviri et al. *(79)*.

Pannus represents the unrestrained growth of fibrous tissue into the orifice and mov-
able components of the valve prosthesis. It usually occurs on the ventricular aspect of
the prosthesis and probably begins at the time of prosthetic valve insertion. It is speculated that pannus may be accelerated with the use of pledgets when they are placed on
the ventricular side of the prosthesis. As demonstrated by Rizolli et al., the hazard
function for obstruction of prosthetic valves by pannus is not linear, but rather expo-
nentially increases with duration of implant *(84)*. Furthermore, pannus is difficult to
distinguish from pure thrombosis with current noninvasive imaging *(85)*. Although it
may be prudent, in select patients, to first pursue thrombolytic therapy for presumed
thrombotic prosthetic occlusion, failure to respond may signify a significant contribution from pannus formation.

Surgical treatment of pannus ingrowth and occlusion of a prosthetic valve will
depend on multiple factors, the most important being the location of the fibrous tissue.
Because most of this fibrous tissue is on the ventricular side of the prosthesis, local
excision (across the prosthesis) is often difficult. More commonly, complete excision
of the prosthesis, debridement of the annulus, and replacement with a new prosthesis
will be required. Although no difference in the degree of pannus development has been
demonstrated between mechanical and bioprostheses, the rapidity with which the valve
will fail may be lower with a bioprosthesis.

ENDOCARDITIS

The true incidence of infective endocarditis with shock is difficult to obtain;
reported rates likely represent an underestimation of the actual incidence resulting
from the difficulty in clinical diagnosis of prior infection contributing to valvular
pathology, an inability to abstract the total denominator, and reporting bias. It can be
stated, however, that the number of patients presenting in shock is small compared to
the total cases of infective endocarditis. In a series from Canada, 16% of patients operated on for active native valve endocarditis in a 16-yr period presented in shock *(86)*. In
a series from England, 12.5% of patients operated on for active endocarditis in a 13-yr
period presented in shock *(87)*. In a 20-yr period, 16 patients have required emergency
operations for active endocarditis at the Mayo Clinic *(88)*. During the same period, 24
patients at the Mayo Clinic in class IV heart failure, without active endocarditis,
required urgent operative intervention.

In the Mayo Clinic series, aortic valve endocarditis accounted for 75% of the cases,
whereas mitral valve infections were present in the remaining four patients *(88)*.
Staphylococcus aureus was cultured in nearly one-third of the cases. Although aortic
annulus abscesses and cusp destruction accounted for the aortic valvular pathology,
75% of the mitral valvular pathology was secondary to chordal rupture. In aortic valve
endocarditis, one must also be cognizant of the possibility of myocardial ischemia secondary to coronary embolism.

Whereas some patients with native valve endocarditis respond to antibiotic therapy, surgical intervention is required in many patients. In the current era, earlier surgical intervention is increasingly advised. Indications for surgery have included the presence of congestive heart failure from valve dysfunction, persistent sepsis, local annular abnormalities (abscesses), conduction abnormalities, fistulas into adjacent cardiac chambers, systemic embolization, progressive renal insufficiency, enlarging vegetations, and prosthetic valve endocarditis.

In general, operation performed in the setting of active infection can be challenging, especially when there is destruction of adjacent tissue (e.g., aortic root abscess with ventricular septal defect or aorta–ventricular discontinuity). Knowledge of abnormalities not only of the valve but also of contiguous structures (e.g., annular abscess) is of great importance to the surgeon prior to going to the operating room. This anatomical information is readily discernible with transesophageal echocardiography. Although valve repair is preferred, it may not be possible, especially if there is significant destruction of cusp or leaflet or subvalvular tissue. If the infection is limited to the cusps of the native valve, complete valvular resection and replacement with a mechanical or biologic prosthesis may suffice. Concomitant annular abnormalities require aggressive debridement and reconstructive procedures. Reconstructive techniques following radical debridement are dependent on the structures resected. Fistulas and chamber defects may be closed with autologous or preserved pericardium *(89,90)*. Alternatively, prosthetic grafts may be used but these may increase the risk of recurrent, or persistent, endocarditis. It has been our practice to locally disinfect the infected annulus and abscess cavity with phenol. Mechanical or biologic valvular prostheses can then be implanted.

Aortic valve homografts have been used following radical debridement of complex aortic valve endocarditis (i.e., presence of root abnormalities) *(91,92)*. Homografts include harvested ascending aorta and a varying amount of attached ventricular myocardium as well as preservation of the anterior leaflet of the mitral valve. This additional tissue, although it is usually trimmed for nonendocarditis aortic valve replacement, can be preserved to reconstruct adjacent defects (Figs. 3 and 4). If there is severe destruction of the aortic root, root excision and subsequent replacement with coronary reimplantation with the aortic valve homograft can be performed. This is often required for prosthetic valve endocarditis. Additionally, aortic homografts appear to be more resistant to infection than other valve substitutes and thus may be ideal for complex aortic infections. In our practice, the aortic valve homograft is the prosthesis of choice for complex aortic valve endocarditis.

In mitral valve endocarditis, valvular replacement is usually required because of the destruction of leaflet tissue. Isolated leaflet destruction without annular involvement may be repaired with autologous pericardium. This is less likely in the acute setting when the tissue is more friable and more likely in a delayed (treated) setting where the tissue is more fibrous and likely to hold sutures. The feasibility of valve repair ultimately depends on the tissue quality and is determined at the time of operation. Although the mitral valve homograft has been used with some success, late follow-up is not yet available *(93–95)*.

In some cases, multiple valve replacements may be required. When aortic valve endocarditis is complicated by annular abscess formation, mitral valve replacement may be necessary. Fully one-tenth of aortic annular abscesses may require mitral valve replacement *(96)*.

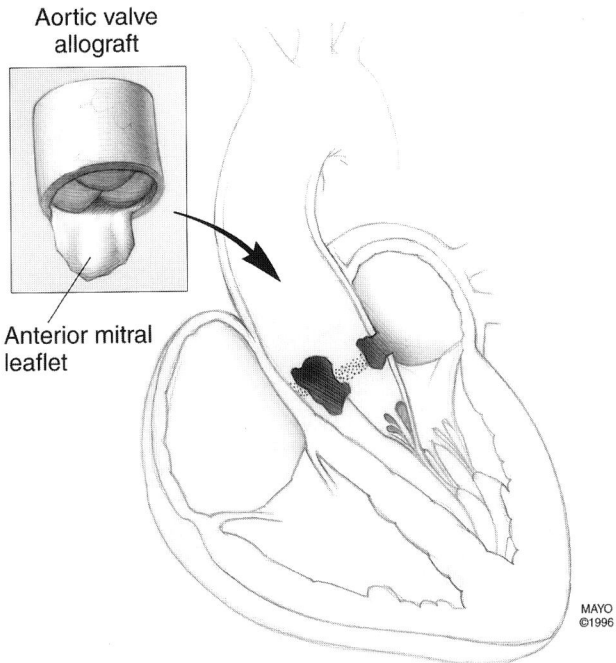

Fig. 3. Aortic homografts have varying amounts of attached ventricular myocardium as well as the anterior leaflet of the mitral valve. Rather than using prosthetic grafts or preserved pericardium to reconstruct defects following radical debridement, this additional tissue (inset) can be used to reconstruct defects produced by annular abscesses. Reproduced with permission from ref. *91*.

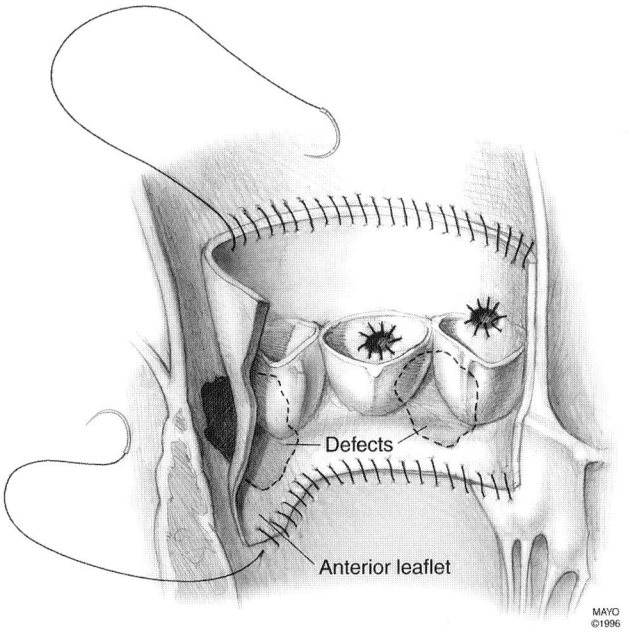

Fig. 4. The relations of the defects produced by endocarditis are shown (dotted lines) to the implanted aortic homograft. The anterior mitral valve leaflet in the aortic homograft was used to cover an annular defect. Reproduced with permission from ref. *91*.

CONCLUSION

Traumatic heart disease, iatrogenic trauma, prosthetic obstructive, and infectious valvular disease may require urgent operative intervention for some hemodynamic compromise. Advances in medical technology have advanced and will continue to advance operative therapies for these conditions.

REFERENCES

1. Karrel R, Shaffer MA, Franaszek JB. Emergency diagnosis, resuscitation, and treatment of acute penetrating cardiac trauma. Ann Emerg Med 1982;11:504–517.
2. Attar S, Suter CM, Hankins JR, Sequeria A, McLaughlin JS. Penetrating cardiac injuries. Ann Thorac Surg 1991;51:711–715.
3. Symbas PN. Cardiac trauma. Am Heart J 1976;92:387–396.
4. Symbas PN. Traumatic heart disease. Curr Probl Cardiol 1991;16:537–582.
5. Demetriades D, VanderVeen PW. Penetrating injuries of the heart: experience over two years in South Africa. J Trauma 1983;23:1034–1041.
6. Carrasquilla C, Wilson RF, Walt AJ, Arbulu A. Gunshot wounds of the heart. Ann Thorac Surg 1972;13:208–213.
7. Tassi AA, Davies AL. Pericardial tamponade due to penetrating fragment wounds of the heart. Am J Surg 1977;118:535–538.
8. Committee on Trauma. American College Advanced Trauma Life-Support Course for Physicians. American College of Surgeons, Chicago, 1997.
9. Estrera AS, Schreiber JT. Management of acute cardiac trauma. Cardiol Clin 1984;2:239.
10. Bolton JW, Bynoe, Lazar HL. Two-dimensional echocardiography in the evaluation of penetrating intrapericardial injuries. Ann Thorac Surg 1993;56:506.
11. Plummer D, Brunette D, Asinger R, et al. Emergency department echocardiography improves outcome in penetrating cardiac injury. Ann Emerg Med 1992;21:709.
12. Brathwaite CE, Weiss RL, Baldino WA, et al. Multichamber gunshot wounds of the heart: the utility of transesophageal echocardiography. Chest 1992;101:287.
13. Hashimi MW, Jenkins DR, McGwier BW, et al. Comparative efficacy of transthoracic and transesophageal echocardiography in detection of an intracardiac bullet fragment. Chest 1994;106:299.
14. Balillot R, Dontigny L, Verdant A, et al. Intrapericardial trauma: surgical experience. J Trauma 1989;30:506.
15. Ludington CG, Bosking AS, Miguel A: Rupture of left ventricle from blunt cardiac trauma. Ann Thorac Surg 1974;18:195.
16. Yener A, Gokgoz L, Soncul H, et al. Nonpenetrating thoracic trauma causing dissection of the interventricular septum and leading to complete heart block. J Thorac Cardiovasc Surg 1992;103:820.
17. Shorr RM, Crittenden M, Indeck M, Hartunian SL. Rodriguez A. Blunt thoracic trauma. Ann Surg 1987;206:200–205.
18. McLean RF, Devitt JH, McLellan BA, Dubbin J, Ehrlich LE, Dirkson D. Significance of myocardial contusion following blunt chest trauma. J Trauma-Injury Infect Crit Care 1992;33:240–243.
19. Sturaitis M, McCallum D, Sutherland G, Cheung H, Driedger AA, Sibbald WJ. Lack of significant long-term sequelae following traumatic myocardial contusion. Arch Int Med 1986;146:1765–1769.
20. Plotnick GD, Hamilton S, Lee YC. The cardiologist and the trauma patient: noninvasive testing. Semin Thorac Cardiovasc Surg 1992;4:168–176.
21. Potkin RT, Werner JA, Trobaugh GB, Chestnut CH, Carrico CJ, Hallstrom A, et al. Evaluation of noninvasive tests of cardiac damage in suspected cardiac contusion. Circulation 1982;66:627–631.
22. Bertinchant JP, Polge A, Mohty D, Nguyen-Ngoc-Lam R, Estorc J, Cohendy R, et al. Evaluation of incidence, clinical significance, and prognostic value of circulating cardiac troponin I and T elevation in hemodynamically stable patients with suspected myocardial contusion after blunt chest trauma. J Trauma-Injury Infect Crit Care 2000;48:924–931.
23. Adams JE, Bodor GS, Davila-Roman VG, Delmez JA, Apple FS, Ladenson JH, et al. Cardiac troponin I. A marker with high specificity for cardiac injury. Circulation 1993;88:101–106.
24. DeMuth WE, Lerner EH, Liedtke AJ. Nonpenetrating injury of the heart: an experimental model in dogs. J Trauma–Injury Infect Crit Care 1973;13:639–644.

25. Parmley LF, Mannion WC, Mattingly TW. Nonpenetrating traumatic injury of the heart. Circulation 1953;18:371–396.
26. Anyanwu CH. Mitral incompetence and ventricular septal defects following non-penetrating injury. Thorax 1976;31:113–117.
27. Reginao E, Speroni F, Riccardi M, Verunelli F, Eufrate S. Post-traumatic mitral regurgitation and ventricular septal defect in absence of left pericardium. Thorac Cardiovasc Surg 1980;28:213–217.
28. Khuddus SA, Bokooki H, Rashid A, Kadivar H, Meyer WH. Successful repair of interventricular septal defect resulting from blunt chest trauma. J Fla Med Assoc 1981;68:438–440.
29. Krajcer Z, Cooley DA, Leachman RD. Ventricular septal defect following blunt, trauma: spontaneous closure of residual defect after surgical repair. Cathet Cardiol Diag 1977;3:409–415.
30. Halstead J, Hosseinpour AR, Wells FC. Conservative surgical treatment of valvular injury after blunt chest trauma. Ann Thorac Surg 2000;69:766–768.
31. Doty JR, Cameron DE, Elmaci T, Salomon NW. Penetrating trauma to the tricuspid valve and ventricular septum: delayed repair. Ann Thorac Surg 1999;67:252–253.
32. Morelli S, Perrone C, Bernardo ML, Voci P. Flail tricuspid valve in a patient with history of stab chest wound. Int J Cardiol 1998;66:111–113.
33. Trotter TH, Knott-Craig CJ, Ward KE. Blunt injury rupture of tricuspid valve and right coronary artery. Ann Thorac Surg 1998;66:1814–1816.
34. Pearson GD, Karr SS, Trachiotis GD, Midgley FM, Eichelberger MR, Martin GR. A retrospective review of the role of transesophageal echocardiography in aortic and cardiac trauma in a level I Pediatric Trauma Center. J Am Soc Echo 1997;10:946–955.
35. Banning AP, Durrani A, Pillai R. Rupture of the atrial septum and tricuspid valve after blunt chest trauma. Ann Thorac Surg 1997;64:240–242.
36. Stahl RD, Liu JC, Walsh JF. Blunt cardiac trauma: atrioventricular valve disruption and ventricular septal defect. Ann Thorac Surg 1997;64:1466–1468.
37. Chirillo F, Totis O, Cavarzerani A, Bruni A, Farnia A, Sarpellon M, et al. Usefulness of transthoracic and transoesophageal echocardiography in recognition and management of cardiovascular injuries after blunt chest trauma. Heart 1996;75:301–306.
38. Bolton JW. Traumatic tricuspid valve injury: leaflet resuspension repair. Ann Thorac Surg 1996;61:721–722.
39. Holper K, Hahnel C, Augustin N, Meisner H. Operative correction of traumatic tricuspid insufficiency. Herz 1996;21:172–178.
40. van Son JA, Danielson GK, Schaff HV, Miller FA Jr. Traumatic tricuspid valve insufficiency: experience in thirteen patients. J Thorac Cardiovasc Surg 1994;108:893–898.
41. FitzGibbon GM, Burton JR. Traumatic tricuspid insuffiencey: a case followed for 32 years, with a note on early sources. Can J Cardiol 1996;12:289–294.
42. Janzing HM, Rommens P, Flameng W, Aerts R, Lauwers P, Broos P. Severe liver rupture and tricuspid valve rupture in a patient with multiple trauma. J Trauma Injury Infect Critical Car 1995;38:828–829.
43. Hige K, Suehiro S, Shibata T, Sasaki Y, Kumano H, Hosono M, et al. Successful repair of tricuspid regurgitation due to blunt trauma. Kyobu Geka–Japan J Thorac Surg 1998;51:1047–1050.
44. McLaughlin JS, Cowley RA, Smith G, Matheson NA. Mitral valve disease from blunt trauma. J Thorac Cardiovasc Surg 1964;48:261–271.
45. McDonald ML, Orszulak TA, Bannon MP, Zietlow SP. Mitral valve injury after blunt chest trauma. Ann Thorac Surg 1996;61:1024–1029.
46. Grinberg AR, Finkielman JD, Pineiro D, Festa H, Cazenave C. Rupture of mitral chorda tendinea following blunt chest trauma. Clin Cardiol 1998;21:300–301.
47. Wilke A, Kruse T, Hesse H, Bittinger A, Moosdorf R, Maisch B. Papillary muscle injury after blunt chest trauma. J Trauma-Injury Infect Crit Care 1997;43:360–361.
48. Wilson WR, Coyne JT, Greer GE. Mitral regurgitation as a late sequela of penetrating cardiac trauma. J Heart Valve Dis 1997;6:171–173.
49. Pellegrini RV, Copeland CE, DiMarco RF, Bekoe S, Grant K, Marrangoni AG, et al. Blunt rupture of both atrioventricular valves. Ann Thorac Surg 1986;42:471–472.
50. McCrory D, Craig B, O'Kane H. Traumatic mitral valve rupture in a child. Ann Thorac Surg 1991;51:821–822.
51. Rashid A, Chandraratna PA, Hilder FJ, Samet P, Yahr WZ, Greenberg J. Papillary muscle rupture following nonpenetrating chest trauma: report of a case with hemodynamic and serial echocardiographic findings and successful surgical treatment. Heart Lung 1978;7:647–651.

52. Araki J, Koizumi S. Emergency surgical repair of massive mitral regurgitation due to ruptured chordae tendineae by blunt chest trauma. Thorac Cardiovasc Surg 1982;30:46–47.

53. Pillai R, Fountain SW, Qureshi SA, Mitchell A, Rees A. Avulsion of the anterior papillary muscle of the mitral valve due to non-penetrating trauma to the chest. Thorax 1982;37:943–944.

54. Fiane AE, Lindberg HL. Delayed papillary muscle rupture following non-penetrating chest injury. Injury 1993;24:690–691.

55. Bromberg BI, Mazziotti MV, Canter CE, Spray TL, Strauss AW, Foglia RP. Recognition and management of nonpenetrating cardiac trauma in children. J Pediatr 1996;128:536–541.

56. Spangenthal EJ, Sekovski B, Bhayana JN, Krawczyk JA, Hajduczok ZD. Traumatic left ventricular papillary muscle rupture: the role of transesophageal echocardiography in diagnosis and surgical management. J Am Soc Echo 1993;6:536–538.

57. Phillips MR, Daly RC, Schaff HV, Dearani JA, Mullany CJ, Orszulak TA. Repair of anterior leaflet mitral valve prolapse: chordal replacement versus chordal shortening. Ann Thorac Surg 2000;69:25–29.

58. Harada M, Osawa M, Kosukegawa K, Usuda T, Nakamura K. Isolated mitral valve injury from non-penetrating cardiac trauma. J Cardiovasc Surg 1977;18:459–464.

59. Van Roye S, Zienkowicz BS. Delayed isolated mitral incompetence after being kicked in the chest by a bull. Thorac Cardiovasc Surg 1989;37:329–331.

60. Loeb T, Matuszczak Y, Petit J, Bessou JP, Pinsard M, Oksenhendler G. Aortic valve rupture—an unsuspected cause of acute cardiac failure after chest trauma. Intensive Care Med 1996;22:714–715.

61. Miralles A, Farinola T, Quiroga J, Obi C, Hernandez J, Granados J, et al. Valvuloplasty in traumatic aortic insufficiency due to subtotal tear of the intima. Ann Thorac Surg 1995;60:1098–1100.

62. Pretre R, Faidutti B. Surgical management of aortic valve injury after nonpenetrating trauma. Ann Thorac Surg 1993;56:1426–1431.

63. Grimball A, Bradham RR, Locklair PR. Traumatic aortic valve rupture. J South Carolina Med Assoc 1987;83:62–64.

64. Haskins CD, Shapira N, Rahman E, Serra AJ, McNicholas KW, Lemole GM. Repair of traumatic rupture of the aortic valve. Arch Surg 1992;127:231–232.

65. Loop FD, Hofmeier G, Groves LK. Traumatic disruption of the aortic valve. Cleveland Clin Q 1971;38:187–194.

66. Katta S, Akosah K, Stambler B, Salter D, Guerraty A, Mohanty PK. Atrioventricular fistula: an unusual complication of endomyocardial biopsy in a heart transplant recipient. J Am Soc Echo 1994;7:405–409.

67. Lazar JM, Uretsky BF. Coronary artery fistula after heart transplantation: a disappearing entity? Cathet Cardiovasc Diag 1996;37:10–13.

68. Wilkins GT, Weyman AE, Abascal VM, Block PC, Palacios I. Percutaneous balloon dilatation of mitral valve: an analysis of echocardiographic variables related to outcome and the mechanism of dilatation. Br Heart J 1988;60:299–308.

69. Padial LR, Abascal VM, Moreno PR, Weyman AE, Levine RA, Palacios IF. Echocardiography can predict the development of severe mitral regurgitation after percutaneous mitral valvuloplasty by the Inoue technique. Am J Cardiol 1999;83:1210–1213.

70. Wyman RM, Safian RD, Portway V, Skillman JJ, McKay RG, Baim DS. Current complications of diagnostic and therapeutic cardiac catheterization. J Am Coll Cardiol 1988;12:1400–1406.

71. Herrmann HC, Lima JA, Feldman T, Chisholm R, Isner J, O'Neill W, et al. Mechanisms and outcome of severe mitral regurgitation after Inoue balloon valvulosplasty: North American Inoue Balloon Investigators. J Am Coll Cardiol 1993;22:783–789.

72. Anonymous. Complications and mortality of percutaneous balloon mitral commissurotomy: a report from the National Heart, Lung, and Blood Institute Balloon Valvuloplasty Registry. Circulation 1992;85:2014–2024.

73. Kannan P, Jeyamalar R. Severe mitral incompetence following balloon mitral valvuloplasty: complete resolution during follow-up. Cathet Cardiovasc Diag 1995;34:220–221.

74. Ramondo A, Chirillo F, Dan M, Sorbara C, Fracasso A, Mazzucco A, et al. Mitral valve disruption following percutaneous balloon valvuloplasty. Cathet Cardiovasc Diagn 1990;21:239–244.

75. Anonymous. Percutaneous balloon aortic valvuloplasty: acute and 30-day follow-up results in 674 patients from the NHLBI Balloon Valvuloplasty Registry. Circulation 1991;84:2383–2397.

76. Renzulli A, DeLuca L, Caruso A, Verde R, Galzerano D, Cotrufo M. Acute thrombosis of prosthetic valves: a multivariate analysis of the risk factors for a lifethreatening event. Eur J Cardio-Thorac Surg 1992;6:412–420.

77. Horstkotte D, Burckhardt D. Prosthetic valve thrombosis. J Heart Valve Ds 1995;4:141–153.

78. Buttard P, Bonnefoy E, Chevalier P, Marcaz PB, Robin J, Obadia JF, et al. Mechanical cardiac valve thrombosis in patients in critical hemodynamic compromise. Eur J Cardio-Thorac Surg 1997;11:710–713.

79. Deviri E, Sareli P, Wisenbaugh T, Cronje SL. Obstruction of mechanical heart valve prostheses: clinical aspects and surgical management. J Am Coll Cardiol 1991;17:646–650.

80. Lengel M, Fuster V, Keltai M, et al. Guidelines for management of left-sided prosthetic valve thrombosis: a role for thrombolytic therapy. J Am Coll Cardiol 1997;30:1521–1526.

81. Jabbour S, Salinger M, Alexander JC. Hemodynamic stabilization of acute prosthetic valve thrombosis using percutaneous catheter manipulation. Cathet Cardiovasc Diagn 1996;39:314–316.

82. Al-Haless Z, Kumar N. Thrombotic obstruction of bileaflet valves: surgical management and fiberoptic thrombectomy. Ann Thorac Surg 1994;58:168–169.

83. Tsai KT, Lin PJ, Chang CH, Chu JJ, Chang JP, Kao CL, et al. Surgical management of thrombotic disc valve. Ann Thorac Surg 1993;55:98–101.

84. Rizzoli G, Guglielmi G, Toscano G, Pistorio V, Vendramin I, Bottio T, et al. Reoperations for acute prosthetic thrombosis and pannus: an assessment of rates, relationship, and risk. Eur J Cardio-Thorac Surg 1999;16:74–80.

85. Barbetseas J, Nagueh SF, Pitsavos C, Toutouzas PK, Quinones MA, Zoghbi WA. Differentiating thrombus from pannus formation in obstructed mechanical prosthetic valves: an evaluation of clinical, transthoracic, and transesophageal echocardiographic parameters. J Am Coll Cardiol 1998;32:1410–1417.

86. d'Udekem Y, David TE, Feindel CM, Armstrong S, Sun Z. Long-term results of surgery for active infective endocarditis. Eur J Cardio-Thorac Surg 1997;11:46–52.

87. Kay PH, Oldershaw PJ, Dawkins K, Lennox SC, Paneth M. The results of surgery for active endocarditis of the native aortic valve. J Cardiovasc Surg 1984;25:321–327.

88. Wilson WR, Geraci JE. Cardiac valve replacement in patients with active infective endocarditis. Herz 1983;8:332–343.

89. David TE. Surgical management of aortic root abscess. J Cardiol Surg 1997;12:262–266.

90. d'Udekem Y, David TE, Feindel CM, Armstrong S, Sun Z. Long-term results of operation for paravalvular abscess. Ann Thorac Surg 1996;62:48–53.

91. Dearani JA, Orszulak TA, Schaff HV, Daly RC, Anderson BJ, Danielson GK. Results of allograft aortic valve replacement for complex endocarditis. J Thorac Cardiovasc Surg 1997;113:285–291.

92. Tuna IC, Orszulak TA, Schaff HV, Danielson GK. Results of homograft aortic valve replacement for active endocarditis. Ann Thorac Surg 1990;49:619–624.

93. Acar C, Farge A, Ramsheyi A, et al. Mitral valve replacement using a cryopreserved mitral homograft. Ann Thorac Surg 1994;57:746–748.

94. Doty DB, Acar C. Mitral valve replacement with homograft. Ann Thorac Surg 1998;66:2127–2131.

95. Acar C, Tolan M, Derrebi A, et al. Homograft replacement of the mitral valve: graft selection, technique of implantation and results in forty-three patients. J Thorac Cardiovasc Surg 1996;111:367–380.

96. Watanabe G, Haverich A, Speier R, et al. Surgical treatment of active infective endocarditis with paravalvular involvement. J Thorac Cardiovasc Surg 1994;107:171–177.

97. Pretre R, Faidutti B. Surgical management of aortic valve injury after nonpenetrating trauma. Ann Thorac Surg 1993;56:1426–1431.

VI CARDIOGENIC SHOCK RELATED TO OTHER CARDIAC CONDITIONS

14 Myocarditis and Cardiogenic Shock

*Mordehay Vaturi, MD, David Hasdai, MD,
and Alexander Battler, MD*

CONTENTS

INTRODUCTION

Myocarditis is a nonischemic inflammatory or immunologic response of the myocardium. The inflammatory process may involve the myocytes, interstitium, cardiac vasculature, and the pericardium. Myocarditis has various causes, the most common being an infectious process. Diagnosing myocarditis and, more so, identifying the specific cause remain a challenge, especially when the course is subclinical, asymptomatic, or self-limiting. In rare cases, myocarditis may take a fulminant and malignant direction, leading to the rapid deterioration of cardiac function and, eventually, to cardiogenic shock. Unlike with extensive myocardial infarction, severe cardiac dysfunction resulting from myocarditis may be totally reversible. Hence, the use of specialized modalities to assist the failing heart until full recovery is of utmost importance. The aim of this chapter is to review the various modalities applied in patients with refractory heart failure resulting from myocarditis.

ETIOLOGY

Various infectious and noninfectious agents are associated with myocarditis (Table 1). In North America, myocarditis is commonly associated with viruses, primarily the Coxsackie B virus *(2),* whereas in South America, myocarditis is most often associated with Chagas' disease, caused by *Trypanosoma cruzi (3).*

From: *Contemporary Cardiology: Cardiogenic Shock: Diagnosis and Treatment*
Edited by: David Hasdai et al. © Humana Press Inc., Totowa, NJ

Table 1
Major Causes of Myocarditis

Infection
Viral
  Coxsackie A
  Coxsackie B
  Influenza A
  Influenza B
  Epstein–Barr virus
  Cytomegalovirus
  Herpes simplex virus
  Varicella zoster virus
  Rubella
  Mumps
  Rabies
  Hepatitis B virus
  Hepatitis C virus
  Human immunodeficiency virus
Bacterial
  Corynebacterium diphtheriae
  Salmonella typhi
  Streptococcus beta-hemolytic
  Neisseria meningitidis
  Legionella pneumophila
  Listeria monocytogenes
  Campylobacter jejuni
  Chlamydia psittaci
  Coxiella burnetti
  Borrelia burgdorferi
  Mycobacterium tuberculosis
Rickettsial
  Rickettsia rickettsii
Protozoal
  Trypanosoma cruzi
  Toxoplasma gondii
Fungal
  Aspergillosis
  Candidiasis
  Blastomycosis
  Coccidioidomycosis
  Histoplasmosis
  Cryptococcosis
  Mucormycosis

Hypersensitivity

Toxic
  Anthracyclines
  Catecholamines
  Interleukin 2
  Alpha interferon

Sources: Modified from ref. *1.*

In the earliest phase of viral myocarditis, the virus replicates in cardiac tissue and elicits a cellular response (predominantly natural-killer cells and macrophages) as well as a humoral response *(4)*. In most cases, the immune response eradicates the virus, leading to a complete recovery. However, if the immune response is ineffective, the residual viral load in the myocardium can lead to further myocardial damage through direct myocardial injury *(5)* or through an autoimmune process mediated primarily by T-cell lymphocytes *(6–8)*.

DIAGNOSIS

Laboratory Evaluation

The following characteristics were reported in one group of 206 acute myocarditis patients: an elevated erythrocyte sedimentation rate (60%), elevated white cell count (25%), or an increased level of creatine kinase MB (12%) *(9)*. Serology studies conducted to identify recent infection by cardiotropic viruses (particularly the common enteroviruses) may enhance the diagnosis. A fourfold rise in IgG titer over a period of 4–6 wk is required for the diagnosis of acute myocarditis, and a rise in IgM titer is of even greater specificity for the diagnosis of acute infection. Abnormalities in the peripheral T- and B-lymphocyte ratio, as well as in the CD4/CD8 T-lymphocyte ratio, may accompany the acute state of this disease. Unfortunately, these and other functional derangements of the immune system (e.g., antibody-dependent cytotoxcity, natural-killer cells, T suppressor cells) are inconsistent and cannot be used as practical diagnostic tools. However, elevated serum levels of soluble Fas (sFas) and soluble Fas ligand (sFasL) have been identified in patients with acute myocarditis. Fuse et al. *(10)* showed that serum levels of sFas and sFasL at hospital admission were significantly higher in patients with predominantly acute lymphocytic myocarditis and fatal outcome.

Electrocardiography

Sinus tachycardia is the most common electrocardiographic feature of myocarditis. Diffuse ST-T changes in the 12-lead electrocardiogram (ECG) during systemic viral infection may imply myocardial involvement *(11)*. Prolongation of the QT-interval and delayed conduction are other possible features *(12)*. Left bundle-branch block is identified in approximately 20% of cases. Complete atrioventricular block (particularly common in Japan) may be present, often manifested as syncopal attacks, but it is usually transient and rarely requires permanent pacing *(13)*. The appearance of ST-T elevations is another electrocardiographic feature suggestive of acute myocardial infarction, possibly reflecting segmental rather than diffuse myocardial injury *(14)*.

Echocardiography

The echocardiographic features are variable. For example, the left ventricle may be normal in function and diameter, or left ventricular dysfunction may be seen either diffusely (Fig. 1) or only with segmental wall motion abnormalities, mimicking acute myocardial infarction *(15,16)*. Either abnormal relaxation or a restrictive pattern of filling also may be detected. In the early stages of acute fulminant myocarditis, echocardiography may reveal increased wall thickness *(17)*. However, these features are nonspecific to the pathogen inducing myocarditis, with the exception of Chagas' dis-

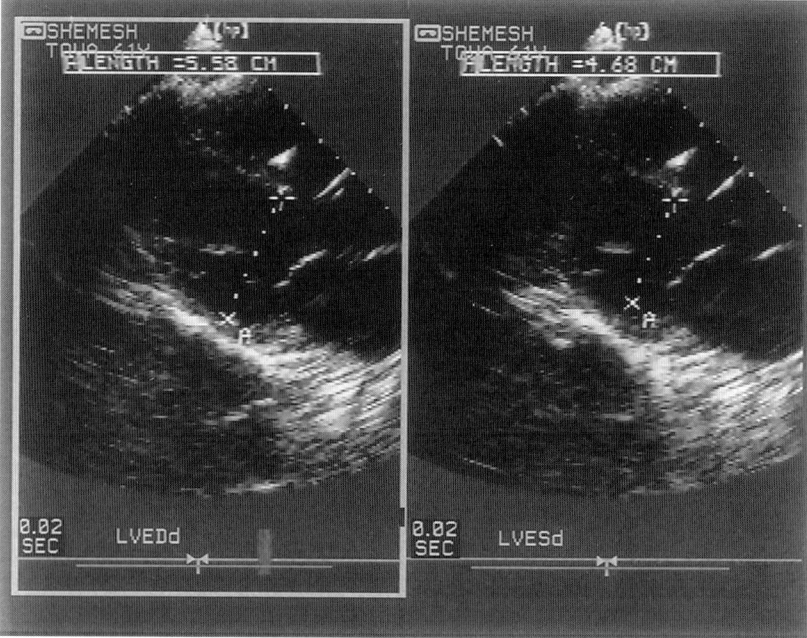

Fig. 1. A transthoracic echocardiogram of a 45-yr-old man in cardiogenic shock because of acute viral myocarditis. Measurements of the left ventricular diameter at end-diastole (LVEDd) and end-systole (LVESd) indicate severe and diffuse systolic dysfunction.

ease, which is characterized by localized aneurysms of the left ventricular apex with a narrow neck *(18).*

Endomyocardial Biopsy

The definitive diagnosis of myocarditis is primarily histological. Although the yield and safety of endomyocardial biopsy (EMB) in adults have been confirmed in large groups of patients *(19,20),* the experience with this procedure in children is less established *(21,22).* Webber et al. *(23)* did report that the biopsy confirmed the diagnosis of myocarditis in 20% of the cases from a study investigating 63 children. Most of the positive biopsies for myocarditis were from children investigated to rule out cardiomyopathy; the remaining positive biopsies were from children evaluated for arrhythmias. In addition, most of the children diagnosed with myocarditis experienced a full recovery. Thus, the diagnostic yield of EMB in children with arrhythmias is low compared with those who present with heart failure. In the latter, the correct diagnosis may avoid premature consideration of heart transplantation.

Several studies have indicated a possible infectious immune etiology in patients with idiopathic cardiomyopathy *(24–28).* Baig et al. *(29)* detected left ventricular dysfunction in nearly one-third of asymptomatic relatives of patients with dilated cardiomyopathy. These findings indicate that dilated cardiomyopathy may be the end stage of myocarditis affecting genetically susceptible patients *(30).*

For the diagnosis of myocarditis, EMB is efficacious, yet its prognostic significance remains controversial. There is a correlation between extensive tissue damage at autopsy and poor outcome, indicating that prognosis of acute myocarditis may be predicted by the histologic characteristics of the initial EMB *(31,32)*. However, in a study of patients with acute dilated cardiomyopathy, there was no correlation between improvement in ventricular systolic function and histologic findings *(33)*. Webber et al. *(23)* indicated a possible role for EMB regarding prognosis in acutely ill children with cardiogenic shock, especially when urgent heart transplantation was considered. The priority to identify acute myocarditis (a potentially reversible condition) changed the therapeutic approach and delayed transplantation in order to allow full recovery to take place. Yet, in less critically ill children, the role of and the need for EMB were less clear.

CLINICAL MANIFESTATIONS

The spectrum of clinical manifestations of myocarditis is wide, ranging from an asymptomatic state (which is, by far, the most common) to cardiogenic shock. Symptoms reflect the severity of left ventricular dysfunction (systolic and/or diastolic) and electrical instability (tachyarrhythmias or heart block).

A typical clue for diagnosing myocarditis is an antecedent flulike syndrome. In one study, this syndrome occurred in approximately 60% of patients with active myocarditis *(9)*. Chest pain appeared in approx 35% of patients with myocarditis and congestive heart failure, suggesting that chest pain may accompany myocarditis *(9)*. Chest pain may be characterized by typical ischemic angina, atypical angina, or pericarditislike pain. The clinical features of myocarditis indicate an acute coronary syndrome when typical chest pain is accompanied by an injury pattern in the ECG and an increased MB fraction of creatine kinase *(14)*. In most autopsy cases, the coronary arteries are patent, although coronary arteritis and coronary spasm have been described during myocarditis *(34–36)*.

In addition, myocarditis is a known cause of sudden death. In a retrospective review of sudden deaths among American Air Force recruits, myocarditis was documented at autopsy in 4 of 19 patients (20%) with structural heart disease *(37)*. Although most patients with acute myocarditis experience a relatively uncomplicated clinical course, a small number may present with cardiogenic shock, which could be refractory to maximal therapy with positive inotropic agents and eventually lead to a fatal outcome *(37)*.

Giant Cell Myocarditis

Idiopathic giant cell myocarditis is a rare and frequently fatal type of myocarditis *(38)*, yet it merits special consideration because of its unique clinical course. Several lines of evidence suggest that giant cell myocarditis is an autoimmune disorder dependent on CD4-positive T-lymphocytes. Histological studies indicate characteristic myocardial infiltration with T-lymphocytes and histiocytes. In experimental models, therapy with cyclosporine and anti-T-lymphocyte antibodies has been shown to prevent this type of myocarditis *(39,40)*.

The clinical course of giant cell myocarditis is usually characterized by progressive congestive heart failure and refractory ventricular arrhythmias. The prognosis of patients with heart failure is often poor. However, there have been reported cases of recovery with long-term survival, often following immunosuppressive therapy but not involving corticosteroids alone *(39,41,42)*. The benefit of heart transplantation in refractory heart failure is questionable because giant cell myocarditis tends to recur in the transplanted heart *(43–48)*, up to 9 yr after the transplantation. In cases of an asymptomatic recurrence (i.e., typical histological features in endomyocardial biopsy without symptoms of heart failure), a short-term increase in the intensity of immunosuppressive therapy may be sufficient. However, symptomatic recurrences are usually fatal despite this therapy *(48)*.

The introduction of EMB rather than autopsy for diagnosing giant cell myocarditis made it possible to investigate the natural history of this unique type of myocarditis. In one study of 63 patients (16–69 yr of age) with documented giant cell myocarditis *(47)*, the presenting symptoms were related to congestive heart failure (75%), ventricular tachycardia (14%), and acute myocardial infarction (6%), accompanied by typical electrocardiographic findings. The combined end point of death or heart transplantation was reached by 89%. Median survival from symptom onset to the end point was 5.5 mo, a finding that did not vary with regard to sex or age. Survival was significantly better among patients who received immunosuppressive therapy.

In conclusion, giant cell myocarditis has a more fulminant course than the more common type of myocarditis, lymphocytic myocarditis. However, the responsiveness to immunosuppressive therapy in pretransplanted patients may improve prognosis, again emphasizing the potential role of EMB in the guidance of therapy for patients with heart failure refractory to usual care.

TREATMENT

The standard therapy for patients with myocarditis complicated by heart failure is similar to that for other causes of heart failure and is described elsewhere in this book. However, the use of digoxin in myocarditis-induced heart failure merits special attention. Digoxin may induce increased expression of proinflammatory cytokines. In murine models of viral myocarditis, the use of digoxin has led to increased mortality *(49)*. Thus, the use of digoxin in this approach, if at all, should be at the lowest possible dosages.

Another unique characteristic of myocarditis is related to the need for specific therapy to halt or repress the inflammatory process in the myocardium. With regard to viral myocarditis, several reports have shown encouraging data supporting the use of antiviral agents in the acute treatment, a trend that may be related to a decrease in the viral load in the infected tissue *(50–56)*. This course of therapy is currently being assessed in a clinical study *(52)*. Another issue is the use of mechanical devices as a bridging therapy in cases of severe refractory (and hopefully transient) heart failure. This new direction emphasizes the need to identify the subgroup of patients in whom the disease is reversible, even though they have severe heart failure. These patients may benefit from "bridging" mechanical support of the heart and avoid the need for heart transplantation.

Immunosuppressive Therapy

Mason et al. *(53)* conducted a multicenter trial designed to evaluate the efficacy of immunosuppressive therapy in myocarditis. Patients (*n* = 111) with left ventricular dysfunction (left ventricular ejection fraction ≤0.45) and documented myocarditis (based on histopathological diagnosis) were randomly assigned to either conventional therapy for heart failure or combined therapy with a 24-wk regimen of immunosuppressive drugs (prednisone with either cyclosporine or azathioprine). The immunosuppressive and control groups did not differ significantly in either survival or left ventricular ejection fraction at 1 yr or throughout the follow-up-period. Furthermore, renal dysfunction was more prevalent in the immunosuppressive group (the cyclosporine–prednisone arm) compared with the control group. In patients with histologic findings of myocarditis associated with dilated cardiomyopathy, improvement was seen in an equal number of patients with and without immunosuppressive therapy *(54)*.

The possible benefit of intravenous immunoglobulins (IVIG) was also examined in a randomized placebo-controlled trial *(49)*. Contrary to a previous report that indicated improvement in left ventricular function *(56)*, treatment with IVIG failed to improve the left ventricular ejection fraction at 6 mo in the control group. Currently, the addition of immunosuppressive therapy in adults with idiopathic or infectious myocarditis and left ventricular dysfunction does not seem to have a beneficial effect. However, this conclusion cannot be generalized. As stated earlier, immunosuppressive therapy may be beneficial in specific types of myocarditis such as idiopathic giant cell myocarditis *(43,44)* and in cases related to autoimmune disorders such as lupus erythematosus, scleroderma, sarcoidosis, and polymyositis *(30)*.

MECHANICAL SUPPORT

Intra-aortic Balloon Pump

In patients with fulminant myocarditis complicated by refractory cardiogenic shock, the use of mechanical devices for hemodynamic support is needed. Intra-aortic balloon pump (IABP) use is mandatory in every case refractory to intravenous inotropic support. The indications and contraindications are similar to those related to cardiogenic shock from other causes.

Ventricular Assist Device

In cases of shock that is refractory to IABP or when IABP use is contraindicated because of comorbidities (peripheral vascular disease, acute ischemia to the lower limbs, etc.), implantation of a ventricular assist device (VAD) is optimal. VADs of various design have been tested over the past three decades for temporary support of the failing heart *(57)*. The use of a VAD should not be based on the findings of endomyocardial biopsy because the correlation between histological findings and recovery of cardiac function with a VAD is controversial. Biopsies from the right ventricle may fail to correlate with the degree of left ventricular dysfunction *(58)*. In fulminant myocarditis, it is also necessary to choose between a left ventricular assist device (LVAD) and biventricular assist device (BVAD). The potentially increased risk of implanting the latter makes LVAD the better option in most cases *(59–61)*. Farrar et al. *(62)* suggested that the earlier the VAD was implanted, the more likely the patient could be supported by LVAD alone. Another possible therapeutic approach suggested by Ueno et al. *(63)* is to implant a LVAD and treat the failing right heart using aggressive pharmacological unloading with inhaled nitric oxide and inotropic agents. (See Chapters 19 and 20 on left ventricular assist devices and artificial hearts.)

Percutaneous Cardiopulmonary Support

Kato et al. *(64)* studied nine patients with acute fulminant myocarditis and cardiogenic shock who were supported by percutaneous cardiopulmonary support (PCPS) for 6.4 ± 2.2 d. The femoral artery and vein were used for cannulation. In seven of the nine patients, PCPS was associated with favorable results. Patients experienced hemodynamic improvement and were successfully weaned from the PCPS without significant side effects *(64)*.

Extracorporeal Membrane Oxygenation

Extracorporeal membrane oxygenation (ECMO) was initially indicated for the treatment of acute pulmonary failure, especially among neonates. Using ECMO in these cases resulted in improved survival. Modest success also has been gained in supporting postbypass heart failure in children *(65)*. During standard venoarterial ECMO cannulation, the patient's right ventricle is effectively decompressed, but decompression of the left ventricle cannot be anticipated. Therefore, the use of ECMO may cause further decompensation of the left ventricle in some patients by increasing afterload and systolic wall stress *(66–70)*. In cases refractory to ECMO alone, LVAD support (aimed for left ventricular decompression) may be added *(69)*. Another option is to place a catheter ("vent") in the left atrium or ventricle, allowing some of the blood return to the left heart to be bypassed into the venous return of the cardiopulmonary bypass *(67)*. Cofer et al. *(70)* reported their experience with ECMO in myocarditis patients. Three children with decompensated heart failure secondary to viral myocarditis were assisted by ECMO, and remarkable decompression of the left heart was noted in each case. One patient died, but successful weaning from ECMO was achieved in the other two children. Chen et al. *(71)* described five patients with myocarditis and cardiogenic shock who were successfully treated with ECMO. Four of them were hemodynamically stabilized, weaned off the ECMO, and resumed functional class I status. The troponin T level that was markedly elevated before initiating ECMO support declined significantly within 3 d. These findings are supported by other reports indicating good outcome in adult patients with fulminant myocarditis rescued by prolonged ECMO support *(72–74)*.

Heart Transplantation

Acute myocarditis associated with cardiogenic shock predicts poor survival. Although this condition may be reversible, thus favoring prolonged use of cardiac support (either medical or mechanical) in a refractory and severely decompensated patient, heart transplantation remains the last choice of therapy. Parisi et al. *(75)* reported their experience of heart transplantation in 65 pediatric patients; for 8 of them, transplantation was indicated because of lymphocytic myocarditis. During the first year, the incidence of acute rejection was higher among patients with myocarditis compared with those with cardiomyopathy and congenital heart disease (3.7 ± 2 episodes/patient/yr, 1.7 ± 1.5 episodes/patient/yr, and 1.58 ± 1.4 episodes/patient/yr, respectively). This report suggests that the stimulation of the immune system during myocarditis may have deleterious effects on the posttransplant course. Calabrese et al. *(76)* examined 45 explanted hearts from patients who underwent orthotrophic heart transplantations for the presence of enterovirus genome using reverse transcriptase–polymerase chain reaction. Among the carriers, further search for the viral genome was performed in biopsies from the transplant. The patients who were studied had various etiologies of heart failure; the enterovirus genome (the most common agent responsible for viral myocarditis) was found in only two patients and was associated with a poor prognosis. Despite the small size of the cohort, this interesting observation may contribute to the understanding of the poor results of heart transplantation in myocarditis.

PERIPARTUM CARDIOMYOPATHY

Peripartum cardiomyopathy is defined clinically as the onset of cardiac failure with no identifiable cause in the last month of pregnancy or within 5 mo after delivery, in the absence of heart disease before the last month of pregnancy *(77)*. Echocardiographically, the diagnosis is supported by left ventricular ejection fraction ≤0.45, fractional shortening <30%, or both, and a left-ventricular end-diastolic dimension of >2.7 cm/m^2 of body surface area *(78)*. In the United States, it is diagnosed in 1 per 3000 or 4000 live births *(79)*. Although some patients improve or remain with stable left ventricular dysfunction and clinical heart failure, others deteriorate rapidly, developing full-blown cardiogenic shock *(80)*. In one series *(81)*, a high proportion of patients with peripartum cardiomyopathy had histologic evidence of myocarditis on EMB (26 of 51 patients). The clinical course of peripartum cardiomyopathy may also mimic that of myocarditis.

Patients with peripartum cardiomyopathy are generally treated in the same way as other patients with heart failure, except for special considerations regarding drug therapy in the pregnant or lactating woman. Because peripartum cardiomyopathy is considered a prothrombotic state, anticoagulation with heparins, heparinoids, or warfarin should be favorably considered. In case of shock, the use of IABP or LVADs should be contemplated as a bridge until myocardial recovery occurs or cardiac transplantation is performed.

CONCLUSION

Acute myocarditis is usually a benign and self-limiting disease, but in some cases, it may result in cardiogenic shock. Early identification of acute myocarditis as the cause of shock may assist clinicians when choosing a proper strategy of therapy. Myocarditis is unique in that the immunosuppressive therapy may be beneficial (in certain subtypes) while the condition may reverse itself. When pharmacological treatment fails, the temporary use of mechanical assist devices to support the failing heart should be encouraged. Heart transplantation should be postponed as much as possible in order to allow a possible recovery in cardiac function. EMB has a certain role in diagnosis as well as in predicting such a recovery, although its benefits are usually limited to distinct etiologies.

REFERENCES

1. O'Connell JB, Renlund DG. Myocarditis and specific myocardial diseases. In: Schlant RC, Alexander RW, eds. Hurst's The Heart. 8th ed. McGraw-Hill, New York, 1994, p. 1592.
2. Hyypia T. Etiological diagnosis of viral heart disease. Scand J Infect Dis 1993;88(Suppl):25–31.
3. Hagar JM. Rahimtoola SH. Chagas' heart disease in the United States. N Engl J Med 1991;325:763–768.
4. Matsumori A, Kawai C. An animal model of congestive (dilated) cardiomyopathy: dilatation and hypertrophy of the heart in the chronic stage in DBA/2 mice with myocarditis caused by encephalomyocarditis virus. Circulation 1982;66:355–360.
5. McManus BM, Chow LH, Wilson JE, et al. Direct myocardial injury by enterovirus: a central role in the evolution of murine myocarditis. Clin Immunol Immunopathol 1993;68:159–169.
6. Woodruff JF. Viral myocarditis: a review. Am J Pathol 1980;101:425–484.
7. Lodge PA, Herzum M, Olszewski J, Huber SA. Coxsackievirus B-3 myocarditis: acute and chronic forms of the disease caused by different immunopathogenic mechanism. Am J Pathol 1987;128:455–463.

8. Rose NR, Neumann DA, Herskowitz A. Coxsackievirus myocarditis. Adv Intern Med 1992;37:411–429.
9. Myocarditis Treatment Trial Investigators. Incidence and clinical characteristics of myocarditis [abstract]. Circulation 1991;84(Suppl 2):II-2.
10. Fuse K, Kodama M, Okura Y, et al. Predictors of disease course in patients with acute myocarditis. Circulation 2000;102:2829–2835.
11. Karjalainen J. Functional and myocarditis-induced T-wave abnormalities. Effect of orthostasis beta-blockade, and epinephrine. Chest 1983;83:868–874.
12. Toshima H, Ohkita Y, Shingu M. Clinical features of acute coxsackie B viral myocarditis. Jpn Circ J 1979;43:441–444.
13. Granath A, Kimby AG, Sodemark T, Volpe U, Zetterquist S. Stokes–Adams attacks requiring pacemaker treatment in three patients with acute nonspecific myocarditis. Acta Med Scand 1980;207:177–181.
14. Costanzo-Nordin Mr, O'Connell JB, Subramanian R, Robinson JA, Scanlon PJ. Myocarditis confirmed by biopsy presenting as acute myocardial infarction. Br Heart J 1985;53:25–29.
15. Laurenceau JL, Cereze P, Dumesnil JG. Echocardiographic monitoring of myocarditis: detection of regional dysfunction. Coeur Med Interne 1979;18:451–459.
16. Pinamonti B, Alberti E, Cigalotto A, et al. Echocardiographic findings in myocarditis. Am J Cardiol 1988;62:285–291.
17. Arvan S, Manalo E. Sudden increase in left ventricular mass secondary acute myocarditis. Am Heart J 1988;116:200–202.
18. Acquatella H, Schiller NB. Echocardiographic recognition of Chagas' disease and endomyocardial fibrosis. J Am Soc Echocardiogr 1988;1:60–68.
19. Herskowitz A, Cambell S, Deckers J, et al. Demographic features and prevalence of idiopathic myocarditis in patients undergoing endomyocardial biopsy. Am J Cardiol 1993;71:982–986.
20. Starling RC, Van Fossen DB, Hammer DF, Unverferth DV. Morbidity of endomyocardial biopsy in cardiomyopathy. Am J Cardiol 1991;68:133–136.
21. Lewis AB, Neustein HB, Takahashi M, Lurie PR. Findings on endomyocardial biopsy in infants and children with dilated cardiomyopathy. Am J Cardiol 1985;55:143–145.
22. Wiles HB, Gilette PC, Harley RA, Upshur JK. Cardiomyopathy and myocarditis in children with ventricular ectopic. J Am Coll Cardiol 1992;20:359–362.
23. Webber SA, Boyle GJ, Jaffe R, Pickering RM, Beerman LB, Fricker FJ. Role of right ventricular endomyocardial biopsy in infants and children with suspected or possible myocarditis. Br Heart J 1994;72:360–363.
24. Sanderson JE, Koech D, Iha D, Ojiambo HP. T-Lymphocyte subsets in idiopathic dilated cardiomyopathy. Am J Cardiol 1985;55:755–758.
25. Caforio ALP, Stewart JT, Bonifacio E, et al. Inappropriate major histocompatability complex expression on cardiac tissue in dilated cardiomyopathy: relevance for autoimmunity? J Autoimmun 1990;3:187–200.
26. Caforio ALP, Goldman JH, Baig MK, et al. Cardiac autoantibodies in dilated cardiomyopathy become undetectable with disease progression. Heart 1997;77:62–67.
27. Magnusson Y, Wallukat G, Waagstein F, Hjalmarson A, Hoebeke J. Autoimmunity in idiopathic dilated cardiomyopathy: characterization of antibodies against the beta 1-adrenoreceptor with positive chronotropic effect. Circulation 1994;89:2760–2767.
28. Podlowski S, Luther HP, Morwinski R, Muller J, Wallukar G. Agonistic anti-betal-adrenergic receptor expression autoantibodies from cardiomyopathy patients reduce the betal-adrenergic receptor expression in neonatal rat cardiomyocytes. Circulation 1998;98:2470–2476.
29. Baig MK, Goldman JH, Caforio ALP, Coonar AS, Keeling PJ, McKenna WJ. Familial dilated cardiomyopathy: cardiac abnormalities are common in asymptomatic relatives and may represent early disease. J Am Coll Cardiol 1998;31:195–201.
30. Feldman AM, McNamara DM. Medical Prognosis: myocarditis. N Engl J Med 2000;343:1388–1398.
31. Fenoglio JJ, Ursell PC, Kellogg CF, Drusin RE, Weiss MB. Diagnosis and classification of myocarditis by endomyocardial biopsy. N Engl J Med 1983;308:12–18.
32. Rockman HA, Adamson RM, Dembitsky WP, Bonar JW, Jaski BE. Acute fulminant myocarditis: long-term follow-up after circulatory support with left ventricular assist device. Am Heart J 1991;121:922–926.
33. Dec GW Jr, Palacios IF, Fallon JT, et al. Active myocarditis in the spectrum of acute dilated cardiomyopathies. Clinical features, histologic correlates, and clinical outcomes. N Engl J Med 1985;312:885–890.

34. Saffitz JE, Schwartz DJ, Southworth W, et al. Coxsackie viral myocarditis causing transmural right and left ventricular infarction without coronary narrowing. Am J Cardiol 1983;52:644–647.

35. Burch GE, Shewey IL. Viral coronary arteritis and myocardial infarction. Am Heart J 1976;92:11–14.

36. Ferguson DW, Farwell AP, Bradley WA, Rollings RC. Coronary artery vasospasm complicating acute myocarditis. West J Med 1988;148:664–669.

37. Phillips M, Robinowitz M, Higgins JR, Boran KJ, Reed T, Virmani R. Sudden cardiac death in Air Force recruits. A 20-year review. JAMA 1986;256:2696–2699.

38. Cooper LT, Berry GJ, Rizeq M, Schroeder JS. Giant cell myocarditis. J Heart Lung Transplant 1995;14:394–401.

39. Hosenpud JD, McAnulty JH, Niles NR. Lack of objective improvement in ventricular systolic function in patients with myocarditis treated with azathioprine and prednisone. J Am Coll Cardiol 1985;6:797–801.

40. Hanawa H, Kodama M, Inomata T, et al. Anti-alpha beta T cell receptor antibody prevents the prognosis of experimental autoimmune myocarditis. Clin Exp Immunol 1994;96:470–475.

41. Zhang S, Kodama M, Hanawa H, Izumi T, Shibata A, Masani F. Effects of cyclosporine, prednisolone and aspirin on rat autoimmune giant cell myocarditis. J Am Coll Cardiol 1993;21:1254–1260.

42. Desjardins V, Pelletier G, Leung TK, Waters D. Successful treatment of severe heart failure caused by idiopathic giant cell myocarditis. Can J Cardiol 1992;8:788–792.

43. Ren H, Poston RS Jr, Hruban RH, Baumgartner WA, Baughman KL, Hutchins GM. Long survival with giant cell myocarditis. Mod Pathol 1993;6:402–407.

44. Kong G, Madden B, Spyrou N, Pomerance A, Mitchell A, Yacoub M. Response of recurrence giant cell myocarditis in a transplanted heart to intensive immunosuppression. Eur Heart J 1991;12:554–557.

45. Gries W, Farkas D, Winters GL, Constanzo-Nordin MR. Giant cell myocarditis: first report of disease recurrent in the transplanted heart. J Heart Lung Transplant 1992;11:370–374.

46. Grant SC. Giant cell myocarditis in a transplanted heart. Eur Heart J 1993;14:1437.

47. Cooper DK, Schlesinger RG, Shrago S, Zuhdi N. Heart transplantation for giant cell myocarditis. J Heart Lung Transplant 1994;13:555.

48. Cooper LT jr, Berry GJ, Shabetai R. Idiopathic giant-cell myocarditis — natural history and treatment. Multicenter Giant Cell Myocarditis Study Group Investigators. N Engl J Med 1997;336:1860–1866.

49. Matsumori A, Igata H, Ono K, et al. High doses of digitalis increase the myocardial production of proinflammatory cytokines and worsen myocardial injury in viral myocarditis: a possible mechanism of digitalis toxicity. Jpn Circ J 1999;63:934–940.

50. McCormack JG, Bowler SD, Donnelly JE, Steadman C. Successful treatment of severe cytomegalovirus infection with ganciclovir in immunocompetent host. Clin Infect Dis 1998;26:1007–1008.

51. Baykurt C, Caglar K, Ceviz N, Akyuz C, Secmeer G. Successful treatment of Epstein–Barr virus infection associated with myocarditis. Pediatr Int 1999;41:389–391.

52. Maisch B, Hufnagel G, Schonian U, Hengstenberg C. The European Study of Epidemiology and Treatment of Cardiac Inflammatory Disease (ESETCID). Eur Heart J 1995;16 (Suppl O):173–175.

53. Mason JW, O'Connell JB, Herskowitz A, et al. and the Myocarditis Treatment Trial Investigators. A clinical trial of immunosuppressive therapy for myocarditis. N Engl J Med 1995;333:269–275.

54. Dec GW, Palacios IF, Fallon JT, et al. Active myocarditis in the spectrum of acute dilated cardiomyopathies. Clinical features, histologic correlates, and clinical outcome. N Engl J Med 1985;312:885–890.

55. McNamara DM, Starling RC, Dec GW, et al. Intervention in myocarditis and acute cardiomyopathy with immune globulin: results from the Randomized Placebo Controlled IMAC Trial [abstract]. Circulation 1999;100(Suppl I):I-21.

56. McNamara DM, Rosenblum WD, Janosko, et al. Intravenous immune globulin in the therapy of myocarditis and acute cardiomyopathy. Circulation 1997;95:2467–2468.

57. Hetzer R, Henning E, Schiessler A, Friedel N, Warnecke H, Adt M. Mechanical circulatory support and heart transplantation. J Heart Lung Transplant 1992;11:S175–S181.

58. Ueno T, Bergin P, Richardson M, Esmore DS. Bridge to recovery with a left ventricular assist device for fulminant acute myocarditis. Ann Thorac Surg 2000;69:284–286.

59. Rockman HA, Adamson RM, Denbitsky WP, Bonar JW, Jaski BE. Acute fulminant myocarditis: long-term follow-up after circulatory support with left ventricular assist device. Am Heart J 1991;121:922–926.

60. Chang AC, Hanley FL, Weindling SN, Wernovsky G, Wessel DL. Left heart support with a ventricular assist device in an infant with acute myocarditis. Crit Care Med 1992;20:712–715.

61. Holman WL, Bourge RC, Kirklin JK. Case report: circulatory support for seventy days with resolution of acute heart failure. J Thorac Cardiovasc Surg 1991;102:932–934.

62. Farrar D, Hill JD, Pennington DG, McBride LR, et al. Preoperative and postoperative comparison of patients with univentricular and biventricular support with the thoratec ventricular assist device as a bridge to cardiac transplantation. J Thorac Cardiovasc Surg 1997;113:202–209.

63. Uneo T, Bergin P, Richardson M, Esmore DS. Bridge to recovery with a left ventricular assist device for fulminant acute myocarditis. Ann Thorac Surg 2000;69:284–286.

64. Kato S, Morimoto SI, Hiramitsu S, Nomura M, Ito T, Hishida H. Use of percutaneous cardiopulmonary support of patients with fulminant myocarditis and cardiogenic shock for improving prognosis. Am J Cardiol 1999;83:623–625.

65. Bartlett RH. Extracorporeal life support for cardiopulmonary failure. Curr Probl Surg 1990;27:623–705.

66. Bavaria JE, Furukawa S, Kreiner G, Gupta KB, Streicher J, Edmunds LH. Effect of circulatory assist devices on stunned myocardium. Ann Thorac Surg 1990;49:123–128.

67. Martin GR, Short BL. Doppler echocardiographic evaluation of cardiac performance in infants on prolonged extracorporeal membrane oxygenation. Am J Cardiol 1988;62:929–934.

68. Bavaria JE, Ratcliffe MB, Gupta KB, Wenger RK, Bogen DK, Edmunds LH. Changes in left ventricular systolic wall stress during biventricular circulatory assistance. Ann Thorac Surg 1988;45:526–532.

69. Kawahito K, Murata SI, Yasu T, et al. Usefulness of extracorporeal membrane oxygenation for treatment of fulminant myocarditis and circulatory collapse. Am J Cardiol 1998;82:910–911.

70. Cofer BR, Warner BW, Stallion A, Ryckman FC. Extracorporeal membrane oxygenation in the management of cardiac failure secondary to myocarditis. J Pediatr Surg 1993;28:669–672.

71. Chen YS, Wang MJ, Chou NK, et al. Rescue for acute myocarditis with shock by extracorporeal membrane oxygenation. Ann Thorac Surg 1999;68:2220–2224.

72. Yasu T, Murata S, Katsuki T, et al. Acutely severe myocarditis successfully treated by percutaneous cardiopulmonary support applied by a newly developed heparin-binding oxygenator and circuits. Jpn Circ J 1997;61:1037–1042.

73. Tsuboi H, Sone T, Sassa H, et al. Rescue of a patient with fulminant myocarditis by percutaneous extracorporeal bypass. Jpn J Med 1990;29:519–522.

74. Morishima I, Sassa H, Sone T, Tsuboi H, Kondo J, Koyama T. A case of fulminant myocarditis rescued by long-term percutaneous cardiopulmonary support. Jpn Circ J 1994;58:433–438.

75. Parisi F, Carotti A, Esu F, Abbattista AD, Cicini MP, Squitieri C. Intermediate and long-term results after pediatric heart transplantation: incidence and role of pretransplant diagnosis. Transplant Int 1998;11(Suppl 1):S493–S498.

76. Calabrese F, Valente M, Thiene G, et al. Enteroviral genome in native hearts may influence outcome of patients who undergo cardiac transplantation. Diagn Mol Pathol 1999;8:39–46.

77. Pearson GD, Veille JC, Rahimtoola S, et al. Peripartum cardiomyopathy: National Heart, Lung, and Blood Institute and Office of Rare Diseases (National Institute of Health) workshop recommendations and review. JAMA 2000;283:1183–1188.

78. Hibbard JU, Lindheimer M, Lang RM. A modified definition for peripartum cardiomyopathy and prognosis based on echocardiography. Obster Gynecol 1999;94:311–316.

79. Ventura SJ, Peters KD, Martin JA, Maurer JD. Births and deaths: United States, 1996. Mon Vital Stat Rep 1997;46(Suppl 2).

80. Aziz TM, Burgess MI, Acladious NN, et al. Heart transplantation for peripartum cardiomyopathy: a report of three cases and a literature review. Cardiovasc Surg 1999;7:565–567.

81. Felker GM, Thompson RE, Hare JM, et al. Underlying causes and long-term survival in patients with initially unexplained cardiomyopathy. N Engl J Med 2000;342;1077–1084.

15 Pericardial Disease and Cardiogenic Shock

Aviv Mager, MD, and David Hasdai, MD

CONTENTS

INTRODUCTION
PATHOPHYSIOLOGY
ETIOLOGY
CLINICAL MANIFESTATIONS
TREATMENT
REFERENCES

INTRODUCTION

Cardiac tamponade is a life-threatening condition caused by external compression of the heart by material, usually fluid, in the pericardial sac. The primary pathophysiological mechanism that leads to alterations in cardiac performance is unique. Clinically, cardiac tamponade is an emergency because it can lead to rapid hemodynamic deterioration, shock, and, eventually, death *(1)*.

The growing availability of echocardiography in recent years has dramatically improved and expedited the bedside diagnosis, evaluation, and treatment of cardiac tamponade. Treatment options have also expanded in recent years with the introduction of safer, echocardiographically guided pericardiocentesis techniques and other catheter-based and surgical interventions.

PATHOPHYSIOLOGY

Principal Mechanism

The pathophysiological mechanism underlying cardiac tamponade has been a subject of controversy; today, several mechanisms are believed to be involved. The principal pathophysiological mechanism is an increase in intrapericardial pressure resulting from an accumulation of material, usually fluid, within the pericardial sac. Because the pericardial sac has sinuses and recesses *(2)*, fluid initially fills the volume reserve and expands the parietal pericardium without increasing the intrapericardial pressure.

The pericardial sac is noncompliant and can stretch in the clinical setting only if distended very slowly. Therefore, if the accumulation of additional fluid exceeds the stretch rate of the parietal pericardium *(3)* or the clearance rate from the pericardial

From: *Contemporary Cardiology: Cardiogenic Shock: Diagnosis and Treatment*
Edited by: David Hasdai et al. © Humana Press Inc., Totowa, NJ

space, then a steep increase in intrapericardial pressure results. Initially, the intrapericardial pressure rises to the level of the right atrial and right ventricular diastolic pressures, reducing the ability of these chambers to distend. Thus, the transmural
(distending) pressures of these chambers are reduced *(4)*. The transmural pressure is
calculated as the intracavitary diastolic pressure minus the pericardial pressure. Loss of
the transmural pressure results in a decrease in end-diastolic volume, a principal determinant of cardiac filling. Loss of transmural pressure also results in a decrease in sar-
comere length; this reduces the heart's ability to contract and results in a reduction in
stroke volume.

The reduction in stroke volume and the decrease in end-diastolic volume hinder the
venous return and this leads to dependence on venous pressure for chamber filling.
Thus, the loss of right atrial and right ventricular distending pressure increases the
impedance to systemic venous return, leading to compensatory elevation in systemic
venous pressure. With further accumulation of fluid in the pericardial sac, the systemic
venous pressure and the diastolic right atrial and right ventricular pressures rise
together with the intrapericardial pressure to reach the level of the left atrial and left
ventricular diastolic pressures. This results in impaired filling of the chambers, a subsequent fall in systemic arterial pressure, and shock.

Ventricular Interdependence

Because the pericardial volume reserve is lost in tamponade and the parietal pericardium and pericardial fluid are noncompliant, the space occupied by the heart in tamponade becomes relatively fixed. An increase in diastolic volume of the ventricle,
particularly the right ventricle, results in a decrease in diastolic volume of the other
ventricle, impairing both filling and contraction of this ventricle. This condition is
known as ventricular interdependence, or coupling.

Dependence on Venous Filling

Because the atria are compressed, atrial contraction may also be impaired, further
increasing the dependence on systemic venous pressure for right ventricular filling and
on pulmonary venous pressure for left ventricular filling. This dependence on venous
pressure becomes particularly important during inspiration because when a patient
breathes in air, the thorax expands and pulmonary venous pressure falls, resulting in
reduced left ventricular stroke volume.

Effects of Respiration

Inspiration creates a negative pressure in the thorax, lowering the pressure in the
pericardial sac and intrathoracic vessels (systemic and pulmonary). Because of the
decreased impedance, the flow from the systemic veins into the right cardiac chambers
increases, increasing right ventricular volume and output. Conversely, the inspiratory
decrease in pulmonary venous pressure reduces left ventricular diastolic volume and
output, producing the physiological inspiratory drop of ≤ 10 mm Hg in systemic arterial pressure.

In cardiac tamponade, the heart is compressed, systemic venous pressure is elevated,
and right and left ventricular pressures are equalized, resulting in the straightening of
the interventricular septum or even in the bulging of the septum into the left ventricular
cavity. The straightening of the normally curved septum shortens its fibers and reduces

its contractility. Therefore, this morphological change may play an important role in reducing left ventricular output during inspiration *(5)*. All of these changes lead to pulsus paradoxus, an exaggerated inspiratory fall in systemic blood pressure characteristic of cardiac tamponade.

The importance of right ventricular overfilling as a cause of pulsus paradoxus was demonstrated by Shabetai et al. *(6)*, who showed that bypass of the right ventricle or strict control of its volume during inspiration prevented the straightening of the septum and the resulting inspiratory fall in blood pressure. This may explain the absence of pulsus paradoxus in conditions where right ventricular filling does not vary significantly with inspiration (e.g., in atrial septal defect, anomalous pulmonary venous connection, and severe hypovolemia).

The reduced intrathoracic pressure during inspiration also decreases pulmonary venous pressure and the diastolic gradient between the pulmonary veins and the left heart chambers. This leads to inspiratory blood pooling in the pulmonary vessels and reduced left ventricular diastolic filling *(7)*. Because in tamponade the distending pressure is lost and the left ventricle is already compressed, the inspiratory decrease in diastolic filling causes a further decrease in left ventricular end-diastolic volume and output. The decrease in intrathoracic pressure is probably similar to normal inspiratory variation; thus, tamponade is not associated with marked dyspnea.

Neurohormones

In tamponade, increased adrenergic tone may initially compensate for the reduction in stroke volume. Increased adrenergic tone causes tachycardia and increased contractility, and these increase the ejection fraction and accelerate myocardial relaxation, which facilitates diastolic filling . β-Adrenergic blockade may, therefore, have a deleterious effect on patients with cardiac tamponade and should not be used. At an advanced stage, left ventricular diastolic pressure becomes elevated, followed by low cardiac output, systemic vasoconstriction, and hypoperfusion. In tamponade, the release of atrial natriuretic factor is inhibited despite the increase in atrial pressure, and sodium retention develops.

Coronary Circulation

In advanced tamponade, reduced blood pressure and increased ventricular diastolic pressure culminate in coronary hypoperfusion and myocardial ischemia, which may further reduce cardiac output.

ETIOLOGY

The underlying causes of cardiac tamponade have varied in recent years, reflecting changes in public health and in the effects and complications of modern medicine. Among reports from different institutions, the variable causes are attributable to differences in caseload, prevalence of disease in the population, and activity of hospital services such as cardiac surgery, interventional cardiology, oncology, and hemodialysis.

Our series *(8)*, which is similar to recent reports *(9)*, identifies the most common causes of cardiac tamponade as malignancy, including the following: lung cancer, breast cancer, lymphoma, and melanoma (44%); idiopathic pericarditis (15%); post-pericardiotomy complications (11%); invasive cardiologic procedures (6%); myocardial infarction (6%); uremia (5%); congestive heart failure (4%); hypothyroidism (2%); purulent pericarditis (2%). Other less common causes of tamponade include tuberculosis, connective tissue disease [scleroderma, systemic lupus erythematosus (SLE), rheumatoid arthritis], postradiation complications, nephrotic syndrome, hypoalbuminemia, pulmonary hypertension, pulmonary embolism, pneumonia, chylous pericarditis, human immunodeficiency virus (HIV) infection *(10),* and anticoagulant use *(11).* In some patients, more than one possible cause of cardiac tamponade can be found.

Cardiac tamponade may occur as a complication of invasive cardiologic procedures, including transcatheter coronary interventions, myocardial biopsies, electrophysiologic procedures (such as pacemaker insertions), and other catheter-based manipulations. In a recent report, 0.2% of 6999 percutaneous coronary interventions were complicated by cardiac tamponade *(12).* In a series of 960 consecutive echo-guided pericardiocentesis procedures, 9.6% were for iatrogenic tamponade *(13).* Cardiac tamponade may occur as late as 36 h after an invasive procedure and often necessitates evacuation of pericardial fluid.

CLINICAL MANIFESTATIONS

Although cardiac tamponade may occur suddenly, it is often a progressive disorder with a spectrum of clinical manifestations. These may vary from a silent accumulation of fluid, detected only by specific physical and echocardiographic findings, to apprehension and shock, depending on the rate of fluid accumulation, extent of cardiac compression, and cardiac and noncardiac comorbidity. Based on representative data, patients with cardiac tamponade present with these clinical manifestations: neck vein distension (80–100%), pulsus paradoxus (100%), tachypnea (80%), tachycardia (80%), hypotension (40%), chest pain (12%), friction rub (10%), and cough (10%).

Beck *(14)* described the classic triad of hypotension, elevated systemic venous pressure, and a small quiet heart. This presentation is typical of sudden-onset tamponade with shock, usually caused by acute intrapericardial bleeding resulting from penetrating trauma, rupture of an aortic dissection, cardiac or coronary perforation during invasive procedures, or cardiac rupture complicating acute myocardial infarction. The predominant signs of sudden-onset tamponade with shock are pulsus paradoxus, neck vein engorgement, and those of shock: diaphoresis, pallor, tachypnea, impaired consciousness with restlessness or stupor, cold and clammy extremities, and anuria. Typically, there are no signs of pulmonary congestion. A small heart is characteristic of patients with sudden-onset tamponade with shock because acute intrapericardial bleeding causes a sudden increase in intrapericardial pressure before the pericardial sac has expanded.

In some patients, tamponade and shock develop at an advanced stage after a large amount of pericardial fluid has gradually accumulated *(15).* Some of these patients become symptomatic before the onset of overt tamponade and complain of chest discomfort, fatigability, dyspnea with effort, or cough. The most consistent physical findings at this stage are elevated systemic venous pressure, mild pulsus paradoxus, mild tachypnea, and mild tachycardia. Often, the predominant manifestations are those of an underlying systemic disease, particularly a malignancy. When severe tamponade develops, the manifestations are indistinguishable from those described in patients with sudden-onset tamponade.

Physical Examination

Pulsus paradoxus (inspiratory decrease in systolic blood pressure of >10 mm Hg) and jugular venous distention are hallmarks of cardiac tamponade. Pulsus paradoxus should be determined during normal breathing because deep breathing may result in a false-positive diagnosis. The extent of the inspiratory decrease in systolic blood pressure may reflect the severity of the hemodynamic compromise. In severe tamponade, the Korotkoff sounds may disappear entirely during inspiration. Jugular venous distention is also essential to the diagnosis of cardiac tamponade unless the patient is severely hypovolemic.

Echocardiography

Transthoracic echocardiography is the most useful method for detecting pericardial fluid in patients with suspected tamponade. Good quality images that show no cardiac tamponade virtually rule out this diagnosis, except for cardiac tamponade that is related to localized cardiac compression. This is particularly important for preventing unnecessary and potentially lethal pericardiocentesis. Once pericardiocentesis is planned, transthoracic echocardiography is also used to delineate the pericardial sac and select the puncture site.

When a pericardial effusion is detected, further echocardiographic investigation may provide important, detailed information on its hemodynamic significance and potential role in the development of shock. Two-dimensional echocardiography often reveals right-atrial compression during late diastole and early systole *(16)*. However, up to 92% of the patients with pericardial effusion, with or without tamponade, have an inversion of ≥ 30% of the right atrial free wall *(15)*. Therefore, this finding is not specific to cardiac tamponade and may simply indicate the accumulation of pericardial fluid around the right atrium when it contracts and empties into the right ventricle.

Another echocardiographic finding, early diastolic right ventricular collapse *(17)*, is considered a more specific and reliable sign of pericardial tamponade. It is more predictive of tamponade than pulsus paradoxus in the context of hypovolemia *(18)*; however, it may be absent in patients with pulmonary hypertension. Dilatation of the inferior vena cava without an inspiratory collapse of > 50% has also been proposed as a sign of tamponade *(19)*.

The typical straightening and leftward shift of the interventricular septum into the left ventricular cavity during inspiration can also be detected by echocardiography *(20)*. In addition, premature closure of the aortic valve and delayed, diminished, or late diastolic mitral valve opening may be detectable on the echocardiogram when tamponade is at an advanced stage and may indicate low output and severe hemodynamic compromise.

Pseudohypertrophy of the left ventricle may be observed during tamponade and may be proportional to the decrease in left ventricular volume. A swinging heart appearance is not necessarily associated with tamponade but is often noted in patients with large pericardial effusions.

In patients with tamponade, Doppler ultrasound typically reveals exaggerated pulmonic and tricuspid flow velocities and markedly increased respiratory variation in transmitral flow velocity, corresponding to the inspiratory decrease and expiratory increase in left ventricular filling and output *(7,21)*. Patients with cardiac tamponade exhibit an approx 43% reduction in E-wave velocity and approx 25% reduction in A-wave velocity during the first inspiratory cardiac cycle and a reduction in the predominantly systolic inflow through the hepatic vein or the superior vena cava (with a predominant X descent and little or no Y descent) *(22)*.

The echocardiographic finding of a left ventricular inflow velocity change of > 22% corresponds with right-sided equalization of pressure *(23)*. In this context, an inspiratory decrease of more than 15% in transmitral flow velocity is often considered significant. However, this "flow paradoxus" change may be the Doppler counterpart of pulsus paradoxus and may have similar limitations *(24)* so that the reliability of a diagnosis made exclusively on this basis is uncertain *(4,24,25)*, particularly in dyspneic patients.

Other typical findings on Doppler ultrasound include an inspiratory decrease and expiratory increase in pulmonary venous diastolic flow, an expiratory increase in hepatic diastolic flow reversal, and a decrease in the diastolic component of the forward flow in the superior vena cava.

Two important pitfalls in the use of echocardiography for diagnosis of pericardial tamponade should be mentioned. First, right ventricular collapse may occur as a result of external compression by a large pleural effusion and may be absent in patients with right ventricular hypertrophy or pulmonary hypertension. Second, transthoracic echocardiography may not identify loculated effusions or localized compressions caused by a thrombus after cardiac surgery.

Nevertheless, the combination of a marked inspiratory decrease in transmitral flow velocity, diastolic right ventricular collapse, abnormal inspiratory septal configuration, right ventricular enlargement, and inferior vena caval plethora is highly suggestive of cardiac tamponade in a patient with pericardial effusion. These findings are important for diagnosis when concomitant conditions associated with a false-positive or false-negative diagnosis of pulsus paradoxus are present (e.g., during atrial fibrillation, hypovolemia, or respiratory distress). Additionally, the echocardiogram may be helpful in the differential diagnosis of cardiac tamponade from other causes of cardiogenic shock, particularly left or right ventricular dysfunction, infarction, and pulmonary embolism.

Transesophageal echocardiography is usually not indicated in patients with cardiac tamponade. However, it may be indicated in postoperative patients in whom tamponade is suspected because it can help detect intrapericardial blood clots or loculated effusions, which are difficult to identify by transthoracic echocardiography.

Electrocardiogram

The appearance of electrical alternans in a patient with a pre-existing effusion may indicate an increase in pericardial effusion and tamponade. Electrical alternans is attributed to the swinging motion of the heart in patients with a large pericardial effusion and may reflect dynamic changes in cardiac filling. However, electrical alternans is not specific to tamponade and may also be observed in constrictive pericarditis, severe heart failure, and tension pneumothorax. Cardiac tamponade usually does not develop during the early stages of pericarditis, and the typical electrocardiographic changes of early pericarditis may be absent.

The electrocardiogram may also show atrial arrhythmia, a common finding in patients with pericardial effusion. Ventricular arrhythmias are rare, but life-threatening ventricular tachycardia may result from metastatic cardiac disease in patients with a pericardial effusion and a present or past history of malignancy *(26)*.

Table 1
Comparison of Clinical and Hemodynamic Changes in Cardiac Tamponade
and Constrictive Pericarditis

	Cardiac tamponade	*Constrictive pericarditis*
Friction rub	Common	Uncommon
Pulsus paradoxus	Common	Mild or absent
Kussmaul's sign	Absent	Present
Pericardial knock	Absent	Present
Neck vein distention	Common	Present
Peripheral edema	Uncommon	Common
Enlargement of cardiac silhouette	Common	Uncommon
X descent	Present	Present
Y descent	Mild or absent	Present
Pericardial effusion	Present	Uncommon
Shock	Common	Uncommon

Chest Roentgenogram

In the presence of pulsus paradoxus, an enlarged cardiac silhouette and clear lung fields on a chest X-ray are highly indicative of cardiac tamponade. The silhouette of a heart in pericardial effusion has a waterbottle, tent, or globular shape, and the normal contour of the left cardiac border is blurred. However, a normal or unchanged cardiac silhouette does not exclude a hemodynamically important pericardial effusion, particularly when an acute accumulation of pericardial effusion is suspected, because enlargement of the cardiac silhouette is usually not observed until at least 250 mL of fluid have accumulated. Additionally, loculated effusions may have a cystlike appearance, and pneumopericardium can be detected when a radiolucent strip of air surrounds the heart.

Fluoroscopy, Computed Tomography, and Magnetic Resonance Imaging

Fluoroscopy is rarely used today for the diagnosis of pericardial effusion. It can, however, be used to find absent or diminished pulsations and respiratory changes of the heart, which may be very useful in confirming cardiac tamponade in the catheterization laboratory.

Computed tomography (CT) and magnetic resonance imaging (MRI) can help identify and characterize pericardial effusions. Although these techniques are rarely used for the diagnosis of pericardial tamponade, they may offer important insights if tamponade is the result of localized cardiac compression. In addition, they may provide information on relevant cardiac, pericardial, and chest pathology such as tumors, inflammatory processes, pericardial thickening, and foreign bodies.

Differential Diagnosis

Pulsus paradoxus and respiratory transmitral flow variation on echocardiography may be symptoms of constrictive pericarditis. Patients with constrictive pericarditis typically present with jugular venous distension and other signs of elevated right atrial pressure, including hepatomegaly and systemic edema (Table 1). Unlike patients with tamponade, patients with constrictive pericarditis have increased systemic venous pressure during inspiration (Kussmaul's sign). Shock is rare in constrictive pericarditis, but hypotension is occasionally observed.

The rigid shell that surrounds the heart in patients with constrictive pericarditis prevents the transmission of respiratory variations in transthoracic pressure into the pericardial sac. In contrast to tamponade, constrictive pericarditis limits only late, and not early, diastolic filling. Because of the rigidity of the pericardial sac, ventricular relaxation is rapid and is followed by a deep fall in early diastolic pressure. This produces an early diastolic dip in ventricular pressure, with a corresponding prominent Y descent in atrial and systemic venous pressures. The early fall in intracardiac pressure is followed by rapid filling, producing the typical dip and plateau configuration of the ventricular diastolic pressure tracing. These findings are easily recognized on intracardiac pressure recordings and are useful for the differential diagnosis between tamponade and constriction. Calcification of the pericardial sac strongly supports the diagnosis of constriction and is better detected by CT or MRI than by echocardiography.

Noninvasive Quantification of Pericardial Fluid Volume

The size of the effusion is a strong predictor of outcome for patients with cardiac tamponade and is superior to other outcome predictors such as right-heart diastolic collapse, distension of the superior vena cava, and respiratory flow variations *(27)*. Noninvasive quantification of pericardial effusion can therefore be beneficial in assessing the need for pericardiocentesis in patients without overt tamponade. However, the commonly used methods for quantification of pericardial fluid volume by echocardiography are not satisfactory, being based on M-mode echocardiographic findings or involving complex calculations *(28,29)*.

We measured the anteroposterior pericardial sac diameter before pericardiocentesis in 83 procedures and found that it correlated well with effusion size *(8)*. Our method was more accurate in predicting the size of larger versus smaller effusions. However, this disadvantage is not clinically important because in patients with smaller effusions, the decision to intervene depends not on size but on the hemodynamic effects of the effusion or other clinical parameters (e.g., suspicion of purulent pericarditis or a need for diagnostic aspiration).

Cardiac Catheterization

Cardiac catheterization can provide important hemodynamic information on stable patients with pericardial effusion, but it is rarely indicated in hemodynamically unstable patients with clinical and echocardiographic findings typical of cardiac tamponade. Tamponade may develop, however, during cardiac catheterization and other invasive procedures in the catheterization laboratory and in patients undergoing balloon pericardiostomy.

The typical findings in patients with cardiac tamponade are elevated intrapericardial and right atrial pressures, which decline during inspiration. Right atrial pressure typically has a systolic X descent, with an absent or nearly absent diastolic Y descent. Normal right atrial pressure in the presence of pericardial effusion suggests a nontense effusion or a low-pressure tamponade.

When the intrapericardial and right atrial pressures are elevated to or above the level of right ventricular diastolic pressure, all three pressures equalize during mid-diastole. When the intrapericardial pressure exceeds the normal left cardiac diastolic pressure, both pressures and the pulmonary wedge pressure become elevated. Thus, in advanced tamponade, pulmonary capillary wedge pressure, intrapericardial pressure, and all the diastolic intracardiac pressures are equalized.

This may not occur, however, in patients with left ventricular hypertrophy, left ventricular dysfunction, or elevated diastolic pressure from other causes, because, in these conditions, the intrapericardial pressure may not reach the level of left ventricular diastolic pressure. Right ventricular and pulmonary arterial systolic pressures can be mildly or moderately elevated but usually do not exceed 50 mm Hg.

During inspiration, all pressures decline. Pulmonary capillary wedge pressure typically declines more than the intrapericardial pressure during inspiration and rises above it during expiration. The inspiratory decline in right cardiac and intrapericardial pressure is followed, after a short delay, by a decline in left ventricular and aortic systolic pressure. Left ventricular stroke volume progressively declines during tamponade, but cardiac output is often preserved until advanced hemodynamic compromise has occurred.

During pericardiocentesis, a normal hemodynamic profile is usually dramatically and promptly restored after the initial 50–100 mL of fluid has been evacuated. The failure of right atrial pressure to decline with intrapericardial pressure is highly suggestive of a concomitant presence of constrictive pericarditis or a pre-existing elevation of right ventricular diastolic pressure. Shock may persist despite fluid evacuation when other cardiac and noncardiac causes are present (e.g., severe left ventricular dysfunction, acute myocardial infarction [usually extensive or complicated by acute mitral regurgitation], acute ventricular septal defect, acute right ventricular infarction, acute or severe hypovolemia, septicemia, pulmonary embolism, and other causes of severe respiratory distress).

False-Negative, False-Positive, and Differential Diagnoses

In otherwise healthy subjects, pulsus paradoxus is highly suggestive of cardiac tamponade and can be regarded as a prerequisite for this diagnosis. However, causes for false-positive or false-negative diagnoses of tamponade are common and necessitate a thorough evaluation.

FALSE-NEGATIVE DIAGNOSES

The inspiratory decrease in diastolic filling caused by decreased pulmonary venous pressure may not occur in patients with severe left ventricular dysfunction or hypertrophy because left ventricular end-diastolic pressure may be elevated depending on the cardiac pathology. Similarly, pulsus paradoxus may not occur in patients with severe aortic valve incompetence because the volume of blood regurgitating from the aorta is sufficient to distend the left ventricle, thereby eliminating the dependence on pulmonary venous return for diastolic filling.

Pulsus paradoxus and jugular venous distention may be absent in patients with severe hypovolemia; the diagnosis of cardiac tamponade in this context is often based on echocardiography. Pulsus paradoxus may also be absent, in spite of cardiac compression, in patients with right ventricular hypertrophy, atrial septal defect, anomalous pulmonary venous return, and positive breathing pressure.

FALSE-POSITIVE DIAGNOSES

An inspiratory fall in systolic blood pressure can result also from pulmonary embolism, restrictive cardiomyopathy, right ventricular infarction, effusive constrictive pericarditis, and dyspnea from any other underlying pulmonary disease.

Respiratory distress is associated with forceful inspiration and negative intrathoracic pressure and can lead to a marked inspiratory decrease in pulmonary venous pressure. Thus, patients who do not have tamponade but are in respiratory distress because of severe lung disease or pulmonary embolism may be diagnosed with cardiac tamponade. The inspiratory decrease in arterial pressure may also result in a false diagnosis of tamponade in patients with nontense pericardial effusion and dyspnea.

Lung involvement is common in patients with pericardial effusion and is often a manifestation of malignancy, scleroderma, pulmonary hypertension, pleural effusion after cardiac surgery, or another underlying disease. In this context, it is often difficult to determine whether dyspnea is a symptom of cardiac tamponade or lung disease and, more important, whether the presence of paradoxical pulse indicates cardiac compression by the effusion or relates to the pulmonary condition.

TREATMENT

The definitive treatment of cardiac tamponade is evacuation of the pericardial fluid. Although much controversy exists as to the exact indications for and timing of pericardiocentesis in patients with pericardial effusion, cardiac tamponade with hemodynamic decompensation is clearly an emergency necessitating prompt intervention, either by catheter-based techniques or surgery.

Echo-Guided Pericardiocentesis

Percutaneous pericardiocentesis has been performed since the nineteenth century. Traditionally, a metal needle is inserted via the subxiphoid route and advanced blindly in the general direction of the pericardial sac. The procedure was associated with considerable morbidity and a mortality rate of up to 6%, even when performed under fluoroscopy in the catheterization laboratory *(9)*. This changed with the introduction of two-dimensional echocardiographic guidance.

The use of two-dimensional echocardiography can help determine where the pericardial sac is closest to the surface of the body and where the distance between the heart and the boundary of the pericardial sac is sufficient to permit safe insertion of a needle. In addition, it can help to identify vital organs such as the liver or the lungs and routes that avoid them.

Pericardiocentesis under echocardiographic guidance (echo-guided pericardiocentesis) has reduced the morbidity and mortality associated with pericardiocentesis to extremely low rates. The reported procedural success rate is more than 95% *(9)*. Death is rare, and major complications are infrequent. The potential complications include cardiac penetration, cardiac vessel injury, pneumothorax, infection, and atrial and ventricular arrhythmias. The risk of a major complication is higher in patients with impaired clotting or unfavorable anatomy or when the needle is inserted at a site where the heart is not sufficiently separated from the pericardial sac throughout the cardiac cycle. Cardiac penetration is particularly dangerous in patients with pulmonary hypertension or impaired clotting.

TECHNIQUE OF ECHO-GUIDED PERICARDIOCENTESIS

In our institution, pericardiocentesis is performed in the intensive care unit after the patient has fasted for 6 h. Before the procedure, the operator determines the anatomic relationships among the heart, the pericardial sac, and the surface of the body, to identify possible access sites. The optimal entry site is the point where (1) the effusion is close to the surface, (2) the route of the needle is short, nonangulated, and avoids vital structures [e.g., the internal mammary artery or the subcostal vascular bundle *(30)*, and (3) the distance between the heart and the pericardial sac throughout the cardiac cycle is sufficient, preferably >1 cm. (4) Criteria 1–3 are still met if the angulation of the needle is not strictly adhered to.

If the anatomy is favorable and there are no contraindications for pericardiocentesis, informed consent is obtained, and the procedure is started. The pericardiocentesis tray, resuscitation equipment, and a syringe containing 1 mg of atropine should be prepared in advance. The patient is placed comfortably at the desired position, connected to a monitor, and given intravenous fluids and mild sedation. The selected entry point and the desired angulation are marked on the skin. The entry point and route should be re-examined to ensure that they are optimal, and the distance between the skin and pericardium should be measured.

The skin is prepared by using antiseptic and is covered with sterile drapes; a transparent sheet is desirable. After a local anesthetic is injected at the predetermined entry point, the skin is penetrated with a plastic sheath or metal needle that is connected to a syringe partially filled with saline. At the predetermined angulation, the needle or sheath is advanced slowly and cautiously with repeated aspirations until fluid appears. The needle is then fixated by hand to avoid further advancement into the pericardial sac. Aspiration is repeated to confirm entry.

A guidewire with a soft J-shaped tip is then inserted through the needle into the pericardial sac while the patient's monitor is watched for arrhythmia. The needle is replaced with a cannula or, if a pigtail catheter is to be used for drainage, with a sheath. To reduce intrapericardial pressure, 50 mL of fluid is initially evacuated. The aspirate is submitted to the laboratory for cytological, hematological, bacteriological, serological, and chemical analysis.

To confirm the position of the sheath in the pericardial space, 5 mL of agitated saline is injected while the pericardial sac is continuously imaged with echocardiography. If the tip of the catheter is in the pericardial space, a contrast effect will immediately appear. The appearance of a contrast effect inside a cardiac chamber indicates cardiac penetration. A rapid disappearance of the contrast effect should also raise the suspicion of inappropriate positioning of the sheath. If the aspirate is bloody, the position of the sheath or catheter should be confirmed and rechecked if the sheath is replaced with another catheter.

After confirming the position of the sheath or catheter in the pericardial space, the intrapericardial pressure is measured with a transducer or a fluid manometer, and they are secured to the skin with sutures and dressings. The effusion should be aspirated intermittently by hand via a three-way stopcock. Drainage by gravitation through a tube into a sterile container is also adequate. Vacuum suction should be avoided. The process should be monitored to detect plugging, catheter entrapment, reaccumulation of fluid, or a change in the color of the aspirate, particularly the appearance of blood. Repeated echocardiograms are necessary to verify the complete evacuation of the effusion. Because congestive heart failure may complicate fluid evacuation, gradual aspiration and continuous monitoring are advisable, particularly in patients with pre-existing heart disease.

After the effusion is evacuated, the catheter should be left in place until the drainage rate decreases to less than 30 mL in 24 h *(30)*. Persistent drainage predicts a rapid recurrence and indicates a need for specific preventive measures.

Pericardial Drainage by Surgery

Subxiphoid pericardiotomy is a minimally invasive surgical procedure that allows urgent access to the pericardium. The relapse rate is higher than for the more extensive surgical procedures because the resection of the pericardial sac is limited. However, thoracotomy is avoided and the procedure can be performed under local anesthesia, rendering it more suitable for critically ill patients who are high risk *(31,32)*.

In *limited pericardiectomy* (pleuropericardial window), a part of the pericardial sac is excised via a left thoracotomy, creating a window between the pericardial and pleural spaces. Extensive pericardiectomy is preferred for treatment of constrictive pericarditis and is carried out via a left thoracotomy or median sternotomy, which provides better exposure and extensive resection of the pericardial sac. These procedures are associated with considerable morbidity and mortality, but the recurrence rate is low *(32)*.

Thoracoscopic pericardial window (video-thoracoscopy) is a minimally invasive method that permits exploration of the thoracic cavity, selection of biopsy sites, and extensive pericardiectomy. The procedure is carried out under general anesthesia with single-lung ventilation and, therefore, is not indicated for patients who are poor candidates for general anesthesia *(33)*.

Choice of Treatment

Table 2 shows recommended approaches for the treatment of pericardial effusion. Several considerations should be taken into account when an intervention is contemplated: the immediate threat to the patient's life, the cause of cardiac tamponade, the patient's general condition, the risk of recurrence, the need for adjuvant therapy, and the advantages, disadvantages, and availability of each of the treatment options. Cardiac tamponade with hemodynamic decompensation is clearly an indication for prompt evacuation of pericardial fluid. With few exceptions, the procedure of choice is echo-guided pericardiocentesis, as this procedure has a high success rate, a low complication rate, and allows immediate decompression of the pericardial sac.

For patients in whom the procedure is contraindicated (e.g., those with inadequate access to the pericardial space or with coagulopathy), supportive medical therapy should be initiated, and surgical evacuation of fluid should be considered. When cardiac tamponade results from a dissecting aortic aneurysm or cardiac rupture complicating acute myocardial infarction, evacuation of pericardial fluid via a catheter may not be sufficient or, according to some investigators, may be lethal. However, in our experience, pericardiocentesis can involve an autotransfusion of blood from the pericardium *(34)* and can stabilize a patient until surgery is performed.

The definitive treatment of purulent pericarditis is early drainage and antibiotics *(35)*. Surgery may have some advantages, but pericardiocentesis can be performed initially to stabilize the patient and to collect the aspirate for analysis and confirmation of the diagnosis. Moreover, purulent pericarditis can be treated successfully with pericardiocentesis only *(36)*.

Table 2
Suggested Approaches to the Treatment of Pericardial Effusion

Approach	Cardiac tamponade	Large symptomatic pericardial effusion	Large asymptomatic pericardial effusion
Echo-guided Pericardiocentesis	Life-threatening hemodynamic decompensation	Severe symptoms, large effusion, Anticoagulant therapy, suspected infectious etiology, diagnostic purposes	Risk of deterioration Concomitant infection
Pericardiocentesis not recommended	C/I,[a] unfavorable conditions	C/I including thickened or calcified pericardium	Same as for symptomatic effusion
Surgery	Hemodynamic stability; specific underlying cause[b]	Constriction, need for biopsy, recurrent effusion	Same as for symptomatic effusion

[a] C/I = contraindications.

[b] Such as purulent pericarditis, trauma, dissection, and rupture.

239

REFERENCES

1. Ball JB, Morrison WL. Cardiac tamponade. Postgrad Med J 1997;73:141–145.
2. Spodick DH. Pathophysiology of cardiac tamponade. Chest 1998;113:1372–1379.
3. Spodick DH. The normal and diseased pericardium: current concepts of pericardial physiology, diagnosis and treatment. J Am Coll Cardiol 1983;1:240–251.
4. Fowler NO. Cardiac tamponade. A clinical or an echocardiographic diagnosis? Circulation 1993;87:1738–1741.
5. Savitt MA, Tyson GS, Elbeery JR, et al. Physiology of cardiac tamponade and paradoxical pulse in conscious dogs. Am J Physiol 1993;265:H1996–H2008.
6. Shabetai R, Fowler NO, Fenton JC, Masangkay M. Pulsus paradoxus. J Clin Invest 1965;44:1882–1898.
7. Gonzalez MS, Basnight MA, Appleton CP. Experimental pericardial effusion: relation of abnormal respiratory variation in mitral flow velocity to hemodynamics and right heart collapse. J Am Coll Cardiol 1991;17:239–248.
8. Mager A, Birnbaum Y, Imbar S, Strasberg B, Herz I, Battler A. Echo-guided pericardiocentesis: a ten year experience and a new method for non-invasive assessment of pericardial fluid volume [abstract]. Eur Heart J 2000;21:419.
9. Tsang TSM, Oh JK, Seward JB. Diagnosis and management of cardiac tamponade in the era of echocardiography. Clin Cardiol 1999;22:446–452.
10. Chen Y, Brennessel D, Walters J, Johnson M, Rosner F, Raza M. Human immunodeficiency virus-associated pericardial effusion: report of 40 cases and review of the literature. Am Heart J 1999;137:516–552.
11. Malouf JF, Alam S, Gharzeddine W, Stefadouros MA. The role of anticoagulation in the development of pericardial effusion and late tamponade after cardiac surgery. Eur Heart J 1993;14:1451–1457.
12. Von Shosten R, Kopistansky C, Cohen M, Kussmaul WG III. Cardiac tamponade in the "new device" era: evaluation of 6999 consecutive percutaneous interventions. Am Heart J 2000;160:2397–2398.
13. Tsang T, Freeman WK, Barnes ME, Reeder G, Packer D, Seward JB. Rescue echocardiographically guided pericardiocentesis for cardiac perforation complicating catheter-based procedures: the Mayo clinic experience. J Am Coll Cardiol 1998;32:1345–1350.
14. Beck CS. Two cardiac compression triads. JAMA 1935;104:714–716.
15. Levine MJ, Lorell BH, Diver DJ, Come PC. Implications of echocardiographically assisted diagnosis of pericardial tamponade in contemporary medical patients: detection before hemodynamic embarrassment. J Am Coll Cardiol 1991;17:59–65.
16. Kronzon I, Cohen ML, Winter HE. Diastolic atrial compression: a sensitive echocardiographic sign of cardiac tamponade. J Am Coll Cardiol 1983;2:770–775.
17. Armstrong WF, Schilt BF, Helper DJ, et al. Diastolic collapse of the right ventricle with cardiac tamponade. Circulation 1982;65:1941–1946.
18. Cogswell TL, Bernath GA, Wann LS, et al. Effects of intravascular volume on the value of pulsus paradoxus and right ventricular diastolic collapse in predicting cardiac tamponade. Circulation 1985;72:1076–1080.
19. Himmelman RB, Kircher B, Rockey DC, Schiller NB. Inferior vena cava plethora with blunted respiratory response: A sensitive echocardiographic sign of cardiac tamponade. J Am Coll Cardiol 1988;12:1470–1477.
20. D'Cruz IA, Cohen HC, Prabhus R, Glick G. Diagnosis of cardiac tamponade by echocardiography. Circulation 1975;52:460–465.
21. Appleton CP, Hattle LK, Popp RL. Cardiac tamponade and pericardial effusion: respiratory variation in transvalvular flow velocities. J Am Coll Cardiol 1988;11:1020–1030.
22. Zhang S, Kerins DM, Byrd BF III. Doppler echocardiography in cardiac tamponade and constrictive pericarditis. Echocardiography 1994;11:507–521.
23. Schutzman JJ, Obarski TP, Pearce GL, Klein AL. Comparison of Doppler and two-dimensional echocardiography for assessment of pericardial effusion. Am J Cardiol 1992;70:1353–1357.
24. Hoit B, Sahn DJ, Shabetai R. Doppler-detected paradoxus of mitral and tricuspid valve flows in chronic lung disease. J Am Coll Cardiol 1986;8:706–709.
25. Simeonidou E, Hamouratidis N, Tzimas K Tsounos J, Roussis S. Respiratory variation in mitral flow velocity in pericardial effusion and cardiac tamponade. Angiology 1994;45:213–218.
26. Mager A, Strasberg B, Zlotikamien E, Kaplinsky C, Sclarovsky S. Life threatening ventricular tachycardia as the presenting symptom of metastatic cardiac disease. Clin Cardiol 1991;14:696–698.

27. Eisenberg MJ, Oken K, Guerrero S, et al. Prognostic value of echocardiography in hospitalized patients with pericardial effusion. Am J Cardiol 1992;70:934–939.

28. Horowitz MS, Schultz CS, Stinson EB, Harrison DC, Popp RL. Sensitivity and specificity of echocardiographic diagnosis of pericardial effusion. Circulation 1974;50:239–247.

29. D'Cruz IA, Hoffman PK. A new cross-sectional echocardiographic method for estimating the volume of large pericardial effusion. Br Heart J 1991;66:448–451.

30. Tsang T, Freeman WK, Sinak L, Seward JB. Echocardiographically guided pericardiocentesis: evolution and state-of-the-art technique. Mayo Clin Proc 1998;73:647–652.

31. Piehler JM, Pluth JR, Schaff HV, Danielson GK, Orzulak TA, Puga F. Surgical management of effusive pericardial disease. Influence of the extent of pericardial resection on clinical course. J Thorac Cardiovasc Surg 1985;90:506–516.

32. Palatianos GM, Thurer RJ, Kaiser GA. Comparison of effectiveness and safety of operations on the pericardium.Chest 1985;88:30–33.

33. Nataf P, Cacoub P, Regan M, et al. Video-thoracoscopic pericardial window in the diagnosis and treatment of pericardial effusions. Am J Cardiol 1998;82:124–126.

34. Proli J, Laufer N. Left ventricular rupture following myocardial infarction treated with streptokinase: successful resuscitation in the cardiac catheterization laboratory using pericardiocentesis and autotransfusion. Cathet Cardiovasc Diagn 1993;29:257–260.

35. Gould K, Barnett JA, Sanford JP. Purulent pericarditis in the antibiotic era. Arch Intern Med 1974;134:923–927.

36. Bouwels L, Jansen E, Janssen J, et al. Successful long-term catheter drainage in an immunocompromised patient with purulent pericarditis. Am J Med 1987;83:581–583.

16 Heart Disease in the Child and Cardiogenic Shock

Amiram Nir, MD, Azaria J.J.T. Rein, MD, and David J. Driscoll, MD

CONTENTS

INTRODUCTION

Heart diseases in infants and children can be classified as either congenital or acquired. The majority of congenital lesions are structural heart defects. Inborn errors of metabolism can produce heart disease that is also, technically, congenital. Acquired heart diseases can be subclassified into myocardial diseases (myocarditis, cardiomyopathy), valvular diseases (rheumatic fever, infective endocarditis), other inflammatory diseases such as Kawasaki's disease, and arrhythmias (tachyarrhythmia and bradyarrhythmias).

CONGENITAL HEART DISEASE

Congenital cardiac disease is more common than acquired heart disease in infants and children. The reported incidence of congenital heart disease in infants and children is about 5–8 per 1000 live births. Many investigators have reported the relative incidence of the different cardiac lesions, most of them in studies performed in the pre-echocardiographic era *(1)*. In the largest study performed in the echocardio-

From: *Contemporary Cardiology: Cardiogenic Shock: Diagnosis and Treatment*
Edited by: David Hasdai et al. © Humana Press Inc., Totowa, NJ

graphic era, Samanek and Voriskova *(2)* studied 815,569 children born between 1980 and 1990 in Bohemia, Czechoslovakia, and found 5030 with congenital heart disease (6.16 per 1000).

Table 1 displays the relative incidence of the different lesions from four combined studies performed in the echocardiographic era *(1–4)*. Lesions causing left-to-right shunt are the most prevalent, accounting for more than 50% of congenital heart diseases. The most common are ventricular septal defect, atrial septal defect, patent ductus arteriosus, and atrioventricular canal defect. Cyanotic lesions make up nearly one-fifth of all lesions. The most common cyanotic lesions are tetralogy of Fallot and transposition of the great arteries. Other less frequent lesions are pulmonary atresia, double outlet right ventricle, totally anomalous pulmonary venous drainage, and single ventricle. The obstructive lesions are the third important group. The most common obstructive lesions are aortic stenosis, pulmonary stenosis, and coarctation of the aorta. Hypoplastic left-heart syndrome is a very important lesion with one of the poorest outcomes.

Prognosis of Congenital Heart Disease

Surgical therapy for congenital heart disease has improved significantly in the last two decades and continues to improve. In the study by Samanek et al. *(2)* reviewing patients born between 1980 and 1990, 77% of the patients survived to age 15 yr. For many lesions, however, survival has improved greatly since the time of that study. Complete repair or palliation is now available for most congenital heart diseases. The mortality figures reported in older natural history studies are much higher than the current surgical mortality for the same lesions. In a recent report, Stark et al. *(5)* reviewed the surgical mortality for the repair of congenital heart lesions in England between 1997 and 1998 (1378 operations). The overall mortality was 4%. A comparison of survival with selected lesions is displayed in Table 2. Another impressive example is the survival of patients with hypoplastic left heart syndrome that was zero in the Samanek report *(2)* and 49%–77% in more recent reports, after surgical repair *(6)* or cardiac transplantation *(7)*. The mortality figures reported by Samanek include about a third of patients who died of noncardiac causes.

ACQUIRED HEART DISEASE

In some countries, acquired heart disease may be more prevalent than congenital heart disease in older children. Rheumatic fever is a major health problem in developing countries, with a prevalence as high as 375/100,000 school children *(8)*. Rheumatic carditis may be associated with significant mortality *(9)*. Kawasaki disease is prevalent in many parts of the world, with an annual incidence of 89.4/100,000 children <5 yr of age in Japan *(10)*. It is the leading cause of acquired heart disease in children in the United States *(11)*. Myocarditis and cardiomyopathies, either primary, familial, or secondary to metabolic disorders or chemotherapy, are important causes of morbidity and mortality in this age group. Rhythm disturbances are much less prevalent in children than in adults, but they may result in cardiomyopathy or heart failure. As repair of congenital heart disease improves, children with these conditions reach older ages and make up a significant proportion of older children and adolescents with heart disease.

Table 1
Relative Prevalence of Congenital Cardiac Lesions Displayed as % of Total Patients with Congenital Heart Disease

Study	Patients	VSD	ASD	AVC	PS	TF	TGA	CoA	AS	PDA	DORV	TAPVR	PA	Tr. Art	HLH
Ferencz et al. (4a)	4390	32.1	7.7	7.4	9	6.8	4.7	4.6	2.9	2.4	2	4	7	2	3.8
Bower and Ramsey (4)	1787	42.6	7.2	6	7.3	3.5	5.8	5.8	3.3	6.8		1	8		2.8
Abu-Harb et al. (3)	1074	24.7		7.4		5.6	7.4	6.2	4.8				4.1	2.7	2.4
Samanek and Voriskova (2)	5030	41.6	8.7	4	5.8	3.4	5.4	5.3	7.8	5.1	1.4	0.8	2.1	1.09	3.4

Abbreviations: AS-aortic stenosis, ASD-atrial septal defect, AVC-atrioventricular canal, CoA-coarctation of the aorta, DORV-double outlet right ventricle, HLH-hypoplastic left-heart syndrome, PA-pulmonary atresia with and without VSD, PDA-patent ductus arteriosus, PS-pulmonary stenosis, TAPVR-total anomalous pulmonary venous return, TF-tetralogy of Fallot, TGA-transposition of the great arteries, Tr. Art-truncus arteriosus, VSD-ventricular septal defect.

245

Table 2
Mortality (%) at 1 yr and 15 yr of Patients with the Various Cardiac Lesions,
Born Between 1980 and 1990, Compared to Recent Surgical Mortality

Type of lesion	VSD	AVC	ToF	TGA	CoA	Tr. Art.
% Recent surgical mortality (5)	0.6	3.6	2.3	0	1	28.6
% 1 yr mortality (2)	8.89	37.8	15.4	38.4	32	87
% 15 yr mortality (2)	10.6	45.8	23.4	46.2	35	93

Abbreviations: AVC-atrioventricular canal defect, CoA-coarctation of the aorta, ToF-tetralogy of Fallot, TGA-transposition of the great arteries, Tr. Art-truncus arteriosus, VSD-ventricular septal defect.

DEVELOPMENTAL ASPECTS OF CARDIAC STRUCTURE AND FUNCTION

Many developmental changes occur in cardiac myocytes. Animal studies show that the immature myocytes are less well organized and occupy relatively less of the muscle mass than mature myocytes. Myocyte division occurs in fetal and early neonatal life. After this period, cell growth (hypertrophy) occurs without cell division. Developmental changes have been observed in the sarcolemma, the sarcoplasmic reticulum, the ion channels, and the contracting proteins. The membranes of the sarcolemma and sarcoplasmic reticulum are less abundant in the fetal than in the adult heart. The sarcoplasmic reticulum has a much smaller role in the regulation of myocyte contraction and relaxation in the newborn than in the adult (12). This was demonstrated by the use of ryanodine, an inhibitor of the sarcoplasmic reticulum calcium release. The inhibitory effect of ryanodine was less prominent in the newborn than in the adult myocyte (13,14). For this reason, the cardiac function of the newborn is thought to be more sensitive to calcium channel blockers (15). Tension development has been shown to be higher in papillary muscle from adult than from newborn rabbits (14). Age-related increase in sarcoplasmic Ca^{2+} ATPase activity has been demonstrated (16). Cardiac relaxation in the immature myocyte may be less dependent on the fast sarcoplasmic reticulum Ca^{2+} ATPase pump and more on slower calcium transport proteins (15). Contractile protein isoforms change with maturation, but the exact contribution of each isoform change to myocyte function remains to be determined (12).

Somewhat contrasting to the animal studies, suggesting less efficient function of young myocytes, are studies in human subjects using echocardiographic measurements of contractility. These studies showed a higher basal contractile state with increased sensitivity to afterload in newborns and young children (17). Left ventricular mass and volume have been shown to increase with age and the left ventricular mass/volume ratio to remain relatively constant (18). Holmgren et al. (19) studied diastolic function in children, demonstrating that isovolumic relaxation time and the deceleration time interval of mitral valve inflow are shorter in young children, suggesting better relaxation but somewhat impaired compliance of young hearts. It is of interest, however, that the normal heart rate in the neonate is roughly twice as fast as in the adult, and there is a gradual decrease in heart rate with increasing age. This suggests that the stroke volume/cardiac output ratio increases with age.

CARDIOGENIC SHOCK IN INFANTS AND CHILDREN WITH HEART DISEASE

The definition of cardiogenic shock varies, and there are no specific criteria for the diagnosis of cardiogenic shock in children. Although the outcome is generally poor, no series of infants and children with cardiogenic shock has been reported and few evidence-based data are available. Thus, assessment of the natural history and the effects of the various therapeutic modalities is only qualitative, depending on the general impression of the treating physicians. A number of investigations have assessed the acute hemodynamic effects of various drugs, but information regarding survival and long-term prognosis is scarce.

Definition

Cardiogenic shock is defined as the inability of the heart to deliver sufficient blood flow to the tissues to meet resting metabolic demands *(20)*. The American Heart Association guidelines *(21)* define decompensated shock as the above definition plus hypotension. Hypotension is defined as systolic blood pressure lower than the 5th percentile for age: systolic blood pressure <60 mm Hg in term neonates (0–28 d of age); <70 mm Hg in infants 1–12 mo; <70+(2 × age in years) in children 1–10 yr; <90 mm Hg beyond 10 yr. The definition of hypotension as blood pressure below the 5th percentile means that 5% of infants and children have hypotension within the range of cardiogenic shock, a number far greater than the subjects with clinically significant hypotension.

Etiology

Table 3 displays causes of cardiogenic shock in infants and children classified by the typical age at presentation. Unlike adults, ischemic heart disease is a very rare cause of shock in the young.

Diagnosis

The diagnosis of shock is based on clinical features and supported by additional tests and examinations. Organ hypoperfusion and compensatory responses can be detected clinically.

The cause of shock should be sought by careful questioning: clues for other causes of shock such as sepsis, hypovolemia, and anaphylaxis; pertinent historical information regarding prior febrile illnesses (myocarditis, Kawasaki's disease, rheumatic fever), congenital heart disease, past cardiac surgery, chemotherapy, drug ingestion, and familial cardiac diseases such as cardiomyopathies. Tachycardia is common in shock, and, in turn, excessive tachycardia may be the cause of shock. Bradycardia is always abnormal in the state of shock and, if present, should be suspected as the cause of shock. Blood pressure usually is maintained in compensated shock. Subsequently, pulse pressure decreases because of a minor decrease in systolic and an increase in diastolic pressure. Eventually, both systolic and diastolic blood pressures fall *(22)*. Lactic acidosis leads to hyperventilation. Poor skin perfusion is evident by decreased skin temperature, long capillary refill time (longer than 3–5 s) and cyanosis. The patient may be distressed and consciousness may be impaired.

Hydration status should be assessed. Femoral or pedal pulses should be checked. One should keep in mind that patients with coarctation of the aorta in shock may have

Table 3
Causes of Cardiogenic Shock in Infants and Children Classified by the Typical Age of Presentation

All ages	First 2 wk	First 2 mo	First year	Older children
• Myocarditis/cardiomyopathy • Arrhythmia • Postoperative • Tamponade	• Critical AS • Critical PS/PA • CoA, IAA • HLH • Obstructive TAPVR • Ebstein anomaly of TV	• Anomalous origin of coronary artery from pulmonary artery • Carnitine deficiency	• Anomalous origin of coronary artery from pulmonary artery • Kawasaki's disease	• Kawasaki's disease • Rheumatic fever • Post chemotherapy • Infective endocarditis

Abbreviations: AS-aortic stenosis, CoA-coarctation of the aorta, HLH-hypoplastic left-heart syndrome, IAA-interrupted aortic arch, PA-pulmonary atresia, PS-pulmonary stenosis, TAPVR-total anomalous pulmonary venous return, TV-tricuspid valve.

Table 4
Clues for Cardiogenic Etiology in Infants and Children with Shock

History	Febrile illness
	Congenital heart disease or cardiac surgery
	Chemotherapy
	Familial cardiac disease
	Drug ingestion
	Chest trauma
Physical examination	Excessive tachycardia
	Bradycardia
	Nonpalpable femoral pulses
	Hepatomegaly/distended jugular veins
	Abnormal cardiac examination
	Rales
ECG	Arrhythmia
	ST-T-wave abnormalities
	Deep Q-waves
Chest X-ray	Cardiomegaly
	Pulmonary congestion

weak or absent arm pulses as well as leg pulses. Liver size and, in older children, jugular venous pressure should be assessed. Abnormal cardiac examination (hyperactive precordium, arrhythmia, gallop, murmur or friction rub) may suggest a cardiac etiology. Apart from the routine laboratory tests, base deficit should be measured as it correlates with tissue hypoperfusion. Oliguria (less than 1 mL/kg/h) often is present. Mixed venous oxygen saturation is an indicator of cardiac output. The electrocardiogram may reveal rhythm abnormalities and signs of myocarditis, pericarditis, or ischemia. The chest X-ray may show cardiomegaly and pulmonary congestion (Table 4). Whenever the cause of the shock is unknown, an echocardiogram should be performed, as it will usually reveal or confirm the cardiac diagnosis.

Management

GENERAL SUPPORT FOR THE PATIENT IN SHOCK

The patient in shock should be stabilized as much as possible. Mechanical ventilation should be instituted if necessary, and hypoxemia should be corrected with oxygen supplementation. The one exception to this rule is the patient with ductus-dependent obstructive lesion who is in shock because of ductal constriction. In this situation, oxygen supplementation may further constrict the ductus arteriosus *(23)*. Oxygen administration is probably safe in these situations when coadministered with prostaglandin E$_1$ (PGE$_1$).

Intravenous access should be established and fluid deficit and metabolic acidosis should be corrected. Bicarbonate supplementation can be given by repeated slow boluses of sodium bicarbonate of 1 to 2 meq/kg, until acidosis is corrected. In the neonate, a solution of 0.5 meq/mL should be used *(22)*.

In general, the baby presenting in cardiogenic shock may have a treatable cause for which early diagnosis and appropriate therapy may be crucial (Table 5).

Table 5
Treatable Causes of Cardiogenic Shock

Cause	Immediate treatment
Ductus-dependent obstructive lesions	PGE_1
Coronary anomalies	Surgical treatment as soon as possible
Arrhythmias	Drugs, cardioversion, pacing
Tamponade	Pericardiocentesis
Carnitine deficiency	Carnitine supplementation

DRUGS

The approach to pump failure is aimed at improving contraction and reducing after-load. This aim has led to the use of drugs that augment contractility in combination with vasodilators (Table 6). Cardiogenic shock may be accompanied by excessive intravascular volume, because of activation of the renin–angiotensin–aldosterone system and low renal perfusion. Diuretic therapy may be required in these cases. Furosemide, a loop diuretic, is generally used.

Dopamine and dobutamine are the main drugs used for sympathomimetic stimulation. A wealth of data is available on the cardiac and hemodynamic effects of dopamine in neonates *(31)* and children *(32)*. Low-dose dopamine (0.5–2 µg/kg/min) stimulates peripheral dopamine receptors in the cardiovascular system, kidneys, and adrenergic nerve endings. This results in vasodilatation of several vascular beds and an increase in coronary, renal, and mesenteric blood flow. At medium doses (2–6 µg/kg/min), it also affects cardiac β1- and β2-adrenergic receptors. This is mediated via dopamine-induced norepinephrine release from cardiac adrenergic nerve endings *(33)*. At these doses, the stimulation of the cardiac β receptors results in enhanced myocardial contractility and some increase in heart rate. At doses higher than 10 µg/kg/min, α1- and α2-adrenergic receptors are stimulated as well. This results in peripheral vasoconstriction and increased afterload and blood pressure *(32)*. Dopamine is also effective in preterm neonates, with blood pressure response evident at lower doses. Dopamine clearance is lower in preterm infants than in older patients *(31)*.

The effect of dobutamine on cardiac contractility is mediated via the β receptors and is not dependent on the release of stored norepinephrine *(34)*. Some believe that dobutamine, possibly in combination with dopamine, is the drug of choice for patients with primary myocardial dysfunction, when norepinephrine stores are likely to be depleted *(32)*. Perkin et al. *(35)* found hemodynamic improvement in children with cardiogenic shock using dobutamine.

Epinephrine infusion may be indicated in the treatment of shock and hypotension unresponsive to fluid resuscitation. It is a potent inotrope and is infused at a rate sufficient to elevate blood pressure. It is also a potent positive chronotrope and thus may be useful in patients with accompanied bradycardia. Epinephrine may be preferable to dopamine in cases with marked circulatory instability, particularly in infants. Epinephrine may cause atrial and ventricular tachyarrhythmias, severe hypertension, and unwanted metabolic changes (hyperglycemia, lactic acidosis, and hypokalemia) *(21)*. There is one report that preoperative administration of epinephrine to infants with congenital heart disease had no effect on outcome *(29)*, but no

Table 6
Drug Therapy for Cardiogenic Shock in Infants and Children

Drug	Dose (µg/kg/min)	Actions	Clinical trials in children
Dopamine	0.5–2 2–10 >10–20	Renal vasodilatation ↑Cardiac index Vasoconstriction	Newborns with shock (31) 2- to 54-mo-old babies after cardiac surgery dopamine effect = dobutamine effect Booker et al. 1995 Preterm infants with low BP. Dopamine more effective than dobutamine for BP elevation Greenough et al. 1993
Dobutamine	1–20	↑Cardiac index Vasodilatation	Cardiogenic shock. More effective in patients > 12 m old (31) 2- to 54-mo-old babies after cardiac surgery dopamine effect = dobutamine effect Booker et al. 1995 Preterm infants with low BP. Dopamine more effective than dobutamine in BP elevation Greenough et al. 1993
Milrinone	Loading 10–50 µg/kg over 10 min; then 0.1–1 µg/kg/min	↑Cardiac index ↓SVR, PVR ↓= Filling pressures Arrhythmia, ↓BP	Neonates with low CO after cardiac surgery (27) 9 mo to 15 y septic shock (36)
Isoproterenol	0.05–0.5	Positive inotrope Vasodilatation ↑O_2 consumption Arrhythmia	None
Epinephrine	0.05–0.3	Positive inotrope ↑HR, ↓ renal flow ↑O_2 consumption Arrhythmia	Infants with congenital heart disease at operation, not in shock (29)
Sodium nitroprusside	0.5–10	Vasodilator Arteries and veins ↑Cardiac index	Infants (2 wk to 17 mo) after cardiac surgery (30)

251

data are available on the effect of epinephrine in cardiogenic shock in the pediatric age group.

Milrinone, a phosphodiesterase inhibitor, increases intracellular cyclic AMP levels, augments contractility, and causes vasodilatation. Chang et al. *(27)* administered milrinone (50 µg/kg loading and then 0.5 µg/kg/min) to neonates with low cardiac output after cardiac surgery and recorded lower filling pressures, systemic and pulmonary arterial pressures, systemic and pulmonary vascular resistances, and improved cardiac index. Barton et al. *(36)* reported the effect of milrinone on 12 patients aged 9 mo to 15 yr with septic shock. They observed an increase in cardiac index and a decrease in systemic and pulmonary resistance, with no change in blood pressure of pulmonary capillary wedge pressure. Milrinone is preferred over amrinone because of its shorter half-life and less thrombocytopenia *(21)*.

No clinical trials of isoproterenol, a β-adrenergic receptor agonist, in infants and children with shock are available. In adults with shock (8 of 12 with cardiogenic shock), Worthley et al. *(37)* found isoproterenol to increase cardiac index and heart rate and to decrease mean pulmonary arterial and wedge pressures.

Nitroprusside, a cyclic GMP generator, has vasodilatory effects and can cause significant hypotension. Appelbaum et al. *(30)* administered the drug to 16 children aged 2 wk to 17 mo immediately after cardiac surgery and observed improved cardiac index and a decrease in filling pressures as well as pulmonary and arterial pressures. No data are available on infants and children with shock. Cotter et al. *(38)* recently reported that N-monomethyl-L-arginine (L-NMMA), which inhibits nitric oxide synthesis, had favorable effects on adults with cardiogenic shock, highlighting the complexity of the cardiogenic shock state and the need for careful assessment of the effect of various agents on this state. The response of infants and children may differ from that of adults.

MECHANICAL CIRCULATORY SUPPORT IN CHILDREN

There are two major indications for the use of mechanical circulatory support in children: (1) to sustain the circulation in the presence of presumed temporary myocardial and/or pulmonary dysfunction (i.e., as a bridge to recovery) and (2) to maintain the circulation in the presence of presumed permanent myocardial and/or pulmonary dysfunction (i.e., as a bridge to cardiac/pulmonary transplantation). A third, but not yet proven, use of mechanical circulatory support is for permanent support of the circulation (i.e., a completely implantable mechanical heart).

Types of Devices and Interface Issues

Mechanical circulatory support systems can be categorized into those that provide left ventricular assistance, right ventricular assistance, biventricular assistance, and cardiopulmonary assistance. The type of assistance required will dictate the support system needed and ways to interface the support system with the patient.

One of the earliest forms of left ventricular assistance is the intra-aortic balloon counterpulsation (IABCP) system. In 1962, Moulopoules *(39)* described the design and in vitro function of the IABCP. He speculated that this system would support cardiovascular function by increasing diastolic coronary blood flow and decreasing end-diastolic pressure, hence decreasing myocardial oxygen demands. This catheter-mounted system usually is inserted through the femoral or iliac artery and positioned in the descending thoracic aorta.

As distinguished from the IABCP system, the left ventricular assistance device (LVAD) and the right ventricular assistance device (RVAD) use an external or internal pump system to propel blood. (See Chapter 19 for a fuller description of these devices.) For the LVAD, the inflow cannula (from patient into device) is placed into the left atrium or left ventricle and the outflow cannula is placed into the aorta. For an RVAD, the inflow cannula is inserted into the right atrium and the outflow cannula is inserted into the right ventricle or pulmonary artery. For a biventricular assistance device (BVAD), both an RVAD and an LVAD can be employed. If only pulmonary support or pulmonary as well as right and/or left ventricular assistance is necessary, a standard extracorporeal membrane oxygenator (ECMO) system can be used. In this situation, a major systemic vein provides inflow to the support system and the outflow cannula can be placed into a major artery. Thoracotomy may or may not be necessary to use ECMO, depending on the flow rates needed to support the patient.

Another form of left ventricular assistance device was the Hemopump™ *(40)*, a catheter-mounted device with an axial flow pump. It was inserted through the femoral artery and advanced across the aortic valve into the left ventricle. Blood was drawn from the left ventricular cavity into the catheter, propelled by the axial flow pump through the catheter, and ejected into the aorta. (As noted in Chapter 19 however, the Hemopump device did not receive FDA approval and is no longer available.)

In small children, there are size and space limitations to cannulation of the cardiovascular system and insertion of the hardware associated with the assist devices. There are also important issues relative to the stroke volume of the ventricular assist device and the flows required to support small children. Thrombosis may be a problem if the flow to the patient is considerably lower than the practical lower limits of the device. Because of this, it is sometimes more practical to use an ECMO system for support of the child with biventricular failure, even in the presence of adequate pulmonary function, simply to reduce the number of cannulation sites needed for support.

Pumps

Several types of pump are used to propel the blood. The oldest is the relatively simple roller pump that is found on most conventional heart/lung bypass machines. Blood flow is unidirectional, making valves unnecessary. Pneumatic pumps are essentially a bellows system activated by changes in air pressure outside the bellows, which use valves to assure unidirectional flow of blood. Centrifugal pumps use a rapidly spinning rotator cone and impeller. The centrifugal force imparted to the blood by the rapidly spinning device propels the blood forward in one direction, making valves unnecessary. Axial flow pumps are small rotor-type devices that spin at very fast rates (7500–12500 rpm) and cause surprisingly little damage to blood cells.

Complications: The major complications of cardiovascular assistance devices are hemorrhage, thrombosis, and infection. The use of a membrane oxygenator in the system substantially increases the risks of thrombosis.

ECMO

Because ECMO has been used for many years to treat newborns with respiratory distress syndrome, considerable data exist regarding the outcome associated with its use in infants and small children. In the past 10–15 yr, ECMO has also been used to support the failing circulation after repair of congenital heart defects. Patients with cir-

Table 7
Results of ECMO for Cardiopulmonary Failure in Children

Authors (ref.)	N	Age (yr)	Died unable to wean		Successfully weaned		Died despite weaning		Total deaths	
			N	%	N	%	N	%	N	%
Anderson et al. (41)	33	0.02–18	21	64	12	36			21	64
Klein et al. (42)	39	0.003–7							14	36
Kanter et al. (43)	13	0.02–17.6	6	46	7	54	1	14	7	54
Rogers et al. (44)	10	0.006–5	2	20	8	80	1	10	3	30
Raithel et al. (45)	65	0.003–14	21	32	44	68	21	32	42	65
Weinhaus et al. (46)	14	0.006–7.4	5	36	9	64	4	29	9	64
Total	174								96	55

Table 8
Results of Intra-aortic Balloon Counterpulsation in Children

Authors (ref.)	N	Age (yr)	Died unable to wean		Successfully weaned		Died despite weaning		Total deaths	
			N	%	N	%	N	%	N	%
Park et al. (48)	9	0.6–15							5	55
Veasy et al. (49)	8	0.1–6	4	50	4	50	2	25	6	75
Pollock et al. (50)	14	5–18							8	57
Webster and Veasy (51)	18	0.1–18	8	44			4	22	13	72
Total	49								32	665

culatory failure after operation for congenital heart defects frequently have biventricular failure and pulmonary dysfunction rather than isolated right or left ventricular dysfunction. Hence, the use of an LVAD or RVAD is not feasible. Six studies of a total of 174 patients are summarized in Table 7. The overall survival for this group of patients was 45%. Complications of ECMO included bleeding, intracranial hemorrhage, thrombosis, and mechanical or circuit failure.

Recently, Ibrahim et al. (47) reported the long-term outcome of children who were hospital survivors of ECMO support for circulatory failure. Of 26 hospital survivors, there was only 1 late death and more than 80% of the survivors were in NYHA class I or II. Moderate-to-severe neurologic impairment was more common for patients supported with ECMO (59%) than for patients supported with VADs (20%).

Intra-aortic Balloon Counterpulsation

There is limited experience with IABCP in infants and children because it is difficult to obtain appropriately sized balloons for small children. The greater compliance of the young aorta makes IABCP less effective than in older patients with stiffer aortas. In addition, improvement of coronary blood flow is less an issue in infants and children than in adults with coronary artery disease. Four studies comprising 49 patients are summarized in Table 8. The overall survival was 35%. Complications included leg ischemia, unintended insertion of the device into the mesenteric artery, sepsis, and thrombocytopenia.

LVAD and RVAD

The LVADs and RVADs have not been used often in pediatric patients. This results both from the limited availability of devices of appropriate size for small patients and, as noted earlier, because infants and children usually have combined right and left ventricular and, frequently, pulmonary failure. An intraoperative algorithm was developed by Karl et al. *(52)* to determine if the child could be supported with a VAD or if an ECMO system would be necessary. While still using cardiopulmonary bypass, a venous return cannula is inserted into the left atrium and the right atrial venous return cannula is clamped, essentially providing only left ventricular assistance. If, while maintaining a flow rate of 150 mL/kg/min, the right atrial pressure remains <12 mm Hg, the pulmonary artery systolic pressure remains one-half or less of systemic pressure, and the right ventricle does not dilate, the patient is ventilated and the oxygenator is temporarily bypassed. If, after these maneuvers, gas exchange, acid–base balance, and hemodynamics remain stable, the patient is recannulated for VAD support; otherwise, ECMO or BVAD is used.

Karl et al. *(53)* reported their experience with a centrifugal pump circuit in 12 children aged 6 d to 12 yr. The patients were supported from 38 to 190 h. Ten patients were weaned from support and six survived to leave the hospital.

Farrar et al. *(54)* used a pneumatic bellows type of ventricular assistance device as a bridge to transplantation in 72 heart transplant candidates. These included a 12-yr-old and a 13-yr-old child, both of whom died. Of the 14 patients who required an LVAD, 10 survived to transplantation and 9 survived after transplantation. Of the 58 patients who required a BVAD, 54 survived to transplantation and 36 survived transplantation. Thus, 63% of the patients survived from the time of device implant.

The results of the first 100 patients who received a Symbion Total Artificial Heart as a bridge to cardiac transplantation were reported by Joyce et al. *(55)*. Five of these patients were between 11 and 20 yr of age. Thirty-two patients died while being supported and 68 survived to transplantation. Forty-seven survived at least 30 d after transplantation and there were 16 late deaths. Either a stroke or transient ischemic attack was noted in 9% of the patients. Age less than or greater than 40 yr did not affect survival, but the investigators did not report if age less than 20 yr affected outcome.

In 1995, a report from the Combined Registry for the Clinical Use of Mechanical Ventricular Assistance Pumps and the Total Artificial Heart in Conjunction with Heart Transplantation summarized the results of 584 patients who ranged in age from 3.9 to 64 yr *(56)*. LVADs were used in 187 cases, RVADs in 5, BVADs in 164, and hybrid BVADs in 37. Survival to hospital discharge was achieved in 274 (68.5%) patients. Survival was 90.6% for LVAD, 0% for RVAD, 68.1% for BVAD, and 50% for hybrid BVAD. Causes of death included bleeding, renal failure, respiratory failure, technical problems, emboli, ventricular failure, infection, and transplantation problems.

Recently, Ibrahim et al. *(47)* reported the long-term outcome of children who were hospital survivors of VAD support for circulatory failure. Of 11 hospital survivors, there was only 1 late death and more than 80% of the survivors were in NYHA class I or II.

The use of the Hemopump axial flow device (which is no longer available) was reported in 20 patients by Frazier et al. *(57)*. Six patients survived more than 30 d after device removal including an 8-yr-old boy with acute cardiac allograft rejection. Meyns et al. *(40)* supported 61 patients with postoperative left ventricular failure using micraxial pumps. Sixty-five percent of the patients were weaned from the device, but only 30% survived to hospital discharge.

DIAGNOSIS, MANAGEMENT, AND PROGNOSIS OF SHOCK IN THE YOUNG CHILD

Cardiogenic Shock in the First 2 Weeks of Life

This period is characterized by dramatic hemodynamic changes. The transition from fetal to neonatal circulation involves a shift in oxygen supply from the placenta to the lungs. This is accompanied by closure of the ductus arteriosus in the first days of life and gradual drastic reduction in pulmonary resistance in the first days to weeks. Patients with cardiac lesions in which these changes lead to inadequate cardiac output and/or oxygenation will present at this period. In many cases, the diagnosis is made prenatally, preventing unexpected shock.

DUCTUS-DEPENDENT LESIONS

A number of lesions in which either the systemic circulation or the pulmonary circulation is dependent on the flow through the ductus arteriosus are severely affected by closure of the ductus. These lesions include stenosis or obstruction of one or more levels in the pulmonary or systemic circulations. Any newborn who deteriorates at age 1–10 d should be suspected of having such a lesion. Prompt diagnosis and therapy with PGE_1 to reopen the ductus arteriosus is lifesaving. Earlier diagnosis, either fetal or following clinical suspicion, and preventive therapy with PGE_1 may improve prognosis.

CRITICAL AORTIC STENOSIS

Newborns with critical aortic stenosis may present in shock when the ductus arteriosus closes. On physical examination, the baby may be ashen, with poor skin perfusion and weak pulses. The precordium may be hyperactive. A systolic murmur is usually, but not always, heard. Echocardiographic examination confirms the diagnosis. The left ventricular (LV) contraction may be poor, and the left ventricular volume should be noted, as small LV volume may prevent two-ventricular repair. The aortic valve is usually thickened, dysplastic, and doming with limited motion. The aortic valve gradient is not a good measure of the severity of the lesion because there may be low flow through the valve producing only a small gradient. The aortic arch should be interrogated, as coarctation of the aorta may coexist. The direction of blood flow through the aortic arch and the ductus arteriosus, if patent, may be reversed in cases with very limited forward flow through the aortic valve.

Stabilization of the patient may require inotropic support and mechanical ventilation. In young infants, prostaglandin E_1 to open the ductus arteriosus may be beneficial *(58)*. Definitive therapy should be aortic valvotomy or valvuloplasty. Open surgical valvotomy has been the procedure of choice in the past. In a recent publication, Howkins et al. *(59)* reported their results in 37 infants operated for critical aortic stenosis between 1986 and 1996. Early mortality was 11%, and 10-yr actuarial survival was 73%. Recently, Alexiou et al. reported better results in a smaller group of neonates with isolated aortic stenosis, who underwent open commissurotomy. They had no operative mortality and 85% freedom from reoperation at 5 yr *(60)*. Transvalvular balloon dilatation of critical aortic stenosis, first reported in 1986 *(61)*, is now used in most centers for initial treatment. It has been shown to be as effective as surgery in terms of gradient relief and appearance of aortic regurgitation. Egito et al. *(62)* reported the results of balloon dilatation of 33 neonates with critical aortic stenosis, performed between 1985 and 1991. Overall mortality was 12%, and midterm results were similar to those of surgery (88% survival at 8 yr). Femoral pulse loss occurred in 65% of patients. Aortic valvotomy was reported through the common carotid artery with encouraging results and few complications *(63,64)*. Balloon dilatation of the aortic valve has been attempted in a fetus with unsatisfactory results *(65)*.

HYPOPLASTIC LEFT-HEART SYNDROME

Hypoplastic left-heart syndrome is a collective term describing a group of cardiovascular malformations in which there is aortic valve hypoplasia, stenosis, or atresia with either hypoplasia or absence of the left ventricle and, as a consequence, hypoplasia of the ascending aorta. The mitral valve usually is stenotic or atretic *(66)*. The patient usually presents when the ductus arteriosus closes. Occasionally, patients with this disease can present soon after birth, when the interatrial communication is obstructive. As the ductus arteriosus closes, systemic and coronary flow are compromised and the baby becomes dusky, tachypneic, and acidotic. This can happen in the first 24–48 h or later. If not treated, cardiogenic shock will ensue and death will follow in a few hours.

The diagnosis is made by two-dimensional echocardiogram; cardiac catheterization is not required routinely. The approach to the newborn with the syndrome historically has been to offer the parents one of three options: (1) do nothing; (2) do a three-stage palliative operation (Norwood procedure); or (3) do a cardiac transplantation. In recent years, because of improved results of the latter two options, many physicians feel that the first option is no longer ethical.

When a surgical approach is elected, prostaglandin E_1 is started and an arterial line should be placed. Because the pulmonary circulation is in series with the systemic circulation while the latter is supplied by the ductus arteriosus, decrease of the pulmonary resistance causes pulmonary overcirculation and may compromise the systemic circulation. Thus, maneuvers to increase pulmonary resistance may be needed. These include hypoventilation or the addition of 2–4% CO_2 to the ventilation mixture. Inotropic drugs may not be necessary or beneficial *(66)*.

Comparable survival data are reported for the Norwood procedure and cardiac transplantation. Hehrlein et al. *(67)* reported better quality of life for patients who had cardiac transplantation. Kern et al. *(68)* reported 67 patients with hypoplastic left-heart syndrome, of whom 47 had the Norwood procedure between 1990 and 1996. Survival was 77% of the surgically treated patients, 61% when including those who did not undergo the operation. The 5-yr actuarial survival for patients who underwent operations was 61%. Others report similar results *(69)*. Jenkins et al. reported the 1-yr survival of 231 patients operated at 4 centers between 1989 and 1994. Patients who were intended for transplantation had 61% 1-yr survival, whereas those intended for staged procedure had 42% 1-yr survival *(70)*. Somewhat better survival (88%) has been reported in recent years for patients who had a cardiac transplantation. The long-term prognosis is uncertain for both procedures. Mental development is a concern in this patient group *(71);* Mahle et al. *(72)* reviewed school-age survivors and found 18% were mentally retarded and 30% required special education.

CRITICAL COARCTATION OF THE AORTA

Coarctation of the aorta can present as an isolated lesion or in association with other cardiac lesions. The baby with coarctation of the aorta may be asymptomatic at birth and discharged from the hospital undiagnosed. When the ductus arteriosus closes in such patients, it results in critical compromise of blood flow to the lower part of the body and a sudden increase in afterload of the left ventricle. Shock may develop in a few hours. In the compensated state, strong right arm pulses and weak or absent femoral pulses may suggest the diagnosis. When cardiac function deteriorates, this classical sign may be absent. The age of the child at presentation should raise the suspicion of a ductus-dependent obstructive lesion. Echocardiography reveals the diagnosis.

Intravenous PGE_1 should be administered immediately to open the ductus arteriosus, and the baby should be stabilized with ventilatory and inotropic support. Gradual improvement usually occurs as the ductus arteriosus opens. Repair of the coarctation is performed after a few days when the patient is stable. Surgical repair is the more commonly used method. The use of balloon dilatation of native coarctation of the aorta is controversial. Fletcher et al. *(73)* reported balloon dilatation in 16 patients up to 1 mo in age. The immediate results were good in 14 (87.5%). In only three (23%) patients, the results remained good at late follow-up. Kain et al. *(74)* reported failure to balloon dilate native coarctation of the aorta in 20 of 21 neonates.

Quaegebeur et al. *(75)* reported a multi-institutional experience of seriously ill neonates with coarctation of the aorta. They reviewed the outcome of 326 neonates born between 1990 and 1992. Survival for at least 24 mo was 84%, and four patients died before an initial procedure was performed.

LESIONS WITH DUCTUS-DEPENDENT PULMONARY CIRCULATION

These lesions include critical pulmonary stenosis and pulmonary atresia with or without ventricular septal defect. In these lesions, the atrial communication is usually adequate; as the ductus arteriosus closes, the major problem is hypoxemia. Prostaglandin E_1 should be administered and usually is sufficient to stabilize the patient. Invasive therapy depends on the lesion. In critical pulmonary stenosis, balloon dilatation is now considered the procedure of choice *(76,77)*. Gournay et al. *(76)* reported 97 infants, 82 with critical pulmonary stenosis and 15 with pulmonary atresia, in whom the valve had been perforated with a wire needle or radiofrequency probe. There were 3 deaths and balloon dilatation was successful in 77 of 81 patients.

Other Causes of Shock in the First Weeks of Life

OBSTRUCTED TOTAL ANOMALOUS PULMONARY VENOUS DRAINAGE

In this lesion, the pulmonary veins drain to the right atrium. Obstruction occurs in cases in which the pulmonary veins drain to a common vein which crosses the diaphragm and joins the portal venous system, the ductus venosus, the hepatic veins, or the inferior vena cava *(78)*. The infant develops cyanosis and respiratory distress in the first hours or days after birth. Pulmonary hypertension develops. Chest X-ray may show increased pulmonary vascular marking with a diffuse linear reticular pattern. The presence of cyanosis and respiratory distress may be incorrectly diagnosed as lung disease. Echocardiography usually reveals the diagnosis. If untreated, most patients die within a few days to weeks of life *(79)*.

Treatment includes stabilization of the patient with ventilatory and inotropic support and correction of acidosis. Inhaled nitric oxide may be used to reduce pulmonary resistance (80,81). A beneficial role of PGE$_1$, which may relax the ductus venosus, has been suggested (82). In severe cases, extracorporal membrane oxygenation (ECMO) may be used as a lifesaving measure.

ANOMALOUS ORIGIN OF THE LEFT CORONARY ARTERY

In this rare, treatable lesion, the left coronary artery originates from the pulmonary artery. As the pressure in the pulmonary artery decreases in the first weeks after birth, perfusion pressure of the anomalous artery decreases. Low perfusion pressure and low oxygen saturation may result in ischemia to the region supplied by the left coronary artery. The whole coronary tree is usually supplied by the large right coronary artery with retrograde flow in the left system via collateral arteries. Ischemia may cause left ventricular dysfunction and mitral valve regurgitation. The presentation can be cardiogenic shock in the infant or it may be more subtle, resulting in cardiomyopathy in older age. Physical examination and chest X-ray do not differ from other forms of myocarditis/cardiomyopathies. The electrocardiogram may reveal deep and wide Q-waves in the left leads (I, avL, V4–6). The diagnosis may be made by echocardiography, where the origin of the left coronary artery and the direction of flow through it can be established. In uncertain cases, catheterization is indicated.

The patient may require preoperative inotropic support. Surgical treatment should not be delayed, because without surgery, the mortality is high (83). A number of surgical techniques have been used. These include ligation of the left coronary artery, creation of an aorto-pulmonary window with a tunnel directing the blood flow from the aorta to the left coronary artery [Takeuchi operation (84),], or reimplantation of the left coronary artery to the aorta (85). Reported surgical results are much better for the Takeuchi and reimplantation techniques (86).

EBSTEIN ANOMALY OF THE TRICUSPID VALVE

Ebstein anomaly of the tricuspid valve is a rare defect in which the septal and posterior leaflets of the tricuspid valve are displaced downward toward the apex of the right ventricle. The right ventricle is divided into an "atrialized" portion above the tricuspid valve and a ventricular portion below the valve. The right atrial pressure is elevated as a result of a combination of low right ventricular compliance, tricuspid regurgitation, and systolic contraction of the atrialized right ventricle. An atrial septal defect or patent foramen ovale is commonly present. Cyanosis results from the right-to-left shunt at the atrial level. The clinical presentation may be hydrops fetalis (87), neonatal cyanosis which may be severe and accompanied by cardiogenic shock, or mild cyanosis in the older child. After birth, when the pulmonary vascular resistance is high, the right ventricle may be incapable of propelling blood antegradely across the pulmonary valve in severe cases, resulting in "functional" pulmonary atresia (88) and ductus-dependent pulmonary circulation. Anatomical pulmonary stenosis or atresia may be present. On physical examination, the baby is cyanotic and may be in shock. A systolic tricuspid regurgitation murmur and a gallop may be heard. Chest X-ray may reveal extreme cardiomegaly resulting from massive enlargement of the right atrium, with diminished pulmonary vascularity. The ECG may reveal large P-waves, and a Wolff–Parkinson–White pattern may be present. Echocardiography is diagnostic.

The sick neonate with Ebstein anomaly may need mechanical ventilation and oxygenation to decrease pulmonary vascular resistance. PGE_1 may be necessary to open the ductus arteriosus and secure pulmonary blood flow. This can be weaned days later when the pulmonary vascular resistance decreases and antegrade flow through the pulmonary valve is demonstrated. Inhaled nitric oxide may be beneficial to reduce pulmonary vascular resistance in severe cases (89). The results of surgical intervention in the neonate with Ebstein anomaly have been poor. Systemic-to-pulmonary shunt is a palliative measure with high mortality (90). Surgical creation of tricuspid atresia is another palliative approach that commits the patient to a single-ventricle repair (91). Tricuspid valvuloplasty or replacement is the definite treatment and is carried out at an older age (92). Recently, Knott-Craig et al. (93) reported successful complete surgical repair in three critically ill neonates with good short- to medium-term results. Celermajer et al. (94) reported 50% intrauterine mortality and 40% postnatal mortality in fetuses presenting with Ebstein anomaly. Neonates presenting with cyanosis had 70% mortality (47% in those born in recent years), compared with 17% mortality for those presenting without cyanosis (87). Postoperative problems include low cardiac output, pulmonary and tricuspid regurgitation, and arrhythmia.

Causes of Cardiogenic Shock That May Appear Later in Life

CARDIOMYOPATHY AND MYOCARDITIS

These poorly distinguishable disorders account for a large proportion of heart failure and cardiogenic shock in pediatric patients. Although many patients presenting with supposed cardiomyopathy have myocarditis on endomyocardial biopsy (95), some patients with myocarditis will develop cardiomyopathy. The diagnosis is made by endomyocardial biopsy, a procedure that is not risk-free in this situation. A recent study reported 1000 consecutive endomyocardial biopsies with 1 death and 9 perforations of the right ventricle. The highest risk for complications was in sick infants with suspected myocarditis receiving inotropic support (96). An alternative method suggested recently used the polymerase chain reaction analysis of tracheal aspirate to detect viral DNA in the myocardium of seven patients with myocarditis (97). The patient presenting in cardiogenic shock with a large cardiac silhouette, pulmonary venous congestion on chest X-ray, poorly contracting left ventricle on echocardiographic examination, and no history of heart disease will often be treated with the working diagnosis of myocarditis/cardiomyopathy.

Myocarditis: Myocarditis, which is in most cases viral, follows a flulike illness. The ECG is highly variable and may reveal generalized low-voltage, left ventricular hypertrophy or ST-T-wave changes. There may be rhythm disturbances with premature atrial or ventricular beats (98–100). Deep Q-waves should raise the possibility of an anomalous left coronary artery. Myocardial enzymes, such as creatinine phosphokinase, may be elevated. Diphtheria still remains endemic in many developing countries with fatality rates of 3% and 10% (101–103); a toxic child with rhythm and conduction abnormalities and typical necrotic throat infiltrate who has not been immunized should be suspected of having diphtheria (103).

In addition to inotropic support, immunosuppressive therapy has been tried in children. Drucker et al. (104) reported treatment with high-dose intravenous gamma-globulin (IVIG, 2 g/kg over 24 h) in 21 children with presumed myocarditis. These were compared to historical controls who did not receive the treatment. The IVIG-treated patients achieved better cardiac function within 3–6 mo and their survival tended to be better by 1-yr follow-up (84% vs 60%, *p*=0.069). In adult patients, Mason et al. *(105)* found that a 24-wk treatment with prednisone together with either cyclosporine or azothioprine had no effect on left ventricular function and survival. Anecdotal reports of treatment with corticosteroids have suggested improvement *(106)*. Recently, extracorporeal membrane oxygenation has been reported as a rescue measure for patients with acute myocarditis and shock. Diphtheria myocarditis should be treated with antitoxin and penicillin or erythromycin.

Lee et al. *(107)* reviewed the outcome of 36 pediatric patients with biopsy-proven lymphocytic myocarditis who were treated with intravenous corticosteroids. Freedom from death or cardiac transplantation was 79% after 2 yr. Most of the deaths occurred in the first 72 h. The prognosis of myocarditis-induced shock is probably much worse, although McCarthy et al. *(108)* reported better prognosis for adult patients with fulminant myocarditis than for those with less fulminant myocarditis.

Cardiomyopathies: As in the adult, cardiomyopathies in children are classified as dilated, hypertrophic, or restrictive. They may be primary, familial, or secondary to metabolic disorders. Dilated cardiomyopathy is characterized by ventricular dilatation and systolic dysfunction. The clinical, radiological, and ECG changes are similar to those described in myocarditis. The ECG is unique in glycogen storage disease type Ia (Pompe's disease), with a short PR interval and signs of marked left ventricular hypertrophy (LVH). The therapeutic approach to most cardiomyopathies is treatment of cardiac failure, as stated earlier. Recently, immunomodulating therapy with immunoadsorption and immunoglobulin substitution has been reported to be hemodynamically beneficial in adults *(109)*.

Carnitine deficiency is important because it is a treatable disease. Carnitine mediates the transport of fatty acids across the inner membrane of the mitochondria for β-oxidation *(109,110)*. Carnitine deficiency is characterized by hypoglycemia, hypotonia, encephalopathy, and cardiomyopathy. There may be a family history of the disease or unexplained deaths *(111)*. The ECG may show LVH, right ventricular hypertrophy, low voltage, or ST-T-wave changes in the left leads. Echocardiography reveals dilated or hypertrophic (less common) cardiomyopathy *(112)*. Free carnitine less than 20 nmol/mL or total carnitine less than 30 nmol/mL are highly suggestive of this disorder *(113)*. Winter et al. *(111)* described 51 patients with carnitine deficiency, 30 of them under 1 yr of age. Ten patients had cardiomyopathy (aged 1 d to 7 mo). All patients with cardiomyopathy, including two with very poor cardiac function, responded to carnitine supplementation. Improvement was evident as early as 2 d after the onset of therapy.

Adriamycin and daunomycin are very effective antineoplastic agents with unfortunate cardiotoxic side effects. Cardiotoxicity consists of myofibrilar loss and vacuolization caused by swelling of the sarcoplasmic reticulum. Toxic effects are usually evident after a cumulative dose of 540 mg/m^2 *(114)*. The cardiac damage may present early as a result of cardiomyocyte damage or death with subsequent diminished left ventricular contractility or it may occur many years after the completion of therapy with signs of inappropriately thin ventricular walls *(115)*. Agents aimed at preventing cardiotoxicity are under investigation with encouraging short-term results *(114)*.

KAWASAKI'S DISEASE

Kawasaki's disease is a generalized vasculitis of unknown etiology, most frequently affecting infants and children under 5 yr of age. The incidence is about 90/100,000 children <5 years of age in Japan *(10),* and about one-tenth of this figure in the United States *(116).* Coronary artery aneurysms are the major cardiac problem, occurring in 15–25% of untreated patients and in about 2.3% in those treated with aspirin and immunoglobulin during the acute phase *(117,118).* Myocardial involvement is evident in the acute phase as demonstrated by elevated cardiac troponin I *(119)* and brain natriuretic peptide *(120).* It may or may not accompany coronary disease as shown by discordance between thallium-201 scintigraphy and coronary angiography *(121).* Cardiogenic shock and death are most commonly a result of myocardial infarction. Kato et al. *(122)* reviewed 195 children with Kawasaki's disease who had myocardial infarction. In their study, myocardial infarction usually occurred within the first year of illness, and 22% of patients died. The common presenting symptoms were shock, crying, chest pain (which was more common in older children), abdominal pain, and vomiting. ECG findings included abnormal Q-waves, usually in leads II, III, and aVF. Rhythm problems were reported as well. Cardiac enzymes are elevated in most patients *(121).*

Treatment of the acute episode of Kawasaki's disease includes intravenous gamma-globulin and aspirin. Intravenous gamma globulin infusion reduces the risk of coronary artery aneurysm formation *(116,123).* The recommended dose is 1–2 g/kg over 10–12 h *(117,124).* High-dose aspirin (80–100 mg/kg/d) is given until the fever subsides and is subsequently reduced to 3–5 mg/kg/d for inhibition of platelet aggregation. This regimen is continued for 8 wk if no or transient coronary artery abnormalities are present, and long term if abnormalities persist. Warfarin may be added to aspirin in the latter case *(117).* Some centers add corticosteroids to the treatment in severe unresponsive cases *(125).* Treatment of myocardial infarction includes optimization of oxygenation, correction of metabolic disturbances, analgesia, inotropic support, and treatment of significant arrhythmia. Anticoagulation with heparin or warfarin is not used routinely for children with myocardial infarction *(126).* Percutaneous transluminal coronary angioplasty (PTCA), percutaneous transluminal coronary rotational ablation (PTCRA), and stent implantation *(127)* have been used in patients with Kawasaki's disease. In one report *(127),* PTCA resulted in 74% immediate success and 24% restenosis, whereas PTCRA resulted in 100% immediate success and no restenosis. Stenting was used in a few patients with 86% immediate success. New aneurysm formation is a worrisome complication. Surgical revascularization has been used with good results *(128).*

RHEUMATIC FEVER

Rheumatic fever is precipitated by group A streptococcal pharyngitis *(129)* and is rare before 5 yr of age. Its incidence has decreased markedly in the last decades in the developed world *(130),* but it is still a major cause for acquired heart disease in developing countries. Richmond et al. *(8)* reported an incidence of 375/100,000 school children-years among the aborigine population in Western Australia. Rheumatic carditis is the major cause of morbidity *(131).* Echocardiographic evidence of valvulitis is present in most patients *(132);* however, the rare involvement of the myocardium in the inflammatory process may be the cause of acute congestive heart failure and shock. Bitar et al. *(9)* reported death from congestive heart failure in 6 of 91 patient with rheumatic fever; all presented with heart failure. Others report a much better prognosis *(133).*

In addition to antistreptococcal and heart failure treatment, anti-inflammatory therapy should be administered. Although the superiority of corticosteroids over salicilates for severe rheumatic carditis has not been proven *(24),* it is advocated by many *(25).*

POSTOPERATIVE CARDIOGENIC SHOCK

Cardiogenic shock is commonly encountered in centers with active cardiac surgery programs for congenital heart disease. The possible causes of hemodynamic deterioration after cardiac surgery include the following:

1. Impaired contractility
2. Structural problem (valve regurgitation, residual stenosis, residual shunt)
3. Tamponade
4. Rhythm problems
5. Pulmonary hypertensive crisis
6. Noncardiac causes: sepsis, inadequate volume status

The management of the postoperative patient with low cardiac output and cardiogenic shock depends on the cause of the problem. Hypovolemia, anemia, and sepsis should be ruled out or treated if present. Myocardial dysfunction could be a result of inadequate myocardial protection, ischemia–reperfusion injury, or cardiopulmonary bypass *(26)*. Management of myocardial dysfunction should be guided by the principles stated earlier with optimization of preload, afterload, contractility, and heart rate. Structural problems such as residual shunt, obstruction, or valve regurgitation may be the cause of failure and may require reoperation. Tamponade from inadequate control of bleeding could cause shock and should be recognized and drained. Dysrhythmia such as junctional ectopic tachycardia or complete heart block are potential causes for failure. Pulmonary hypertension is a cause of right ventricular failure and low cardiac output. This is sometimes seen in patients with preoperatively elevated pulmonary vascular resistance, as in infants with Down syndrome and atrioventricular canal defect or patients with large shunts operated at an older age. Pulmonary vascular resistance could be supra-systemic. Moderately elevated pulmonary vascular resistance could be detrimental in situations in which right ventricular function is compromised as in Ebstein anomaly of the tricuspid valve. Management includes assessing and treating lung problems, oxygenation, hyperventilation and correction of metabolic acidosis. Inhaled nitric oxide is an effective selective pulmonary vasodilator *(28)*.

CONCLUSION

It is important to understand the potential causes of shock when dealing with young patients with suspected cardiogenic shock, as the causes of cardiogenic shock in infants and children are unique. Although the prognosis is generally poor, many treatable causes exist and thus should be sought and treated appropriately. A systematic approach to cardiogenic shock in the young must include practical diagnostic criteria.

A greater understanding of the best treatment of shock in infants and children is needed. Gathering evidence-based data regarding the outcomes of various treatment strategies in these patients is a fertile field for future research.

REFERENCES

1. Rosenthal G. Prevalence of congenital heart disease. In: Garson A, Jr, Bricker JT, Fisher DJ, Neish SR, eds. The Science and Practice of Pediatric Cardiology. 2nd ed. Williams & Wilkins, Baltimore, MD, 1998, pp. 1625–1645.
2. Samanek M, Voriskova M. Congenital heart disease among 815,569 children born between 1980 and 1990 and their 15-year survival: a prospective Bohemia survival study. Pediatr Cardiol 1999;20:411–417.

3. Abu-Harb M, Hey E, Wern C. Death in infancy from unrecognized congenital heart disease. Arch Dis Child 1994;71:3–7.

4. Bower C, Ramsey JM. Congenital heart disease: a 10 year cohort. J Pediatr Child Health 1994;30:414–418.

4a. Ferencz C, Rubin JD, Loffredo CA, Magee C, eds. Perspectives in Pediatric Cardiology. Vol 4. Epidemiology of Congenital Heart Disease: The Baltimore–Washington Infant Study, 1981–1989. Futura, Mount Kisco NY, 1993.

5. Stark J, Gallivan S, Lovegrove J, et al. Mortality rates after surgery for congenital heart defects in children and surgeon's performance. Lancet 2000;355:1004–1007.

6. Kern JH, Hayes CJ, Michler RE, Gersony WM, Quaegebeur JM. Survival and risk factor analysis for the Norwood procedure for hypoplastic left heart syndrome. Am J Cardiol 1997;80:170–174.

7. Hehrlein FW, Yamamoto T, Orime Y, Bauer J. Hypoplastic left heart syndrome: Which is the best operative strategy? Ann Thorac Cardiovasc Surg 1998;4:125–132.

8. Richmond P, Harris L. Rheumatic fever in the Kimberely region of Western Australia. J Trop Pediatr 1998;44:148–152.

9. Bitar FF, Hayek P, Obeid M, Gharzeddine W, Mikati M, Dhaibo GS. Rheumatic fever in children: a 15-year experience in a developing country. Pediatr Cardiol 2000;21:119–122.

10. Yanagawa H, Nakamura Y, Sakatak K, Yashiro M. Use of intravenous gamma-globulin for Kawasaki disease: effect on cardiac sequelae. Pediatr Cardiol 1997;18:19–23.

11. Taubert KA, Rowley AH, Shulman ST. Seven-year national survey of Kawasaki disease and acute rheumatic fever. Pediatr Infect Dis J 1994;13:704–708.

12. Fisher DJ. Perinatal maturation of the cardiomyocyte: An integrated view of the molecular basis of the perinatal maturation of cardiac function. In: Garson A Jr, Bricker JT, Fisher DJ, Neish SR, eds. The Science and Practice of Pediatric Cardiology. 2nd ed. Williams & Wilkins, Baltimore, MD, 1998, pp. 201–209.

13. Seguchi M, Harding JA, Jarmakani JM. Developmental changes in the function of sarcoplasmic reticulum. J Mol Cell Cardiol 1986;18:189–195.

14. Klitzner TS. Maturational changes in excitation-contraction coupling in mammalian myocardium. J Am Coll Cardiol 1991;17:218–225.

15. Epstein ML, Keil EA, Victoria BE. Cardiac decompensation following verapamil therapy in infants with supraventricular tachycardia. Pediatrics 1985;75:737–740.

16. Mahony L, Jones LR. Developmental changes in cardiac sarcoplasmic reticulum calcium pump in sheep. J Biol Chem 1986;261:15,257–15,265.

17. Crepaz R, Pitscheider W, Radetti G, Gentili L. Age-related variation in left ventricular myocardial contractile state expressed by stress velocity relation. Pediatr Cardiol 1998;19:463–467.

18. Rowland DG, Gutgessel HP. Noninvasive assessment of myocardial contractility, perload and afterload in healthy newborn infants. Am J Cardiol 1995;75:818–821.

19. Holmgren SM, Goldberg SJ, Donnerstein RL. Influence of age, body size and heart rate on left ventricular diastolic indexes in young subjects. Am J Cardiol 1991;68:1245–1247.

20. Califf RM, Bengtson JR. Cardiogenic shock. N Eng J Med 1994;330:1724–1730.

21. The American Heart Association in Collaboration with the International Liaison Committee on Resuscitation. Pediatric advanced life support. Guidelines of the American Heart Association. Circulation 2000;102(Suppl I):I-291–I-342.

22. Tobin JR, Wetzel RC. Shock and multiorgan failure. In: Rogers MC, Nichols DG, eds. Texbook of Pediatric Intensive Care. Williams & Wilkins, Baltimore, MD, 1996, pp. 555–605.

23. McMurphy DM, Heyman MA, Rudolph AM, Melmin KL. Developmental changes in constriction of the ductus arteriosus: response to oxygen and vasoactive substances in the isolated ductus arteriosus of the fetal lamb. Pediatr Res 1972;6:231–238.

24. Albert DA, Harel L, Karrison T. The treatment of rheumatic carditis: a review and meta-analysis. Medicine Baltimore 1995;74:1–12.

25. Booker PD, Evans C, Franks R. Comparison of the haemodynamic effects of dopamine and dobutamine in young children undergoing cardiac surgery. Br J Anaesth 1995;74:419–423.

26. Greenough A, Emery EF. Randomized trial comparing dopamine and dobutamine in preterm infants. Eur J Pediatr 1993;152:925–927.

27. Chang AC, Atz AM, Wernovsky G, Burke RP, Wessel DL. Milrinone: systemic and pulmonary hemodynamic effects in neonates after cardiac surgery. Crit Care Med 1995;23:1907–1914.

28. Haydar A, Mauriat P, Pouard P, et al. Inhaled nitric oxide for postoperative pulmonary hypertension in patients with congenital heart defects. Lancet 1992;340:1545.

29. Jonmaker C, Olsson AK, Jogi P, Forsell C. Hemodynamic effects of tracheal and intravenous adrenaline in infants with congenital heart disease. Acta Anaesthesiol Scand 1996;99:65–72.

30. Appelbaum A, Blackstone EH, Kouchoukos NT, Kirklin JW. Afterload reduction and cardiac output in infants after intracardiac surgery. Am J Cardiol 1977;39:445–451.

31. Seri I, Rudas G, Bors Z, Kanycska B, Tulassay T. Effect of low-dose dopamine infusion on cardiovascular and renal functions, cerebral blood flow, and plasma catecholamine levels in sick preterm neonates. Pediatr Res 1993;34:742–749.

32. Seri I. Cardiovascular, renal, and endocrine actions of dopamine in neonates and children. J Pediatr 1995;126:333–344.

33. Lass NA, Glock D, Goldberg LI. Cardiovascular and renal hemodynamic effects of intravenous infusion of the selective DA_1 agonist, fenoldopan, used alone or in combination with dopamine and dobutamine. Circulation 1988;78:1310–1315.

34. Tuttle RR, Mills J. Dobutamine: development of a new catecholamine to selectively increase cardiac contractility. Circ Res 1975;36:185–196.

35. Perkin RM, Levin DL, Webb R, Aquino A, Reedy J. Dobutamine: a hemodynamic evaluation in children with shock. J Pediatr 1982;100:977–983.

36. Barton P, Garcia J, Kouatli A, et al. Hemodynamic effects of iv milrinone lactate in pediatric patients with septic shock. A prospective, double-blinded, randomized, placebo-controlled, interventional study. Chest 1996;109:1302–1312.

37. Worthley LI, Tyler P, Moran JL. A comparison of dopamine, dobutamine and isoproterenol in the treatment of shock. Intensive Care Med 1985;11:13–19.

38. Cotter G, Kaluski E, Blatt A, et al. L-NMMA (a nitric oxide synthase inhibitor) is effective in the treatment of cardiogenic shock. Circulation 2000;101:1358–1361.

39. Moulopoulos S, Topaz S, Lolff W. Diastolic balloon pumping (with carbon dioxide) in the aorta–a mechanical assistance to the failing heart. Circulation 1962;63:669–675.

40. Meyns B, Sergeant P, Wouters P, et al. Mechanical support with microaxial blood pumps for postcardiotomy left ventricular failure: can outcome be predicted? J Thorac Cardiovasc Surg 2000;120:393–400.

41. Anderson H, Attorri R, Custer J, Chapman R, Bartlett R. Extracorporeal membrane oxygenation for pediatric cardiopulmonary failure. J Thorac Cardiovasc Surg 1990;99:1011–1012.

42. Klein M, Shahedn K, Whittlesey G, Pinsky W, Arciniegas E. Extracorporeal membrane oxygenation for the circulatory support of children after repair of congenital heart disease. J Thorac Cardiovasc Surg 1990;100:498–507.

43. Kanter K, Pennington G, Weber T, Zambie M, Braun P, Martychenko V. Extracorporeal membrane oxygenation for postoperative cardiac support in children. J Thorac Cardiovasc Surg 1987;93:27–35.

44. Rogers A, Trento A, Siewers R, et al. Extracorporeal membrane oxygenation for postcardiotomy cardiogenic shock in children. Ann Thorac Surg 1989;47:903–906.

45. Raithel S, Pennington G, Boegner E, Fiore A, Weber T. Extracorporeal membrane oxygenation in children after cardiac surgery. Circulation 1992;86:(Suppl II):II-305–II-310.

46. Weinhaus L, Canter C, Noetzel M, McAlister W, Spray T. Extracorporeal membrane oxygenation for circulatory support after repair of congenital heart defects. Ann Thorac Surg 1989;48:206–212.

47. Ibrahim AE, Duncan BW, Blume ED, Jonas RA. Long-term follow-up of pediatric cardiac patients requiring mechanical circulatory support. Ann Thorac Surg 2000;69:189–192.

48. Park J, Hsu D, Gersony W. Intraaortic balloon pump management of refractory congestive heart failure in children. Pediatr Cardiol 1993;14:19–22.

49. Veasy L, Blalock R, Orth J, Boucek M. Intra-aortic balloon pumping in infants and children. Circulation 1983;68:1095–1100.

50. Pollock J, Charlton M, Williams W, Edmonds J, Trusler G. Intraaortic balloon pumping in children. Ann Thorac Surg 1980;29:522–528.

51. Webster H, Veasy L. Intra-aortic balloon pumping in children. Heart Lung 1985;14:548–555.

52. Karl T, Horton S. Options for mechanical support in pediatric patients. In: Goldstein D, Oz M, eds. Cardiac Assist Devices. Futura, Armonk, NY, 2000, pp. 37–62.

53. Karl T, Sano S, Horton S, Mee R. Centrifugal pump left heart assisted pediatric cardiac operations: Indications, techniques, and results. J Thorac Cardiovasc Surg 1991;102:624–630.

54. Farrar D, Lawson J, Litwak P, Cederwall G. Thoratec VAD system as a bridge to heart transplantation. J Heart Transplant 1990;9:415–423.

55. Joyce L, Johnson K, Toninato C, et al. Results of the first 100 patients who received Symbion total artificial hearts as a bridge to cardiac transplantation. Circulation 1989;80(Suppl III):III-192–III-201.

56. Mehta S, Aufiero T, Pae W, Miller C, Pierce W. Combined Registry for the Clinical Use of Mechanical Ventricular Assistance Pumps and the Total Artifical Heart in Conjunction with Heart Transplantation: Sixth Official Report–1994. J Heart Lung Transplant 1995;14:585–593.

57. Frazier, O., Nakatani, T., Duncan, M., Parnis, S., Fuqua, J. Clinical experience with the Hemopump. Trans Am Soc Artif Intern Organs 1989;35:604–606.

58. Artman M, Boucek RJ Jr, Hammon J Graham TP Jr. Emergency palliation of critical valvar aortic stenosis. Am J Dis Child 1983;137:339–340.

59. Howkins JA, Michin LL, Tani LY, et al. Late results and reintervention after aortic valvotomy for critical aortic stenosis in neonates and infants. Ann Thorac Surg 1998;65:1758–1763.

60. Alexiou C, Langley M, Dalrymple-Hay MJR, et al. Open commissurotomy for critical isolated aortic stenosis in neonates. Ann Thorac Surg 2001;71:489–493.

61. Lababidi Z, Weinhous L. Successful balloon valvuloplasty for neonatal critical aortic stenosis. Am Heart J 1986;12:913–916.

62. Egito EST, Moore P, O'Sullivan T, Colan S, Perry SB, Lock JE. Transvascular balloon dilatation for neonatal aortic stenosis: early and midterm results. J Am Coll Cardiol 1997;29:442–447.

63. Weber HS, Mart CR, Kupferschmid J, Myers JL, Cyran SE. Transcarotid balloon valvuloplasty with continuous transesophageal echocardiographic guidance for neonatal critical aortic valve stenosis: An alternative to surgical palliation. Pediatr Cardiol 1998;19:212–217.

64. Maeno M, Akagi T, Hashino M, et al. Carotid artery approach to balloon aortic valvuloplasty in infants with critical aortic valve stenosis. Ped Cardiol 1997;18:288–291.

65. Kohl T, Sharland G, Allan LD, et al. World experience of percutaneous ultrasound-guided balloon valvuloplasty in human fetuses with severe aortic valve obstruction. Am J Cardiol 2000;85:1230–1233.

66. Barber G. Hypoplastic left heart syndrome. In: Garson A Jr, Bricker JT, Fisher DJ, Neish, SR, eds. The Science and Practice of Pediatric Cardiology. 2nd ed. Williams & Wilkins, Baltimore, MD, 1998, pp. 1625–1645.

67. Hehrlein FW, Yamamoto T, Orime Y, Bauer J. Hypoplastic left heart syndrome: which is the best operative strategy? Ann Thorac Cardiovasc Surg 1998;4:125–132.

68. Kern JH, Hayes CJ, Michler RE, Gersony WM, Quaegebeur JM. Survival and risk factor analysis for the Norwood procedure for hypoplastic left heart syndrome. Am J Cardiol 1997;80:170–174.

69. Williams DL, Gelijns AC, Moskowitz AJ, et al. Hypoplastic left heart syndrome: valuing the survival. J Thorac Cardiovasc Surg 2000;119:720–731.

70. Jenkins PC, Flanagan MF, Jenkins KJ, et al. Survival analysis and risk factors for mortality in transplantation and staged surgery for hypoplastic left heart syndrome. J Am Coll Cardiol 2000;36:1178–1185.

71. Cohen DM, Allen HD. New developments in the treatment of hypoplastic left heart syndrome. Curr Opin Cardiol 1997;12:44–50.

72. Mahle WT, Clancy RR, Moss EM, Gerdes M, Jobes DR, Wernovsky G. Neurodevelopmental outcome and lifestyle assessment in school-aged and adolescent children with hypoplastic left heart syndrome. Pediatrics 2000;105:1082–1089.

73. Fletcher SE, Nihill MR, Grifka RG, O'Laughlin MP, Mullins CE. Balloon angioplasty of native coarctation of the aorta: midterm follow-up and prognostic factors. J Am Coll Cardiol 1995;25:730–734.

74. Kain SF, Smith EO, Mott AR, Mullins CE, Geva T. Quantitative echocardiographic analysis of the aortic arch outcome of balloon angioplasty of native coarctation of the aorta. Circulation 1996;94:1056–1062.

75. Quaegebeur JM, Jonas RA, Weinberg AD, Blackstone EH, Kirklin JW, and the Congenital Heart Surgeons' Society. Outcome of seriously ill neonates with coarctation of the aorta. A multiinstitutional study. J Thorac Cardiovasc Surg 1994;108:841–854.

76. Gournay V, Piechaud JF, Delogu A, Sidi D, Kachaner J. Balloon valvotomy for critical stenosis or atresia of pulmonary valve in newborns. J Am Coll Cardiol 1995;26:1725–1731.

77. Wang JK, Wu MH, Lee WL, Cheng CF, Lue HC. Balloon dilatation for critical pulmonary stenosis. Int J Cardiol 1999;69:27–32.

78. Ward KE, Mullins CE. Anomalous pulmonary venous connections, pulmonary vein stenosis, and atresia of the common pulmonary vein. In: Garson A, Jr, Bricker JT, Fisher DJ, Neish SR, eds. The Science and Practice of Pediatric Cardiology. 2nd ed, Williams & Wilkins, Baltimore, MD, 1998, Vol. 1, pp. 1431–1461.

79. Duff DF, Nihill MR, McNamara DG. Infradiaphragmatic total anomalous pulmonary venous return: review of clinical and pathological findings and results of operation in 28 cases. Br Heart J 1977;39:619–626.

80. Okamoto K, Sato T, Kurose M, Kukita I, Fujii H, Taki K. Successful use of inhaled nitric oxide for treatment of severe hypoxemia in an infant with total anomalous pulmonary venous return. Anesthesiology 1994;81:256–259.

81. Atz AM, Wessel DL. Inhaled nitric oxide in neonates with cardiac disease. Semin Perinatol 1997;21:441–455.

82. Bullaboy CA, Johonson DH, Azar H, Jennings RB Jr. Total anomalous pulmonary venous connection to portal system: a new therapeutic role for prostaglandin E1? Pediatr Cardiol 1984;5:115–116.

83. Vouhe PR, Baillot-Vernant F, Trinquet F, et al. Anomalous left coronary artery from the pulmonary artery in infants. J Thorac Cardiovasc Surg 1987;94:192–199.

84. Takeuchi S, Imamura H, Katsumoto K, et al. New surgical method for repair of anomalous left coronary artery from pulmonary artery. J Thorac Cardiovasc Surg 1979;78:7–11.

85. Chang AC, Hanely FL. Anomalous origin of the left coronary artery from the pulmonary artery (ALCAPA). In: Chang AC, Hanely FL, Wernovsky G, Wessel DL, eds. Pediatric Cardiac Intensive Care. Lippincott Williams & Wilkins, Philadelphia, 1998:312–316.

86. Turley K, Szamicki RJ, Flachsbart KD, Richter RC, Popper RW, Tarnoff H. Aortic implantation is possible in all cases of anomalous origin of the left coronary artery from the pulmonary artery. Ann Thorac Surg 1995;60:84–89.

87. Hsieh YY, Lee CC, Chang CC, Tsai HD, Yeh LS, Tsai CH. Successful prenatal digoxin therapy for Ebstein anomaly with hydrops fetalis. A case report. J Reproduct Med 1998;4:710–712.

88. Yetman AT, Freedom RM, McCrindle BW. Outcome of cyanotic neonates with Ebstein's anomaly. Am J Cardiol 1998;81:749–754.

89. Bruckheimer E, Bulbul Z, Pinter E, Gailani M, Kleinman CS, Fahey JT. Inhaled nitric oxide therapy in a critically ill neonate with Ebstein's anomaly. Pediatr Cardiol 1998;19:477–479.

90. Roberson DA, Silverman NH. Ebstein anomaly: echocardiographic and clinical features in the fetus, and neonate. J Am Coll Cardiol 1989;14:1300–1307.

91. Chang AC, Hanely FL, Ebstein anomaly of the tricuspid valve. In: Chang AC, Hanely FL, Wernovsky G, Wesse DL, eds. Pediatric Cardiac Intensive Care. Lippincott Williams & Wilkins, Philadelphia, 1998, pp. 316–321.

92. Augustin N, Schmidt-Habelmann P, Wottke M, Meisner H, Sebening F. Results after surgical repair of Ebstein's anomaly. Ann Thorac Surg 1997;63:1650–1656.

93. Knott-Craig CJ, Overholt ED, Ward KE, Razook JD. Neonatal repair of Ebstein's anomaly: indications, surgical technique, and medium-term follow-up. Ann Thorac Surg 2000;69:1505–1510.

94. Celermajer DS, Bull C, Till JA, et al. Ebstein anomaly: presentation and outcome from fetus to adult. J Am Coll Cardiol 1994;23:170–176.

95. Camargo PR, Snitcowsky R, Da Luz PL, et al. Favorable effect of immunosuppressive therapy in children with dilated cardiomyopathy and active myocarditis. Pediatr Cardiol 1995;16:61–68.

96. Pophal SG, Sigfusson G, Booth KL, et al. Complications of endomyocardial biopsy in children. J Am Coll Cardiol 1999;34:2105–2110.

97. Akhtar N, Stomberg D, Rosenthal GL, Bowles NE, Towbin JA. Tracheal aspirate as a substrate for polymerase chain reaction detection of viral genome in childhood pneumonia and myocarditis. Circulation 1999;99:2011–2018.

98. Taliercio CP, Seward JB, Driscoll DJ, Fisher LD, Gersh BJ, Tajik AJ. Idiopathic dilated cardiomyopathy in the young: clinical profile and natural history. J Am Coll Cardiol 1985;6:1126–1131.

99. Wiles HB, Gillette PC, Harley RA, Upshur JK. Cardiomyopathy and myocarditis in children with ventricular ectopic rhythm. J Am Coll Cardiol 1992;20:359–362.

100. Leatherbury L, Chandra RS, Shapiro SR, Perry LW. Value of endomyocardial biopsy in infants, children and adolescents with dilated cardiomyopathy and myocarditis. J Am Coll Cardiol 1988;12:1547–1554.

101. Chen RT, Broome CV, Weinstein RA, Weaver R. Diphtheria in the United States, 1971–1998 Am J Public Health 1985;75:1393–1397.

102. Kadirova R, Kartoglu HU, Strebel PM. Clinical characteristics and management of 676 hospitalized diphtheria cases, Kyrgyz republic, 1995. J Infect Dis 2000;Suppl:S110–S115.

103. Perles Z, Nir A, Cohen E, Bashary A, Engelhard D. Atrio-ventricular block in a toxic child. Do not forget the diphtheria. Pediatr Cardiol 2000;21:282–283.

104. Drucker NA, Colan SD, Lewis AB, et al. Gamma-globulin treatment of acute myocarditis in pediatric population. Circulation 1994;89:252–257.

105. Mason JW, O'Connell JB, Herskowitz A, et al. A clinical trial of immunosuppressive therapy for myocarditis. N Engl J Med 1995;333:269–275.

106. Zales VR, Deal BJ, Pahl E, Wright KL, Alboliras ET, Crawford S. High-dose steroids therapy for acute myocarditis in pediatric patients. Circulation 1994;90:I–50.

107. Lee KJ, McCrindle BW, Bohn DJ, et al. Clinical outcome of acute myocarditis in childhood. Heart 1999;82:226–233.

108. McCarthy RE, Boehmer JP, Hutchins GM, Kasper EK, Hare JM, Baughman KL. Long-term outcome of fulminant myocarditis as compared with acute (nonfulminant) myocarditis. N Engl J Med 2000;342:690–695.

109. Felix SB, Staudt A, Dorffel WV, et al. Hemodynamic effect of immunoadsorption and subsequent immunoglobulin substitution in dilated cardiomyopathy. J Am Coll Cardiol 2000;35:1590–1598.

110. Pepine CJ. The therapeutic potential of carnitine in cardiovascular disorders. Clin Ther 1991;13:2–21.

111. Winter SC, Szabo-Aczel S, Curry CJR, Hutchinson HT, Hogue R, Shung A. Plasma carnitine deficiency. Am J Dis Child 1987;141:660–665.

112. Ino T, Sherwood WG, Benson LN, Wilson GJ, Freedom RM, Rowe RD. Cardiac manifestations of disorders of fat and carnitine metabolism in infancy. J Am Coll Cardiol 1988;11:1301–1308.

113. Lewis AB. The failing myocardium. In: Chang AC, Hanely FL, Wernovsky G, Wesse DL, eds. Pediatric Cardiac Intensive Care. Lippincott Williams & Wilkins, Philadelphia, 1998, pp. 483–496.

114. Wexler LH. Ameliorating anthracycline cardiotoxicity in children with cancer: clinical trials with dexrazoxane. Semin Oncol 1998;25(Suppl 10):86–92.

115. Grenier MA, Lipshultz SE. Epidemiology of anthracycline cardiotoxicity in children and adults. Semin Oncol 1998;25(Suppl 10):72–85.

116. Laupland KB, Davis HD. Epidemiology, etiology, and management of Kawasaki disease: state of the art. Pediatr Cardiol 1999;20:177–183.

117. Dajani AS, Taubert KA, Takahashi M, et al. Guidelines for long-term management of patients with Kawasaki disease. Report from the committee on rheumatic fever, endocarditis, and Kawasaki disease, council on cardiovascular disease in the young, American Heart Association. Circulation 1994;89:916–922.

118. Durongpisitkul K, Guruaj VJ, Park JM, Martin CH. The prevention of coronary artery aneurysm in Kawasaki Disease: a meta-analysis on the efficacy of aspirin and immunoglobulin treatment. Pediatrics 1995;96:1057–1061.

119. Kim M, Kim K. Elevation of cardiac troponin I in the acute stage of Kawasaki disease. Pediatr Cardiol 1999;20:184–188.

120. Kawamura T, Wago M, Kawaguchi H, Tahara M, Yuge M. Plasma brain natriuretic peptide concentrations in patients with Kawasaki disease. Pediatr Cardiol 2000;42:241–248.

121. Fukazawa M, Fukushige J, Takeuchi T, et al. Discordance between thallium-201 scintigraphy and coronary angiography in patients with Kawasaki's disease: myocardial ischemia with normal coronary angiogram. Pediatr Cardiol 1993;14:67–74.

122. Kato H, Ichinnose E, Kawasaki T. Myocardial infarction in Kawasaki disease: clinical analysis in 195 cases. J Pediatr 1986;108:923–927.

123. Yanagawa H, Nakamura Y, Sakata K, Yashiro M. Use of intravenous gamma-globulin for Kawasaki disease: effect on cardiac sequelae. Pediatr Cardiol 1997;18:19–23.

124. Newburger JW, Takahashi M, Beiser AS, et al. A single intravenous infusion of gamma globulin as compared with four infusions in the treatment of Kawasaki syndrome. N Engl J Med 1991;324:1633–1639.

125. Dale RC, Saleem, Daw S, Dillon MJ. Treatment of severe complicated Kawasaki disease with oral prednisolone and aspirin. J Pediatr 2000;137:723–726.

126. Johnsrude CL, Towbin JA. Myocardial infarction in childhood. In: Garson A, Jr, Bricker JT, Fisher DJ, Neish, SR, eds, The Science and Practice of Pediatric Cardiology. 2nd ed. Williams & Wilkins, Baltimore, MD, 1998, pp. 1933–1982.

127. Akaji T, Ogawa S, Ino T, et al. Catheter interventional treatment in Kawasaki disease: a report from the Japanese pediatric interventional cardiology investigation group. J Pediatr 2000;137:181–186.

128. Kitamura S, Kameda Y, Seki T, et al. Long-term outcome of myocardial revascularization in patients with Kawasaki coronary artery disease. A multicenter cooperative study. J Thorac Cardiovasc Surg 1994;107:663–673.

129. Catanzaro FJ, Stenson CA, Morris AJ, et al. The role of the streptococcus in the pathogenesis of rheumatic fever. Am J Med 1954;17:749–756.

130. Gordis L. The virtual disappearance of rheumatic fever in the United States: lessons in the rise and fall of disease. Circulation 1985;72:1155–1162.

131. Dajani AS, Ayub E, et al. The special writing group of the committee on rheumatic fever, endocarditis, and Kawasaki disease of the council on cardiovascular disease in the young of the American Heart Association. Guidelines for the diagnosis of rheumatic fever. JAMA 1992;268:2069–2073.

132. Veasy LG, Wiedmeier SE, Orsmond GS, et al. Resurgence of acute rheumatic fever in the intermountain area of the United States. N Engl J Med 1987;316:421–427.

133. Karaaslan S, Oran B, Reisli I, Erkul I. Acute rheumatic fever in Konya, Turkey. Pediatr Int 2000;42:71–75.

134. Albert DA, Harel L, Karrison T. The treatment of rheumatic carditis: a review and meta-analysis. Medicine (Baltimore) 1995;74:1–12.

135. Human DG, Hill ID, Fraser CB. Treatment choice in acute rheumatic fever. Arch Dis Child 1984;59:410–413.

136. Roth SJ. Postoperative care. In: Chang AC, Hanely FL, Wernovsky G, Wessel DL, eds: Pediatric Cardiac Intensive Care. Lippincott Williams & Wilkins, Philadelphia, 1998, pp. 163–187.

137. Haydar A, Mauriat P, Pouard P, et al. Inhaled nitric oxide for postoperative pulmonary hypertension in patients with congenital heart defects. Lancet 1992;340:1545.

17 Congenital Heart Disease in the Adult and Cardiogenic Shock

Rafael Hirsch, MD

CONTENTS

INTRODUCTION

With the advent of modern cardiovascular surgery, adult survival of congenital heart disease has become the rule, with more than 85% of affected newborns expected to reach adulthood *(1)*. With the exception of patients with anomalies for which adult survival is common and a few patients with complex malformations that allow survival without intervention, an ever-growing number of adults owe their lives to surgical or catheter intervention early in life. For example, division of the patent arterial duct (PDA), surgical closure of a secundum atrial septal defect (ASD) and balloon valvoplasty of a stenosed pulmonary valve in early childhood are usually curative.

Even with advanced methods of treatment, however, truly curative therapy is rare for most malformations. For some malformations, residua and sequelae are the rule and will gradually express themselves with advancing age. Adults treated with evolving medical knowledge may not have long-term outcomes as good as would be expected of children treated today for the same conditions. In adult "natural sur-

From: *Contemporary Cardiology: Cardiogenic Shock: Diagnosis and Treatment*
Edited by: David Hasdai et al. © Humana Press Inc., Totowa, NJ

vivors," who were either undiagnosed or untreated in childhood, the natural history is an accumulation of adverse effects on the cardiovascular system imposed by the morphology and pathophysiology of their congenital anomaly. Another great challenge to those taking care of adults with congenital heart disease is the interaction between congenital heart disease and acquired diseases of adulthood, such as coronary artery disease, hypertension, and diabetes, with very little information in the medical literature to date.

Cardiogenic shock is defined as a hemodynamic state in which there is inadequate organ perfusion as a result of malfunction of the heart. In acquired heart disease, events leading to shock are often abrupt, with dramatic changes in cardiac function leading to rapid clinical deterioration. Few adaptive and compensatory mechanisms are efficient under those circumstances. In contrast, chronic cardiac conditions, of which congenital heart disease is the utmost example, allow the development of efficient adaptive mechanisms. Generally, the hemodynamic derangement is more gradual and the full-blown clinical picture of cardiogenic shock is rare, even in the face of very low cardiac output. However, having exhausted the compensatory mechanisms, cardiac reserves are limited and make the patients more vulnerable to conditions usually regarded as benign in healthier populations (e.g., an intercurrent febrile disease, dehydration, atrial dysrhythmias, negative inotropic drugs, contrast material, high altitude, and pregnancy).

This chapter will concentrate on mechanisms of hemodynamic decompensation that are typical and often unique to congenital anomalies in adults. It will highlight the groups of patients with borderline hemodynamics who are at risk for developing cardiogenic shock, and it will attempt to focus on the measures taken by the clinician to try and avoid such mishaps. Finally, the treatment of cardiogenic shock in these unique conditions will be discussed. This chapter cannot encompass all possible anomalies and clinical settings. Representative conditions have been chosen.

THE MORPHOLOGICALLY RIGHT VENTRICLE AS THE SYSTEMIC VENTRICLE

Three groups of anomalies will be discussed under this heading: congenitally corrected transposition of the great arteries (CTGA), transposition of the great arteries (TGA) after atrial-switch repair (Mustard, Senning), and "single ventricle" of right ventricular morphology (mitral atresia). Common to these malformations is a hypertrophied, globular-shaped right ventricle, ejecting blood to the aorta through an infundibulum and guarded by a tricuspid valve.

The natural history of these anomalies depends on associated lesions. In patients with a large ventricular septal defect (VSD) and unrestricted pulmonary blood flow, severe pulmonary hypertension gradually develops. They will be discussed under the Eisenmenger syndrome. Patients with a large VSD and restricted pulmonary flow resulting from pulmonary stenosis behave clinically like Fallot's tetralogy (TOF) and will be discussed under cyanotic malformations. This section discusses the remaining patients; those without pulmonary hypertension and without right-to-left shunting.

Three major factors influence the outcome of these patients: myocardial function, tricuspid insufficiency and rhythm and conduction disorders.

Myocardial Function

The right ventricle may not be ideally structured to perform as a systemic ventricle. Some case reports describe patients with CTGA without associated anomalies surviving to the seventh and eighth decade before the appearance of cardiac symptoms *(2–4)*. Larger series suggest that most patients with this rare disease develop myocardial dysfunction severe enough to cause heart failure around the fifth to sixth decades of life *(5,6)*. These reports may be heavily biased toward symptomatic patients, as those who do not develop heart failure may easily go unrecognized in an entire lifetime.

Patients who have had an atrial switch repair for simple transposition are followed from early childhood, and right ventricular function can be monitored over the years. To date, the oldest people who have had these operations are 40 yr old, the majority being 20–30 yr old (the younger ones would have had an arterial switch operation). At present, despite the concern inherent to this method of surgery leaving a systemic right ventricle, patients who had a good surgical result have reasonable although not normal right ventricular systolic function and good functional capacity *(7–10)*.

What should one recommend to a young patient with CTGA or TGA after a successful atrial switch operation who wants to engage in competitive sports or get pregnant? Should vasodilators be prescribed to all patients in an attempt to delay deterioration of myocardial function? The data needed to answer these questions do not yet exist. There is reasonable concern that in a decade or two, we may be confronted with a population of middle-aged patients in heart failure and shock.

Treatment of the patient in heart failure and shock resulting from a failing right systemic ventricle is basically the same as for the patient with a failing left ventricle in a normal heart. In the case of failure of pharmacological treatment, mechanical support with intra-aortic balloon counterpulsation and assist devices can be used as a bridge to transplantation, which is feasible with some technical modifications *(11,12)*. Mee has described a surgical approach specific for failing systemic right ventricles after Mustard or Senning operations for transposition: the double-switch operation. This consists of two stages: preparation of the left ventricle to pump at systemic pressures by graded pulmonary artery banding first, and removal of the atrial baffle, resepation of the atria, and arterial switch procedure as the final stage. Reported mortality is relatively high and the left ventricle may fail because of the sudden increase in afterload, requiring heart transplantation or immediate progression to arterial switch, using an assist device for the left ventricle *(13–16)*.

"Single right ventricle" (e.g., mitral atresia) is rare. When compared to a "single left ventricle" with similar hemodynamics (pulmonary stenosis or pulmonary hypertension), the natural history is worse because of a more rapid deterioration of myocardial function *(17,18)*. Little can be done in the face of a failing ventricle because of the anatomical complexity and often-associated pulmonary hypertension, necessitating heart–lung transplantation.

Tricuspid Insufficiency

Some patients with CTGA have an associated Ebstein's malformation of the systemic tricuspid valve with severe tricuspid insufficiency from the onset. Many more patients with CTGA and an anatomically normal tricuspid valve or those after atrial switch operation may develop important tricuspid regurgitation with time. The hypotensive subpulmonary left ventricle contributes to the dilatation and distortion of the tricuspid annulus, resulting in regurgitation. Patients who have concomitant left ventricular outflow tract obstruction have less tricuspid regurgitation *(19)*. The systemic right ventricle poorly tolerates tricuspid regurgitation *(20)*. Patients not promptly treated for this condition deteriorate rapidly and develop severe congestive failure and shock, dying before cardiac transplantation can be performed. We advocate vasodilators even for moderate regurgitation and prompt replacement of the valve for severe regurgitation *(21)*.

Our results of early replacement of the valve are encouraging. The valve tissue is often thickened and myxomatous and not suited for repair. After replacement, we continue treatment with vasodilators indefinitely. As in the case of myocardial dysfunction, a double-switch procedure may be the solution for severe tricuspid regurgitation, as it almost always improves when the right ventricle becomes subpulmonary *(14,22)*.

Rhythm and Conduction Disturbances

Patients with CTGA have a high incidence of congenital or acquired advanced atrioventricular block *(6,23,24)*. Those after atrial-switch repair of TGA have a high incidence of sinus node dysfunction with slow nodal rhythms taking over *(25,26)*. Bradycardia at rest or on exertion is a cause of poor exercise tolerance, diastolic myocardial dysfunction, and low cardiac output. We recommend dual-chamber rate-responsive pacing for poor exercise tolerance. A transvenous system can be used, with the ventricular screw-in electrode in the left ventricular myocardium.

Atrial tachyarrhythmias are not uncommon after atrial-switch operations because of extensive surgical scars. The hemodynamic effects may be devastating because of the very rapid heart rate, sometimes unveils a previously unrecognized abnormal systemic right ventricular function. Degeneration of a rapid atrial rhythm into ventricular fibrillation may be the cause of sudden cardiovascular collapse and death *(25)*. In treatment of these conditions, negative inotropic drugs such as verapamil and β-blockers should be used with care, bradycardia-induced tachyarrhythmias should be prevented by pacing, and ablation therapy should be used where applicable.

CYANOTIC AND NONCYANOTIC ANOMALIES WITH HYPERTROPHY OF THE SUBPULMONARY VENTRICLE

The classic nomenclature of congenital heart disease is based on the pathophysiology early in life. In adulthood, patients who were born with a noncyanotic shunt lesion (e.g., VSD) may have severe cyanosis resulting from the development of the Eisenmenger syndrome. In order to prevent confusion, we will analyze the different groups of patients who have in common a hypertrophied subpulmonary ventricle:

1. Pulmonary stenosis without cyanosis—valvar, subvalvar
2. Pulmonary stenosis with cyanosis (e.g., unoperated Fallot's tetralogy)
3. Pulmonary vascular disease with cyanosis—the Eisenmenger syndrome
4. Pulmonary vascular disease without cyanosis—after late repair of a shunt lesion (e.g., ASD, VSD, PDA)

Congenital cardiac malformations with essentially one pumping chamber, often referred to as "single ventricle" (e.g., tricuspid atresia, double inlet ventricle), present disease. For practical purposes, they will be discussed together with groups 2 or 3, according to the nature of pulmonary physiology. Those after a Fontan-type operation will be discussed in a later section.

PULMONARY STENOSIS

Tight pulmonary valve stenosis with suprasystemic pressures in the right ventricle is poorly tolerated and manifests in childhood. Lesser degrees of stenosis are usually well tolerated until adult life, when it presents with symptoms of low cardiac output, angina, and syncope. The same applies to other anomalies with similar physiology (e.g., double-chambered right ventricle and congenitally corrected transposition [CTGA] with subpulmonary stenosis). Valvar stenosis is amenable to balloon valvoplasty at any age, with excellent immediate results and little recurrence long term *(27,28)*. Most adults with long-standing pressure load of the subpulmonary ventricle have some degree of diastolic dysfunction, expressed by an increase of ventricular filling pressure. The degree of dysfunction correlates poorly with age and severity of stenosis and is an individual response of the myocardium.

After successful balloon valvoplasty or surgery, many patients report an immediate improvement in their well-being, especially improved exercise tolerance. However, it is not uncommon that after a latency period of as little as several months to many years after successful alleviation of pulmonary stenosis, patients present with signs and symptoms of "right-heart failure." Those with a patent foramen ovale become cyanosed, especially on exertion. These manifestations are the result of restrictive right ventricular physiology. On echocardiography, the right ventricle is often hypertrophied (despite the successful relief of stenosis), with normal or near-normal systolic function, the right atrium is dilated, the atrial septum is deviated to the left, and there is "smoke" (i.e., spontaneous contrast). On transesophageal echocardiography (TEE) or contrast study, one can demonstrate right-to-left shunting through a patent foramen ovale. Provided there is no residual pulmonary stenosis and pulmonary artery pressure is normal, one can appreciate the degree of myocardial restriction from the timing of premature forward flow in the pulmonary artery *(29,30)*. The shorter the duration of pulmonary regurgitation and the earlier the opening of the pulmonary valve, the more severe is myocardial restriction (Fig. 1). In extreme cases, the right ventricle becomes an almost passive conduit between the systemic veins and the pulmonary arteries. All patients with this degree of diastolic dysfunction who we catheterized had very low cardiac output (1.3–1.8 L/min km^2), were in functional class III–IV and had a very poor prognosis, most dying within 5 yr from diagnosis.

Are there therapeutic options for this condition? Patients without an existing interatrial communication can benefit from a small-diameter septostomy (around 4 mm) produced by transcatheter technique, to allow right-to-left shunting and decompression of the right atrium. The cost is mild systemic arterial desaturation and a risk of paradoxical emboli. The surgical performance of a bidirectional cavo-pulmonary anatomosis (Glenn shunt) to divert systemic venous blood from the right heart may be a reasonable approach, but, to date, we have had no experience with it.

Dynamic ventricular outflow tract obstruction can be a rare but important mechanism of syncope or near-syncope in adult patients with operated Fallot's tetralogy or similar malformations that had inadequate resection of obstructing muscle bundle at

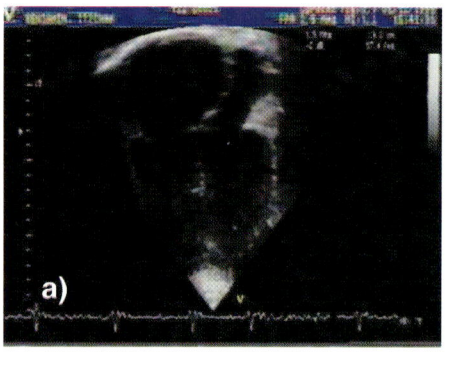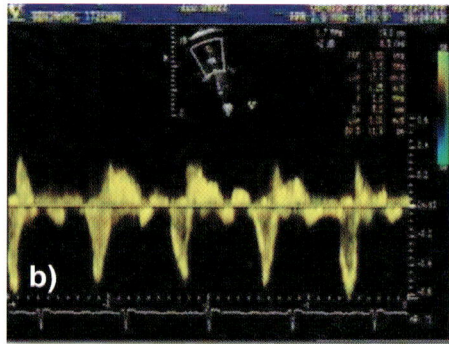

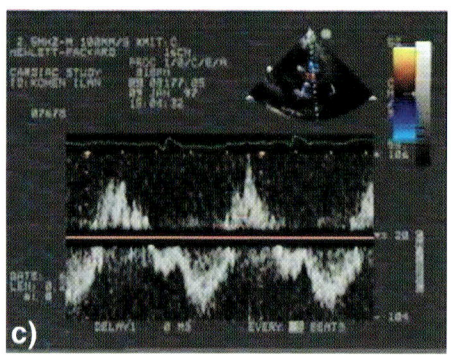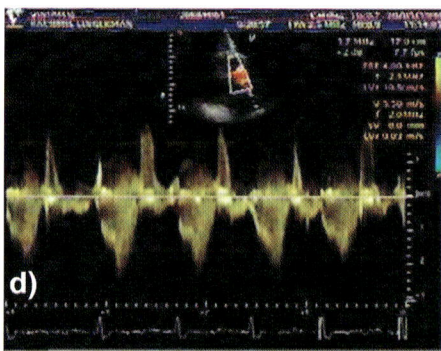

Fig. 1.　The restrictive right ventricle. (a) The right atrium is dilated and the septum is deviated to the left. (b) Hepatic venous flow shows a short rapid flow in diasotle compatible with the prominent venous Y descent. (c) Pulmonary flow in mild–moderate restriction. There is premature forward flow coinciding with the P-wave. (d) Pulmonary flow in severe restriction. The duration of pulmonary regurgitation is very short due to the abrupt rise of diastolic pressure which then drives the blood forward.

surgery. β-Blockers are effective in eliminating or markedly reducing these troublesome symptoms, which are sometimes wrongly attributed to rhythm disorders.

CYANOTIC HEART DISEASE

Cyanosis is the clinical manifestation of systemic arterial desaturation. Many congenital anomalies cause cyanosis and they all share the same two pathophysiological properties: the mixing of systemic with pulmonary venous blood and restriction of pulmonary blood flow. Those with an anatomical obstruction to pulmonary flow (e.g., pulmonary valvar or subvalvar stenosis) will be cyanosed from infancy. The most common representative of this group is Fallot's tetralogy. Those without obstruction have initially increased pulmonary flow and become cyanosed later in life, when the cumulative damage to the pulmonary vascular tree significantly restricts pulmonary blood flow. These are the patients with the Eisenmenger syndrome.

Adult patients with unoperated Fallot's tetralogy are rare. They usually represent the group with milder restriction to pulmonary blood flow ("pink Fallot's") or have had a palliative shunt operation in childhood. Children with extreme cyanosis rarely survive to adulthood without intervention.

Cyanosis with its accompanying compensatory erythrocytosis is a multiorgan disease with gradual deterioration of renal function, risk of paradoxical embolism and cerebral abscess formation, osteoarthropathy, cholelithiasis, and more. Therefore, adult patients with this physiology should be encouraged to have corrective surgery where feasible or palliation to improve oxygen saturations (e.g., a Fontan or Glenn operation for "single ventricle").

Patients with the Eisenmenger syndrome have a chronic and progressive disorder without a surgical or medical solution. Over the years, it has become clear that unnecessary medical intervention and other management mistakes have been the cause of deterioration and death in many. It is important that medical personnel who are familiar with this complex pathophysiology take care of these patients.

THE EISENMENGER SYNDROME

Eisenmenger syndrome results from congenital anomalies with a large communication between systemic and pulmonary circulations and unobstructed pulmonary flow. These communications can be intracardiac (e.g., VSD, ASD, "single ventricle"), extracardiac (e.g., patent ductus arteriosus, aorto-pulmonary window), or combined (e.g., common arterial trunk). A predominantly left-to-right shunt early in life gradually turns into a right-to-left shunt in adolescence or early adulthood, due to a reduction of the cross-sectional area of the arteriolar tree and resultant increased resistance. The major exception is atrial septal defect (ASD), which is a cause of severe pulmonary vascular disease in only around 5% of patients *(31,32)*, even if left untreated until old age. Because of the large communication between the pulmonary and systemic circulations, the driving pressure across the two vascular beds is the same for most malformations (ASD, again, being the exception), and the relative flow into each vascular bed is directly dependent on the vascular resistance.

Shock in the Eisenmenger patient is related to inadequate supply of oxygen to the target organs because of the low oxygen content of blood bypassing the lungs, rather than organ hypoperfusion. The goal of treatment is to act favorably on the two vascular beds, increasing the systemic and decreasing the pulmonary vascular resistances. Such actions improve pulmonary blood flow and decrease right-to-left shunt and cyanosis. In practice, the means that are available to us to improve hemodynamics in these patients are very limited, as most vasodilating agents are not selective and will have an equal or stronger effect on the healthy peripheral vascular bed than on the diseased pulmonary vessels. Nitric oxide, prostacycline analogs (epoprostenol, iloprost), and oxygen may be useful, but there is little information regarding the benefit of their use in the Eisenmenger syndrome *(33,34)*.

At present, the major role of physicians taking care of these patients is to prevent and treat conditions that have adverse hemodynamic effects (i.e., systemic vasodilatation and/or pulmonary vasoconstriction). These result in reduced pulmonary flow and increased cyanosis and may start a vicious cycle, when the heart, perfused with blood containing very little oxygen, deteriorates in function and further reduces pulmonary blood flow, culminating in shock and death, sometimes within minutes. In the face of these dramatic events, little if anything can be done to prevent the fatal outcome. A patient of ours became hypoxemic and gradually went into shock after delivery by cesarean section. She was treated with nebulized prostacyclin inhalations, and when she continued to deteriorate, nitric oxide was administered through a mechanical ventilator, but to no avail. A similar case has been described in ref. *(35)*.

As little can be done once rapid deterioration occurs, avoidance and, where possible, quick correction of the following lifestyle and management mistakes is probably the most effective way to improve survival:

1. Hypovolemia: exposure to heat and overexcitement (hot climate, disco, sauna, and hot baths), long-distance flights, diarrhea, vomiting, and phlebotomy without prompt and adequate fluid replacement. Abrupt changes of blood volume may be one of the reasons, together with hypoxemia and hormonal influences, for the extremely high incidence of maternal mortality and morbidity associated with pregnancy and delivery in Eisenmenger syndrome *(36)*.
2. Hypoxemia: high altitude and conditions responsible for systemic vascular dilatation like strenuous exercise, sepsis, and pregnancy.
3. Arrhythmia: atrial flutter and fibrillation and nonsustained ventricular tachycardia are often associated with rapid clinical deterioration.
4. Excessive phlebotomies may result in an increased incidence of hemoptysis and iron deficiency, in itself a cause of exacerbation of hyperviscosity symptoms and increased cerebral complications *(36)*.
5. Noncardiac surgery, sometimes trivial, like extraction of a tooth under anesthesia, may be the cause of shock and death. The factors involved are probably mental stress, hypoxemia, and/or hypercarbia during induction of anesthesia, and negatively inotropic drugs. Procedures should be avoided whenever possible or performed under the strictest measures by an experienced team of anesthetist and cardiologist.
6. The use of anticoagulants to prevent thromboembolic complications is not warranted. Most patients with compensatory erythrocytosis have thrombocytopenia and intrinsic coagulation abnormalities, and anticoagulants may increase the incidence and severity of hemoptysis *(36)*. At the very late stages of the disease, thrombosis *in situ* in the pulmonary tree is common and may be the nidus for distal embolization and increasing hypoxemia. The diagnosis is made by angio-CT (computed tomograph). Whether anticogulants are effective in preventing further thrombus formation is questionable, and the risk of hemoptysis increases. Estrogens may dramatically increase the risk of thromboembolic complications and should be avoided. Progestins cause fluid retention, but may be used carefully in small doses to regulate menstruation, as menometrorhagia is common and could be the cause of significant discomfort and iron deficiency.

End-stage Eisenmenger syndrome patients are candidates for heart–lung transplantation, but results are poor. In a large recent retrospective series *(36)*, 8 of 12 patients referred for transplantation had the operation, 5 of whom died at a mean of 16 mo posttransplantation. Referral for transplantation should be considered only in those in functional class IV with evidence of poor ventricular function, intractable arrhythmia, or massive pulmonary thrombosis and hemoptysis.

CYANOTIC ANOMALIES WITH PULMONARY STENOSIS

As mentioned earlier, patients with these anomalies in adulthood are rare, and, if suitable, they are usually referred to corrective surgery soon after presenting at a specialized center. Those not suited for corrective surgery but with optimal hemodynamics may be considered for a Fontan-type palliation (discussed later).

Patients unsuited for corrective surgery or Fontan may benefit from partial palliation, such as a venous shunt (e.g., Glenn anastomosis), arterial shunt (e.g., Blalock Taussig anastomosis), or dilatation of collaterals and stenosed pulmonary valve at catheterization. These procedures improve blood oxygenation but leave the basic physiology unchanged. Cyanotic anomalies with pulmonary stenosis have a physiology similar to that in the Eisenmenger syndrome, as here, too, pulmonary blood flow decreases with systemic vasodilatation. However, obstruction to pulmonary blood flow is fixed and is not subject to reactive vasospasm, the most vicious and fatal mechanism in pulmonary hypertensive patients. In general, the precautions and recommendations regarding the Eisenmenger syndrome apply to cyanotic patients with pulmonary stenosis, except for a generally better prognosis and less prohibitive risk in some activities, especially pregnancy *(37)*. In those with resting oxygen saturations above 85%, the likelihood of successful pregnancy for the mother and fetus is good *(34)* if the pregnancy is watched carefully throughout and the expecting mother instructed to rest.

Patients with complex pulmonary atresia (i.e., Fallot's tetralogy with pulmonary atresia, underdeveloped or absent central pulmonary arteries, and major aorto-pulmonary collaterals) form a heterogeneous group ranging from severe pulmonary stenosis, on one hand, to pulmonary vascular disease, on the other. Sometimes, both coexist in different lung segments of the same patient. Care of these patients in adulthood can be extremely difficult and should be individualized according to the hemodynamics of each patient.

PULMONARY HYPERTENSION WITHOUT SHUNT

Congenital heart disease causing a left-to-right shunt is considered repairable when calculated pulmonary vascular resistance is less than 7–8 Woods × ms^{2}q, at baseline or after pulmonary vasodilatation with oxygen and drugs. Nevertheless, the evolution of pulmonary vascular disease postoperatively is unpredictable and probably genetically determined; some will have regression to near-normal values and others will gradually develop severe pulmonary vascular disease to the degree seen in primary pulmonary hypertension. The pathophysiology of this condition differs markedly from that in the Eisenmenger syndrome, despite an identical pulmonary vascular pathology. In the absence of a right-to-left shunt, no blood can bypass the high-resistance pulmonary vascular bed, which becomes the flow-limiting factor for the entire circulation. Cardiac output is fixed and inadequate, particularly on exertion. Under conditions that further raise pulmonary vascular resistance, as mentioned in the section on the Eisenmenger syndrome, cardiac output becomes extremely low and is often the cause of loss of consciousness.

The rate of clinical deterioration in this kind of pulmonary hypertension is faster than seen in the Eisenmenger syndrome but not as malignant as in primary pulmonary hypertension (PPH). Treatment for advanced disease should be the same as for PPH: warfarin, calcium channel blockers (if responsive), and prostacycline analogs intravenously or by inhalation *(34,38)*. Those who experience recurrent syncope and dizziness should be considered for atrial septostomy *(39)*. A hole around 4 mm in diameter usually delivers around 500 mL/min of blood directly into the systemic circulation, bypassing the lungs, at the price of mild systemic arterial desaturation and an increased risk of paradoxical embolism. One should not oversize the interatrial communication, as patients unaccustomed to low oxygen saturation (an abrupt reduction by more than 10%) become extremely symptomatic and may not survive the procedure.

THE FONTAN CIRCULATION

The original operation described by Fontan et al. *(40)* and its many surgical modifications are used for separating the pulmonary and systemic circulations in hearts that have only one functional ventricle. The pulmonary circulation becomes "pumpless." After a successful Fontan operation, patients usually perform well in everyday life and have a subnormal but reasonable exercise capacity *(41)* and uneventful pregnancies and deliveries are not rare *(42)*.

Proper function of the Fontan circuit requires the uncompromised fulfillment of the following physiologic conditions:

1. The systemic ventricle should have normal systolic and diastolic function. Increased filling pressure results in decreased transpulmonary gradient and reduced flow.
2. Pulmonary vascular resistance should be within the normal range. The pumpless pulmonary circulation does not have the ability of increasing pulmonary pressure to overcome a high-resistance circulation.
3. The negative intrathoracic pressure of inspiration is an important contributor of forward flow in the passive pulmonary circuit, by exertion of a sucking mechanism. An increase of intrathoracic pressure by positive pressure ventilation or large effusions results in decreased flow.
4. The hydrostatic pressure in the systemic veins drives blood through the lungs. Conditions that lower systemic venous pressure (e.g., dehydration) reduce pulmonary flow.
5. There should be minimal energy loss in the Fontan circuit. Flow dynamics can be compromised by the construction of a circuit with sharp angles, large saclike spaces, and unnecessary valves. The formation of clot and tachyarrhythmia are important causes of reduced flow.

Low cardiac output and shock can be encountered in the post-Fontan patient, either in the immediate postoperative period or many years after an initially successful operation. Often, there are several mechanisms acting in concert, causing clinical deterioration. Some clinical settings are discussed with emphasis on the pathophysiology and possible solutions.

In the early postoperative period, there is a marked reduction in the preload of the enlarged hypertrophied ventricle that used to supply both systemic and pulmonary circulations. It diminishes in size and its wall thickness increases. This is a cause of discoordinate wall motion, relaxation abnormalities, and increased filling pressure. The coexistence of subaortic stenosis (e.g., a narrowed bulbo-ventricular foramen in "single ventricle") may further aggravate the hemodynamic conditions *(43)*. The low transpulmonary gradient that ensues is a cause of a protracted recovery period with low cardiac output. The shifts in volume and abrupt rise in systemic venous pressure often results in accumulation of effusions, mainly pleural, sometimes chylos, which increase intrathoracic pressure and further compromise the transpulmonary gradient, creating a vicious cycle. Often, positive-pressure ventilation is a contributing factor. It has been shown that negative-pressure ventilation using a cuirass significantly augments stroke volume and output in these patients *(44)*. Nitric oxide to reduce pulmonary resistance in the immediate postoperative period has been found useful in children *(45)*. Creation of a small fenestration at the atrial level for decompression has significantly reduced the convalescence period from the Fontan operation, and a protracted period of profuse effusions and low output state is rarely seen nowadays *(46)*. There is still a debate whether these fenestrations should be closed after several months, when adaptive homeostatic mechanisms of fluid balance have been established. Those with a permanent fenestration have mild chronic arterial desaturation and an increased risk of paradoxical embolism but may be less vulnerable to future events that may compromise the Fontan circuit. Another approach is to stage the operation by first performing a bidirectional cavopulmonary anastomosis (Glenn). This results in a gradual rather than abrupt reduction of ventricular preload *(46)*.

What are the concerns in adults many years after palliation with a Fontan circuit? One important concern is the systemic ventricle. In children studied serially, diastolic function does not normalize over the years. Not only do relaxation abnormalities persist, but also a decrease in ventricular compliance is noted *(47)*. Left ventricular filling pressure rises with age. To date, most patients with Fontan circuits are less than 40 yr of age, but this may become a major problem in the future in long-term survivors. Arterial hypertension, valvar disease, diabetes mellitus, and coronary artery disease are common diseases in middle-aged people that could further contribute to diastolic dysfunction. It is likely that even a small myocardial infarction could have a devastating effect resulting from the abrupt rise in diastolic ventricular pressure. There are no data regarding the prophylactic use of vasodilators in young, well patients in order to prevent deterioration of ventricular function. However, it seems reasonable to recommend that preventive cardiology should be meticulously applied to these patients and that the threshold for pharmacological and surgical intervention should be lower than in the normal population.

To be eligible for a Fontan operation, patients must have normal or near-normal pulmonary vascular resistance. The main mechanism that could in later years cause an increase of pulmonary pressure and resistance is thromboembolic disease *(48)*. The long venous circuit without a pumping chamber is prone to thrombus formation, especially in the sometimes huge right atrium. Rhythm disorders further increase the risk. Platelet antiaggregants are often prescribed, and some people advocate the routine use of anticoagulants, especially in adults. Thrombogenic substances like estrogens are relatively contraindicated. Patients who had a large left-to-right shunt preoperatively may be at risk of a significant rise in pulmonary pressure at high altitudes or intensive physical activity, even when normal at rest.

The importance of a negative intrathoracic pressure for the Fontan circuit should always be kept in mind. In consultation for noncardiac surgery, anesthesists should be aware of the possible damage of positive-pressure ventilation. Negative-pressure ventilation, as mentioned earlier, is a valid and proven method in children in the postoperative period. We tried to use a cuirass negative-pressure ventilator (modern iron lung) in a patient in shock who was in need of mechanical ventilation, but it was not effective.

The development of a pleural effusion from any etiology reduces pulmonary blood flow resulting in fluid retention. This, in turn, causes a further rise in systemic venous pressure and increases the amount of effusion, resulting in a vicious cycle. We had a patient who went into intractable shock from an accumulation of massive effusions despite repeated drainage. The driving force of the Fontan circuit is the hydrostatic pressure in the systemic veins. Hypovolemia as a result of dehydration, bleeding, vomiting, and diarrhea results in an immediate reduction of pulmonary and systemic blood flow. Diuretics should be used as little as possible in these patients, even at the cost of some discomfort from elevated venous pressure, such as edema. The abrupt change in blood volume postpartum is a risk to Fontan patients, and patients should be given a generous regime of intravenous fluids.

Protein-losing enteropathy (PLE) is a serious complication of the Fontan circuit, thought to be indicative of a suboptimal hemodynamic result. Patients with PLE carry a grave prognosis. The hypoalbuminemia contributes to edema and intravascular hypovolemia, thus further aggravating the fluid dynamics in a vicious cycle. It has been suggested that some patients respond to subcutaneous heparin *(49)* or prednisone *(50)*, but information on adults is scarce. Some patients with suboptimal Fontans, especially a right-atrium-to-pulmonary-artery anastomosis, benefit from conversion to a total cavopulmonary anastomosis *(51)*. It has been our experience that decisions have to be made at an early stage of deterioration. Any intervention, be it "conversion," "take down" of the Fontan circuit, or even heart transplantation, has been unsuccessful when performed at an advanced stage of the disease.

THE POSTOPERATIVE PERIOD

This section will highlight postoperative complications typical to adult congenital heart disease.

Bleeding

Cyanotic patients with compensatory erythrocytosis have an increased incidence of postoperative bleeding. This is because of a larger cross-sectional area of the capillary bed and abnormal coagulation functions, making intraoperative hemostasis more difficult. Phlebotomy preoperatively to a hematocrit level of around 65% improves hemostasis *(52)*.

Excessive postoperative bleeding can result in hemodynamic decompensation directly from hypovolemia but, more importantly, by accumulation of blood clots behind the heart, causing cardiac decompensation by tamponade.

Tamponade

This may result from clot formation as mentioned earlier but also from rapid accumulation of fluid, especially after the performance of a peripheral or central shunt using synthetic material, because of serous leakage *(53)*.

Restrictive Physiology

The development of restrictive physiology in the hypertensive subpulmonary ventricle many years after surgical relief of pulmonary stenosis has been described in detail earlier. Once severe restriction has developed, this condition carries a grave prognosis, and in our experience, further cardiac surgery in these patients carries a prohibitive risk.

One of the common management mistakes in the immediate postoperative period is excessive use of inotropic drugs for low cardiac output. Inotropes should be used sparingly, if it all, in patients with predominantly diastolic dysfunction, as they further aggravate myocardial diastolic dysfunction and result in further reduction of cardiac output. Instead, colloid and fluid should be generously infused, even at the cost of aggravation of systemic venous congestion and edema. In one of our patients, we performed a fenestration of the atrial septum for decompression at the time of aortic valve replacement, but this did not prevent rapid deterioration and death. A Glenn cavo-pulmonary anastomosis could be a better means of reducing preload of the subpulmonary ventricle, but requires normal pulmonary vascular resistance.

When a cyanotic congenital malformation is first operated on in adulthood, it is not uncommon to have a restrictive physiology of both ventricles. That of the subpulmonary ventricle has been discussed in length. However, occasionally, the systemic ventricle (usually the left) has a severe restrictive reaction postoperatively with pulmonary congestion and hypotension. The following mechanisms may be involved:

1. Preoperative volume overload from a long-standing left-to-right shunt in patients with relatively milder obstruction to pulmonary flow (pink Fallot)
2. Changes in ventricular morphology and interventricular relations resulting from abrupt reduction of a lifelong subpulmonary pressure load
3. Increased preload resulting from a sudden postoperative increase in pulmonary flow in patients who had severe obstruction to pulmonary blood flow preoperatively

The most effective means of controlling this complication is by delaying extubation for at least 24 h and using positive-pressure ventilation. This is the exact opposite approach to that applied for restriction of the subpulmonary ventricle. Balancing between the two problems and avoidance of low cardiac output by positive-pressure ventilation needs a careful and tailored approach to the individual patient.

THE PROBLEM OF ASD AND LEFT VENTRICULAR FILLING

The shunt through an atrial septal defect increases with age. This is a well-known phenomenon attributed to the gradual decrease of left ventricular compliance. In normal hearts, an increased left ventricular filling pressure because of various mechanisms compensates for the reduced compliance so that stroke volume remains normal and can further increase with demand. In elderly patients with large ASDs undergoing catheterization, we often measure borderline low and even below-normal cardiac output despite good left ventricular function. Left ventricular diastolic pressure remains low, as the normal compensatory increase of left atrial pressure cannot exist as long as the nonrestrictive ASD diverts the blood to the right heart. This chronic low cardiac output is often well tolerated by the elderly with a sedate lifestyle. However, the inability to adequately increase cardiac output during conditions like sepsis and blood loss results in rapid clinical deterioration and the development of organ hypoperfusion and shock. Myocardial systolic function is usually preserved and inotropes are not helpful. In the present era, when a large majority of secundum ASDs can be closed percutaneously, this can be performed during such a crisis provided infection has been addressed. We performed ASD closure with an Amplatzer device in an 82-yr-old woman in shock. Blood pressure went up 40 mm Hg immediately upon ASD closure, and on the same day, she needed *hypotensive* drugs to control her blood pressure.

Conditions like acute myocardial infarction that cause a sudden deterioration of left ventricular function result in a similar problem. The normal compensatory increase of left ventricular filling pressure does not occur, resulting in low systemic flow and an abrupt increase of left-to-right shunt. In the small number of patients with ASD and acute myocardial infarction we have encountered to date, the clinical outcome was considerably worse than that expected from the size of infarction *per se*. ASD closure in this setting has not yet been reported and its usefulness is questionable. There is a potential risk that the elimination of a long-standing left-to-right shunt, forcing all pulmonary venous return into the diseased left ventricle may cause an abrupt rise of diastolic pressure and pulmonary edema.

CONCLUSION

In general cardiology, cardiogenic shock is almost synonymous with severe deterioration of the pumping action of the left ventricle, often in the context of myocardial infarction.

Congenital heart disease is different. The anatomic and hemodynamic complexity of the numerous malformations results in an almost endless combination of variables that can lead to inadequate organ perfusion. Those culminating in left ventricular dysfunction were left out of this chapter, which concentrated on mechanisms with which the general cardiologist is less familiar. In adults with congenital heart disease, clinical signs and symptoms suggesting deterioration can be subtle until very advanced stages. At that time, little if anything can be done. This chapter draws to basic principles that apply to relatively large groups of patients, emphasizing the complications that should be anticipated in each group and the triggering events for deterioration so that these can be avoided whenever possible.

REFERENCES

1. Perloff Jk. Congenital heart disease in adults, a new cardiovascular specialty. Circulation 1991;84:1881–1890.
2. Lieberson AD, Schumacher RR, Childress RH, Genovese PD. Corrected transposition of the great vessels in a 73-year-old man. Circulation 1969;39:96–100.
3. Attie F, Rijlaarsdam M, Zabal C, Buendia A, Vargas-Barron J. Corrected transposition of the great arteries in patients over 65. Arch Inst Cardiol Mex 1995;65:57–64.
4. Melero-Pita A, Alonso-Pardo F, Bardaji-Mayor JL, Higueras J. Corrected transposition of the great arteries. N Engl J Med 1996;334:866–877.
5. Graham TP, Bernard YD, Mellen BG, et al. Long-term outcome in congenitally corrected transposition of the great arteries: a multi-institutional study. J Am Coll Cardiol 2000;36:255–261.
6. Presbitero P, Somerville J, Rabajoli F, Stone S, Conte MR. Corrected transposition of the great arteries without associated defects in adult patients: clinical profile and follow up. Br Heart J 1995;74:57–59.
7. Oechslin E, Jenni R. 40 Years after the first atrial switch procedure in patients with transposition of the great arteries: long-term results in Toronto and Zurich. J Thorac Cardiovasc Surg 2000;48:233–237.
8. Parrish MD, Graham TP, Bender HW, Jones JP, Patton J, Partain CL. Radionuclide angiographic evaluation of right and left ventricular function during exercise after repair of transposition of the great arteries. Comparison with normal subjects and patients with congenitally corrected transposition. Circulation 1983;67:178–183.
9. Lubiszewska B, Gosiewska E, Hoffman P, et al. Myocardial perfusion and function of the systemic right ventricle in patients after atrial switch procedure for complete transposition: long-term follow-up. J Am Coll Cardiol 2000;36:1365–1370.
10. Labbe L, Douard H, Barat JL, et al. Alteration of myocardial viability and systemic ventricular dysfunction after Senning procedure. Arch Mal Coeur Vaiss 1997;90:631–637.
11. Lamour JM, Addonizio LJ, Galantowicz ME, et al. Outcome after orthotopic cardiac transplantation in adults with congenital heart disease. Circulation 1999;100(Suppl II):II-200–II-205.
12. Speziali G, Driscoll DJ, Danielson GK, et al. Cardiac transplantation for end-stage congenital heart defects: the Mayo Clinic experience. Mayo Cardiothoracic Transplant Team. Mayo Clin Proc 1998;73:923–928.

13. Mee RB. Severe right ventricular failure after Mustard or Senning operation. Two-stage repair: pulmonary artery banding and switch. J Thorac Cardiovasc Surg 1986;92:385–390.

14. Imamura M, Drummond-Webb JJ, Murphy DJ, et al. Results of the double switch operation in the current era. Ann Thorac Surg 2000;70:100–105.

15. Cochrane AD, Karl TR, Mee RB. Staged conversion to arterial switch for late failure of the systemic right ventricle. Ann Thorac Surg 1993;56:854–861; discussion 861–862.

16. Carrel T, Pfammatter JP. Complete transposition of the great arteries: surgical concepts for patients with systemic right ventricular failure following intra-atrial repair. Thorac Cardiovasc Surg 2000;48:224–227.

17. Moodie DS, Ritter DG, Tajik AJ, O'Fallon WM. Long-term follow-up in the unoperated univentricular heart. Am J Cardiol 1984;53:1124–1128.

18. Sano T, Ogawa M, Yabuuchi H, et al. Quantitative cineangiographic analysis of ventricular volume and mass in patients with single ventricle: relation to ventricular morphologies. Circulation 1988;77:62–69.

19. Acar P, Sidi D, Bonnet D, Aggoun Y, Bonhoeffer P, Kachaner J. Maintaining tricuspid valve competence in double discordance: a challenge for the paediatric cardiologist. Heart 1998;80:479–483.

20. Prieto LR, Hordof AJ, Secic M, Rosenbaum MS, Gersony WM. Progressive tricuspid valve disease in patients with congenitally corrected transposition of the great arteries. Circulation 1998;98:997–1005.

21. Numata S, Uemura H, Yagihara T, Kawahira Y, Yoshikawa Y, Kitamura S. Replacement of the morphologically tricuspid valve in children with discordant atrioventricular connections. J Heart Valve Dis 1999;8:649–654.

22. Van Son JA, Reddy VM, Silverman NH, Hanley FL. Regression of tricuspid regurgitation after two-stage arterial switch operation for failing systemic ventricle after atrial inversion operation. J Thorac Cardiovasc Surg 1996;111:342–347.

23. Connelly MS, Liu PP, Williams WG, Webb GD, Robertson P, McLaughlin PR. Congenitally corrected transposition of the great arteries in the adult: functional status and complications. J Am Coll Cardiol 1996;275:1238–1243.

24. Yeh T, Connelly MS, Coles JG, et al. Atrioventricular discordance: results of repair in 127 patients. J Thorac Cardiovasc Surg 1999;117:1190–1203.

25. Puley G, Siu S, Connelly M, et al. Arrhythmia and survival in patients > 18 years of age after the Mustard procedure for complete transposition of the great arteries. Am J Cardiol 1999;83:1080–1084.

26. Helbing WA, Hansen B, Ottenkamp J, et al. Long-term results of atrial correction for transposition of the great arteries. Comparison of Mustard and Senning operations. J Thorac Cardiovasc Surg 1994;108:363–372.

27. Lip GY, Singh SP, de Giovanni J. Percutaneous balloon valvuloplasty for congenital pulmonary valve stenosis in adults. Clin Cardiol 1999;22:733–737.

28. Jarrar M, Betbout F, Farhat MB, et al. Long-term invasive and noninvasive results of percutaneous balloon pulmonary valvuloplasty in children, adolescents, and adults. Am Heart J 1999;138:950–954.

29. Wann LS, Weyman AE, Dillon JC, Feigenbaum H. Premature pulmonary valve opening. Circulation 1977;55:128–133.

30. Cullen S, Shore D, Redington A. Characterization of right ventricular diastolic performance after complete repair of tetralogy of Fallot. Restrictive physiology predicts slow postoperative recovery. Circulation 1995;91:1782–1789.

31. Vogel M, Berger F, Kramer A, Alexi-Meshkishvili V, Lange PE. Incidence of secondary pulmonary hypertension in adults with atrial septal or sinus venosus defects. Heart 1999;82:30–33.

32. Steele PM, Fuster V, Cohen M, Ritter DG, McGoon DC. Isolated atrial septal defect with pulmonary vascular obstructive disease—long-term follow-up and prediction of outcome after surgical correction. Circulation 1987;76:1037–1042.

33. McLaughlin VV, Genthner DE, Panella MM, Hess DM, Rich S. Compassionate use of continuous prostacyclin in the management of secondary pulmonary hypertension: a case series. Ann Intern Med 1999;130:740–743.

34. Rosenzweig EB, Kerstein D, Barst RJ. Long-term prostacyclin for pulmonary hypertension with associated congenital heart defects. Circulation 1999;99:1858–1865.

35. Goodwin TM, Gherman RB, Hameed A, Elkayam U. Favorable response of Eisenmenger syndrome to inhaled nitric oxide during pregnancy. Am J Obstet Gynecol 1999;180:64–67.

36. Daliento L, Somerville J, Presbitero P, et al. Eisenmenger syndrome. Factors relating to deterioration and death. Eur Heart J 1998;19:1845–1855.

37. Presbitero P, Somerville J, Stone S, Aruta E, Spiegelhalter D, Rabajoli F. Pregnancy in cyanotic congenital heart disease. Outcome of mother and fetus. Circulation 1994;89:2673–2676.

38. Hoeper MM, Schwarze M, Ehlerding S, et al. Long-term treatment of primary pulmonary hypertension with aerosolized iloprost, a prostacyclin analogue. N Engl J Med 2000;342:1866–1870.

39. Kerstein D, Levy PS, Hsu DT, Hordof AJ, Gersony WM, Barst RJ. Blade balloon atrial septostomy in patients with severe primary pulmonary hypertension. Circulation 1995;91:2028–2035.

40. Fontan F, Mounicot FB, Baudet E, Simonneau J, Gordo J, Gouffrant JM. "Correction" of tricuspid atresia. 2 cases "corrected" using a new surgical technic. Ann Chir Thorac Cardiovasc 1971;10:39–47.

41. Rosenthal M, Bush A, Deanfield J, Redington A. Comparison of cardiopulmonary adaptation during exercise in children after the atriopulmonary and total cavopulmonary connection Fontan procedures. Circulation 1995;91:372–378.

42. Canobbio MM, Mair DD, van der Velde M, Koos BJ. Pregnancy outcomes after the Fontan repair. J Am Coll Cardiol 1996;28:763–767.

43. Freedom RM. Subaortic obstruction and the Fontan operation. Ann Thorac Surg 1998;66:649–652.

44. Shekerdemian LS, Bush A, Shore DF, Lincoln C, Redington AN. Cardiopulmonary interactions after Fontan operations: augmentation of cardiac output using negative pressure ventilation. Circulation 1997;96:3934–3942.

45. Gamillscheg A, Zobel G, Urlesberger B, et al. Inhaled nitric oxide in patients with critical pulmonary perfusion after Fontan-type procedures and bidirectional Glenn anastomosis. J Thorac Cardiovasc Surg 1997;113:435–442.

46. Mott AR, Spray TL, Gaynor JW, et al. Improved early results with cavopulmonary connections. Cardiol Young 2001;11:3–11.

47. Cheung YF, Penny DJ, Redington AN. Serial assessment of left ventricular diastolic function after Fontan procedure. Heart 2000;83:420–424.

48. Jahangiri M, Ross DB, Redington AN, Lincoln C, Shinebourne EA. Thromboembolism after the Fontan procedure and its modifications. Ann Thorac Surg 1994;58:1409–1413.

49. Kelly AM, Feldt RH, Driscoll DJ, Danielson GK. Use of heparin in the treatment of protein-losing enteropathy after Fontan operation for complex congenital heart disease. Mayo Clin Proc 1998;73:777–779.

50. Therrien J, Webb GD, Gatzoulis MA. Reversal of protein losing enteropathy with prednisone in adults with modified Fontan operations: long term palliation or bridge to cardiac transplantation? Heart 1999;82:241–243.

51. Conte S, Gewillig M, Eyskens B, Dumoulin M, Daenen W. Management of late complications after classic Fontan procedure by conversion to total cavopulmonary connection. Cardiovasc Surg 1999;7:651–655.

52. Perloff JK, Rosove HR, Sietsema KE, Territo MC. Cyanotic congenital heart disease: a multisystem disorder. In: Perloff JK, ed. Congenital Heart Disease in Adults. 2nd ed. Saunders, Philadelphia WB, 1998, pp. 203–210.

53. LeBlanc J, Albus R, Williams WG, et al. Serous fluid leakage: a complication following the modified Blalock–Taussig shunt. J Thorac Cardiovasc Surg 1984;88:259–262.

VII TRANSPORT, ASSIST DEVICES, AND FUTURE PERSPECTIVES

18   Transport of the Patient with Cardiogenic Shock

Eric R. Bates, MD, Michael J. Lim, MD, and Mark J. Lowell, MD

CONTENTS

INTRODUCTION

Hospital facilities vary widely, with some providing 24-h full tertiary cardiac services, others having cardiac catheterization laboratories but lacking interventional cardiology or cardiac surgery services, and still others having no tertiary cardiac services. Although all hospitals can offer aspirin, β-blockers, angiotensin-converting enzyme inhibitors, and fibrinolytic therapy to patients with acute myocardial infarction (MI), fewer hospitals have intra-aortic balloon pump (IABP) counterpulsation capability, and only tertiary-care hospitals offer coronary angioplasty and coronary artery bypass graft surgery. This raises the question of whether all high-risk acute MI patients should be initially transported to hospitals with full tertiary cardiac services *(1)*.

The highest-risk patients with MI are those with cardiogenic shock. It is not clear that standard medical therapy, fibrinolytic therapy, or IABP reduces mortality in these patients *(2)*. Recently, the SHOCK (SHould we emergently revascularize Occluded Coronaries for cardiogenic shocK?) Trial *(3,4)* conclusively demonstrated that early coronary revascularization reduces mortality in patients with cardiogenic shock. Therefore, selected patients (i.e., those without progressive hemodynamic collapse or life-threatening comorbid diseases or complications) will need to be transferred from hospitals without coronary revascularization programs to tertiary-care hospitals with this capability. This chapter will review the limited data available regarding transport of the patient with MI and, specifically, cardiogenic shock.

From: *Contemporary Cardiology: Cardiogenic Shock: Diagnosis and Treatment*
Edited by: David Hasdai et al. © Humana Press Inc., Totowa, NJ

RISK STRATIFICATION

Determining which patients are high-risk for death from MI can quickly be ascertained by simple clinical criteria. Lee and colleagues *(5)* found that 90% of the deaths in patients treated with fibrinolytic therapy were related to older age, systolic blood pressure <100 mm Hg, heart rate > 100 bpm, higher Killip class, and anterior infarct location. In a meta-analysis of randomized trials comparing fibrinolytic therapy with angioplasty, the superiority of angioplasty was seen in the high-risk patients who were defined as having age >70 yr, anterior infarction, previous myocardial infarction, or diabetes mellitus *(6)*.

Patients with large MIs may go though a period of preshock with nonhypotensive peripheral hypoperfusion before they develop cardiogenic shock *(7)*. The clinical manifestations are oliguria (urine output < 30 cc/h) or cold extremities despite a systolic blood pressure >90 mm Hg. In the SHOCK Trial Registry *(7)*, these patients had an in-hospital mortality rate of 43% compared with a rate of 66% in patients with classic cardiogenic shock. Early recognition and treatment may prevent the onset of hypotension and tissue hypoperfusion.

In the prethrombolytic era, the development of cardiogenic shock was predicted by age >65 yr, left ventricular ejection fraction <35%, larger infarction as measured by cardiac enzyme levels, history of diabetes mellitus, and prior myocardial infarction *(8)*. Additionally, age, female sex, prior angina, prior stroke, and peripheral vascular disease were adverse markers *(9)*. In the thrombolytic population, Hasdai et al. *(10)* developed an algorithm to predict the occurrence of shock. Age, elevated heart rate, reduced blood pressure, and congestive heart failure provided 85% of the information needed to predict cardiogenic shock.

AMBULANCE TRANSPORT

Ambulance Staffing

Before examining the interhospital transfer of cardiac patients, it is important to consider the organization of Emergency Medical Services (EMS). There exists great variability in both the type and staffing of ambulances as well as the services they are able to provide. In the United States, there are over 12,000 ambulance services with more than 35,000 ground ambulances *(11)*. The U.S. Department of Transportation has established four different levels of EMS ambulance personnel: (1) the first responder; (2) the basic emergency medical technician (EMT); (3) the intermediate EMT; and (4) the paramedic EMT *(6)*. First responders have 40 h of training, but do not transport patients. They provide first aid and may be trained to use automated external defibrillators. They are often firefighters, policemen, security guards, or volunteers. The basic EMT has 120–150 h of training, including CPR, oxygen therapy, and additional first aid skills. In the United States, most ambulance personnel are basic EMTs. The intermediate EMT receives 450–600 h of training and is trained in intravenous therapy, limited drug therapy, defibrillation, and endotracheal intubation. These individuals often provide services in rural areas. The paramedic EMT trains for 900–1500 h, approximately 200 of which are spent in a clinical setting. They are trained to recognize and treat most medical emergencies, interpret electrocardiographic rhythms, defibrillate, administer cardiac drugs (especially those used in cardiac arrest), infuse intravenous fluids, and perform endotracheal intubation. Of note, they receive little training in the use of invasive monitoring devices, mechanical ventilation, and the titration of drugs in patients with changing hemodynamic parameters.

Prehospital Versus Interhospital Care

Federal patient transfer laws (commonly referred to as "COBRA laws" after the Consolidated Omnibus Budget Reconciliation Act that established them), dictate that during the interhospital transfer of a patient, the responsibility for that patient's care rests with the sending physician until the patient is turned over to another physician or arrives at the receiving hospital. Therefore, the decision on how to send a patient has important medical and legal implications.

Emergency medical technician training at all levels is geared mostly toward the provision of prehospital care, not interhospital transfers. As a result, a locally based ambulance service may not be appropriate to transport an unstable or potentially unstable cardiac patient. In an effort to overcome this, a staff member from the referring facility (usually a nurse or, less commonly, a physician) may be recruited to accompany the patient to avoid a diminution in the level of care. This can be problematic in that these personnel are usually unfamiliar with the intricacies of transport medicine. They are not used to caring for patients in an unstable environment where noise, vibration, and tight working conditions limit the ability to identify and manage changes in a patient's condition. They may be unfamiliar with the operation of the equipment on the ambulance. Moreover, their absence will impair the performance of their assigned hospital duties.

In response to the growing need for interhospital transfers, the past several years have seen the development and marketing of "Mobile Intensive Care Units" by many ambulance providers. Importantly, the training, experience level, and licensure of the caregivers on these units have not yet been standardized in most states. Staffing can range from basic EMTs to nurses and, in some locales, to physicians. Thus, it is important that the sending physician be aware of the capabilities of the transportation service prior to agreeing to the transport of the patient.

Fortunately, most tertiary facilities have some type of specialty transport team available for this situation. These teams are usually based at the receiving facility, so the patient must wait for the team to arrive. Although time is lost in waiting, there are advantages to this type of transport. The teams usually have personnel dedicated to the transport of critically ill patients. They have the necessary training and expertise to stabilize the patient before and during the transport, and they are prepared to recognize and attend to any problems that arise en route. The sending physician must decide if the benefit of waiting for the expertise of a specialized transport team outweighs the risk of sending the patient with potentially underqualified personnel.

AMBULANCE TRANSPORT MODES

Ground Ambulance

Motorized vehicles were first used to transport patients in the early 1900s. Since that time, EMS ground vehicles have evolved from hearselike vehicles (many ambulance companies originated as a division of funeral homes) to the current modular-type vehicle in common use today. The federal government has developed minimal equipment lists for ambulances, based on the level of care provided by the EMTs on board. State and local authorities have the ability to develop specific protocols and equipment lists. The amount of equipment needed for caring for critically ill patients is variable. Many ambulances now carry noninvasive sphygmomanometers and pulse oximeters. Inverter systems, used for the generation of 110 v electrical power, are not standard equipment, and, if present, may not be powerful enough for multiple devices or even a single high-demand device such as an IABP. Although much progress has been made in the later-generation ambulances, patients and caregivers in the rear compartment are still subjected to vibrations and changes in velocity that can dislodge devices and equipment, cause erroneous readings, damage instrumentation, or result in motion sickness of the patient and/or crew.

Helicopter Ambulance

The first helicopter flight took place on September 14, 1939, and the first medical emergency flight was January 15, 1945 when a test pilot flew a physician to a snow-bound farm house in upstate New York to treat an injured patient *(12)*. Medical helicopter services have evolved to the point where they have become a routine, integral part of tertiary-care hospital emergency services. They offer the capability of transporting critical-care specialists and equipment to remote areas or small peripheral hospitals, as well as transporting seriously ill or injured patients to tertiary-care hospitals. Helicopters offer the advantage of speed and maneuverability. They are usually staffed with advanced practice paramedics, nurses, or physicians. Disadvantages include cramped working quarters, vibration, and noise. In most areas of the country, helicopters fly at altitudes that will not adversely affect the patient (see below).

Fixed-Wing Ambulance

Fixed-wing aircraft (airplanes) provide longer range, greater speed, and greater cabin capacity than rotor-wing aircraft. However, patient accessibility is frequently difficult, as the long, narrow fuselage usually necessitates the placement of the patient adjacent to the wall, limiting access to one side of the patient. Loading and unloading is often difficult, as most aircraft doors are narrow and their height off the ground may require a large amount of lifting and maneuvering to get the patient on board.

Several different types of aircraft are used as air ambulances. Single-engine, piston-driven airplanes are usually nonpressurized, noisy, and leave little room for patient care. Turboprop aircraft are used for medium-distance transports, are usually pressurized, and have adequate space. Small jets are faster, have less cabin noise, and are pressurized.

Special consideration must be given to physiologic changes that occur at altitude. According to Boyle's law, the volume of a gas is inversely proportional to pressure. So, as altitude increases, atmospheric pressure decreases, and the volume of enclosed gas expands. Thus, changes in the size of any gas-containing cavity, such as a hollow viscus or endotracheal tube, must be considered during transport. For example, at 8,000 ft (the usual altitude to which commercial jets are pressurized), the volume of a gas expands by 25%. At 10,000 ft, it expands by 50%, and at 18,000 ft it expands by 100%. A corollary to Boyle's law is Dalton's law, which states that the total pressure is equal to the sum of the partial pressures of each gas in the mixture. This becomes important when considering tissue oxygenation and the oxygen–hemoglobin saturation curve. Normal individuals will have a compensatory increase in respiratory rate and heart rate in response to the decreased oxygen tension at altitude. Patients with cardiopulmonary compromise may become hypoxic when brought to altitude, leading to additional ischemia. For example, a patient with a PaO_2 of 60 mm Hg may have an oxygen saturation of 90% at sea level, but because the PaO_2 declines with altitude, oxygen saturation may drop to 70% at 5,000 ft *(13)*.

In contrast to medical helicopters, few airplanes are dedicated solely to patient transport because of the relatively small demand. Many charter operators will reconfigure an aircraft from other uses (such as cargo transport) when hired as an air ambulance. Crews will be of varying experience. When choosing a fixed-wing air ambulance, the physician must ensure that the aircraft is suitable for the type of transport requested and that it is staffed by appropriate crew. One should look for accreditation by a national agency such as the Commission on Accreditation of Medical Transport Services.

Choosing the Method of Transport

Although a few studies have shown the safety of transporting patients with acute ischemic coronary syndromes, none has demonstrated a beneficial effect of air transport. According to a personal communication from the Association of Air Medical Services, cardiac patients account for approximately 25% of all air medical transports in the United States. Most of these patients have an acute ischemic coronary syndrome and are being transferred to a facility for cardiac catheterization. To date, we know of no data addressing the air transport of patients in cardiogenic shock. The choice of air transport instead of ground transport involves several considerations, including the distance between facilities, options for stopping at other facilities should problems arise during transport, total transport time, personnel availability, vehicle availability, weather, traffic, terrain, safety, cost, and the ability of the vehicle to accommodate any external devices.

Helicopter transportation has some advantages over ground transportation. First, helicopter units are dedicated to interhospital transfer, and highly trained nurses are included in the flight crew. Second, constant radio communication with a physician is available. Third, out-of-hospital transport time is shorter, although total transfer times are similar. Our twin-engine Bell 430 helicopters fly at an average speed of 172 mph and serve an air mile radius of 200 nautical miles.

Limitations include aircraft noise and vibration, and safety is a major concern *(14)*. From 1980 to 1986, there were 66 aeromedical helicopter crashes, with 21 deaths and 16 injuries. In 1986, the accident rate for medical helicopters was 17.7/100,000 patient transfers. This experience has led to improved guidelines for personnel and aircraft safety standards. A summary of the types of ambulances and their advantages and disadvantages appears in Table 1.

CLINICAL REPORTS

Fibrinolysis

Alteplase was the first recombinant drug approved for clinical use. It was first cautiously introduced into clinical practice at large medical centers. We initially demonstrated the importance of early time to treatment with this fibrinolytic agent and the safety of administering it in a community hospital *(15)*. In the beginning, patients were treated with alteplase only after interhospital transfer. Later, the drug was sent with a

Table 1
Advantages and Disadvantages of Transport Modes

Advantages	*Disadvantages*
Ground	
Usually readily available	Lengthy travel times over long distances
Only two patient transfers required	Limited by geographic, traffic, and weather conditions
Adequate working environment	Variable capacity and capability for additional specialized equipment
Easily diverted and adaptable to destination changes	Potential for limited AC power source
Low maintenance costs	Potential for motion sickness
Door-to-door service	
Ready availability of backup units in case of mechanical problems	
Helicopter	
Rapid transport time	Adequate landing zone required
Trained nurses and/or paramedics and/or physicians	Multiple patient transfers may be necessary if landing is remote from the referring facility
Smoother transport	Prone to weather restrictions
	Limited working space
	Noise and vibration may limit evaluation and monitoring
	Potential for limited AC power source
	Potential for motion sickness
	High maintenance costs
Fixed wing	
Rapid transport time	Multiple patient transfers may be necessary if landing area is remote from the referring facility
Able to fly around or over weather, especially in a pressurized aircraft	Requires airport with appropriate service available at each end
Cabin size usually adequate	High maintenance costs
	Potential for adverse patient effects from altitude changes
	Potential for limited AC power source
	Potential for motion sickness
	May require lengthy "scramble time"

nurse and a physician to the community hospital, where therapy was begun before transport to our hospital. Still later, the drug was administered in the community hospital by the emergency department physician before transport to our hospital for subsequent care. Now, community hospitals regularly administer fibrinolytic therapy, and patients are routinely emergently referred to tertiary-care hospitals for treatment of complications or for rescue angioplasty *(16)*.

Many ambulance companies are now equipped with cardiac monitors capable of performing and interpreting a 12-lead electrocardiogram, the results of which can be relayed via radio or faxed via cellular telephone to the emergency department. The performance of a prehospital electrocardiogram has been demonstrated to assist in reducing time-to-treatment. Prehospital fibrinolytic therapy by emergency personnel has been shown to be safe and effective and to decrease time-to-treatment, but it has logistical and legal limitations *(17)*.

Primary or Rescue Percutaneous Transluminal Coronary Angioplasty

Zijlstra et al. initially reported on 104 patients transferred for primary percutaneous transluminal coronary angioplasty (PTCA) *(18)*. Ten patients had cardiogenic shock, and one died during transport. One patient required intubation during transport. Two required treatment for hypotension, and three were treated for ventricular arrhythmias. The referral network in Zijlstra's study now includes 13 hospitals with a mean travel distance of 45 km. By emphasizing early diagnosis, immediate ambulance mobilization, and telephone activation of the interventional laboratory, transfer patients have similar door-to-balloon times as patients reporting directly to the hospital.

Strauman and colleagues transported 68 patients within 24 h of MI for primary PTCA *(19)*. Ground transport in 54 patients averaged 8 (5–68) km and 50 (18–100) min. Helicopter transport in 14 patients averaged 42 (24–122) km and 63 (40–115) min. Eight patients were on ventilators, 15 were resuscitated before transfer, and 17 were in cardiogenic shock. There were no deaths during transfer, although five of the patients in cardiogenic shock died before hospital discharge. Hospital and 1-yr outcomes were not different from 78 patients who reported directly to the hospital, despite a longer ischemic time of 1 h.

Oude Ophius and co-workers transferred 165 patients for rescue PTCA from a community hospital 20 miles away *(20)*. Median time delays included 61 min from symptom onset to hospital, 53 min in the emergency department, 16 min for transport, and 36 min from hospital arrival to arrival in the interventional laboratory. One patient in cardiogenic shock died as he was being placed in the ambulance, eight required ventricular defibrillation, three had complete atrioventricular block, and four were treated for severe hypotension. Reperfusion was noninvasively diagnosed in 66 (40%) patients and they were immediately returned to the referring hospital. The other 98 patients underwent coronary angiography, where 41 were found to have patent infarct arteries and 57 were treated with rescue PTCA. Only 10 patients died during hospitalization and 2 died in the subsequent year.

Vermeer and colleagues randomized 224 patients with large MIs to alteplase in the community hospital, alteplase and transfer for possible rescue PTCA, or tansfer for primary PTCA *(21)*. Transfer distances ranged from 25 to 50 km and transfer time averaged 20 min. Two patients were cardioverted for ventricular arrhythmias, two patients received atropine for bradyarrhythmias, and the nitroglycerin infusion was decreased in six patients because of hypotension during transfer. There were no deaths. Time to fibrinolytic therapy was 10 min, whereas time to angiography was 100 min in the rescue PTCA group and 85 min in the primary PTCA group. The primary PTCA patients had insignificantly lower rates of morbidity and mortality.

The PRAGUE (PRimary Angioplasty in patients transferred from General community hospitals to specialized PTCA Units with or without Emergency thrombolysis) study randomized 300 patients to streptokinase therapy in the community hospital, streptokinase therapy during transportation to a referral hospital for angioplasty, or transfer to the hospital for primary angioplasty without pretreatment with streptokinase

(22). Transport distances in 201 patients ranged from 5 to 74 km and and mean transfer time was 37 min. There were no deaths during transfer, two patients were successfully defibrillated for ventricular fibrillation, and two patients had worsening congestive heart failure. Patients treated in the four tertiary-care centers by cardiologists had better outcomes than the patients who remained in the 17 community hospitals with primary care physicians, but factors other than PTCA probably explain some of the outcomes. The PRAGUE-II study will expand the time window from 6 to 12 h and randomize 1200 patients to streptokinase in the community hospital or transfer to a tertiary-care hospital for primary PTCA. The logistical goal is <30 min from decision to departure, <30 min transport time, and <30 min to balloon inflation in the interventional laboratory after arrival in the tertiary-care hospital.

The Air-PAMI trial studied lytic-eligible, high-risk patients (age >70 yr, anterior MI, Killip class II–III, heart rate >100 bpm, or blood pressure <100 mm Hg) within 12 h of symptom onset *(23).* The study was stopped prematurely after 3 yr when only 138 of the anticipated 430 patients had been enrolled. Time-to-treatment in the PTCA group was prolonged by 100 min by transfer (120 ± 69 vs 20 ± 16 min; p <0.0001). Transport time averaged 34 ± 30 min. No patient died or required CPR during transfer. Thirty-day events in the PTCA and lytic-treated groups, including death (10.0% of vs 12.5%), recurrent MI (1.7% vs 3.6%), and disabling stroke (0%), were not statistically different. When the 71 transfer patients undergoing PTCA were subsequently compared with 500 patients undergoing immediate PTCA, a 67-min delay (187 ± 75 vs 120 ± 69; $p = 0.001$) in time from emergency department to balloon inflation was documented, and 30-d and 1-yr mortality were higher *(24).*

The DANAMI-II study is randomizing 1200 patients to front-loaded alteplase versus PTCA/stent *(25).* The PTCA/stent patients will include patients randomized at community hospitals but transported emergently to the tertiary-care hospital for PTCA. A preliminary report on the complications during transfer documented six patients with ventricular fibrillation, six patients with atrial fibrillation, and six patients with third-degree atrioventricular heart block, but no deaths during transfer. The in-door-to-outdoor time averaged 45 min, the transfer time was 40 min, and the door-to-balloon time was 30 min for a 115-min time-to-treatment result.

Cardiogenic Shock

Impressed by the improved outcomes we were seeing in patients with cardiogenic shock undergoing emergency coronary revascularization *(26),* we explored alternative treatment strategies for treating these patients in the community hospital *(27).* We retrospectively reviewed the records from 64 patients with cardiogenic shock complicating MI treated at a community teaching hospital from 1985 to 1991. Treatment strategies were determined by the attending cardiologist. Patients were divided into three groups: 13 patients received thrombolytic therapy, 29 patients received IABP support, and 22 patients were treated with combined thrombolytic therapy and IABP support (Table 2). Hospital survival was 23%, 28%, and 68%, respectively. Importantly, survival was 7% for those remaining in the community hospital compared with 69% for those transferred to the tertiary-care hospital. Moreover, survival was 17% for medical therapy versus 71% for revascularization therapy in these patients. This study suggested that a treatment strategy of early stabilization and transfer to a tertiary-care center for emergency revascularization could result in

Table 2
Survival Data

	TT (n=13)	IABP (n=29)	TT/IABP (n=22)
Survival	3 (23%)	8 (28%)	15 (68%)
Medical therapy	1/10 (10%)	1/16 (6%)	4/10 (40%)
PTCA	2/3 (66%)	4/5 (80%)	3/4 (75%)
CABG	—	3/8 (38%)	8/8 (100%)

Abbreviations: CABG = coronary artery bypass graft surgery; IABP = intra-aortic balloon pump; PTCA = percutaneous transluminal coronary angioplasty; TT = thrombolytic therapy.

better survival rates for patients presenting at community hospitals with MI complicated by cardiogenic shock.

In a study conducted over a 10-yr period (1985–1995), we reviewed the results of 46 patients treated with fibrinolytic therapy within 12 h of MI who developed cardiogenic shock *(28)*. Twenty-seven patients were treated with IABP and 19 were not. Patients treated with IABP had a significantly higher rate of community hospital survival (93% vs 37%), and more of them were transferred for revascularization (85% vs 37%). Of 30 transfer patients, 27 were revascularized; the hospital survival rate was 74%. Therefore, this study also suggested that survival is enhanced when patients can be hemodynamically stabilized and transferred for emergency revascularization.

The SHOCK Trial Registry enrolled 1,190 patients; 44% were transferred to tertiary-care centers *(29)*. They had a lower mortality rate than direct admissions to those centers (54% vs 67%). This underscores the selection bias present when clinicians choose treatment strategies based on clinical situations and patients survive long enough to undergo those treatments.

Helicopter Transport

Between May 1983 and December 1984, 104 patients with suspected MI were transferred to our hospital *(30)*. Before transfer, 22 were Killip class II, 5 were Killip class III, and 9 were Killip class IV. During transport, 82 required intravenous antiarrhythmics and 11 required pressors. There were nine episodes of serious hypotension, four new arrhythmias requiring treatment, and no deaths. After arrival, 69 patients underwent a reperfusion procedure. Ninety patients (87%) survived to discharge.

Bellinger et al. subsequently reported on 250 patients with MI transported to Duke University Medical Center from within a 150-mile radius *(14)*. The majority were receiving fibrinolytic therapy. Flight time ranged from 12 to 77 (median 31) min. Complications during transport included hypotension, third-degree atrioventricular heart block, and ventricular tachycardia. Cardioversion, defibrillation, or intubation were not necessary during the flight, although five patients received CPR and three were treated with an external pacemaker. There were no deaths during transfer and all patients underwent emergency cardiac catheterization. Similarly, Gore et al. successfully transferred 34 patients by helicopter without major complications *(31)*.

More recently, Barron et al. reported on 1,059 (0.8%) patients from the Second National Registry of Myocardial Infarction who were transported by helicopter *(32)*. Compared to those transported by ground ambulance, patients were younger, had fewer comorbid conditions, had less severe MI, and were more likely to receive reperfusion therapy. There was no difference in adjusted mortality rates.

SUPPORT DEVICE TRANSPORT

Intra-aortic Balloon Pump

Many patients in cardiogenic shock will need access to cardiac support devices during transportation. Almost always, the device will be an IABP. A perfusionist or nurse competent in all phases of IABP operation will be part of the transport team and responsible for the safety of the patient. Transport of patients with an IABP in place has been demonstrated to be safe and feasible *(33)*. The newest IABP consoles weigh less than 90 lbs, and have 2-h batteries. Before transporting a patient with an IABP, one must ensure that the team is familiar with troubleshooting the device and that adequate supplies and equipment are available to correct any situation that may arise. Suggested additional equipment and supplies for IABP patients are as follows:

1. IABP with charged battery
2. Additional ECG monitoring electrodes
3. Automatic defibrillator/pacer pads
4. ECG monitoring cables compatible with IABP
5. Pressure monitoring cables compatible with IABP
6. IAB connects compatible with IABP
7. Slave cables as necessary
8. Strip-chart paper for IABP
9. Additional helium tank
10. Syringe and adapters for manual inflation of IAB catheter
11. Appropriate dressings
12. Extra PVC extension tubing
13. Vehicle power inverter compatible with IABP (and any other electrical device)

Certain precautions are necessary before and during transport. Before leaving, the IABP catheter must be correctly and securely placed, as the amount and degree of maneuvering that takes place may dislodge or move it. If going to altitude, the IABP operator must determine if the pump will automatically compensate for Boyle's law and adjust the balloon inflation volume appropriately or whether manual purging of the system will be required. This should be done at every 2000 ft of altitude change. If the balloon becomes dormant, manual inflation should be performed at predetermined intervals to prevent a thrombus from forming on the catheter.

Extracorporeal Life Support

Since the 1980s, extracorporeal life support (ECLS) (still commonly referred to as extracorporeal membranous oxygenation, or ECMO) has been successfully used in newborns with severe, reversible respiratory or cardiac failure. More recently, this technology has been applied to adults with cardiac emergencies *(34)*. Only a few centers in the United States use ECLS on adults, and even fewer have the ability to transport a patient on ECLS. The development of an ECLS transport team requires months of planning and procurement of specialized equipment.

Extracorporeal life support should be considered for patients who, despite appropriate medical management, have hemodynamic collapse but the potential to reverse myocardial stunning if they can be supported for several days. Essentially, ECLS supports the patient by functioning as the heart and lungs while these organs rest and heal. ECLS can also be used as a bridge to left ventricular assist device implantation. Exclusion criteria include contraindication to anticoagulation, terminal disease with short expected survival, underlying moderate to severe lung disease, advanced multiorgan system failure, central nervous system injury, or severe immunosuppression. Relative contraindications include, but are not limited to, mechanical ventilation greater than 7 d, severe pulmonary hypertension, and age greater than 60 yr. Potential candidates for ECLS should be discussed with the regional provider to determine if they are appropriate candidates. The regional providers will determine whether an attempt should be made to transport the patient to the referral center first, or whether the ECLS team needs to be deployed to the referring hospital. A list of providers can be found at the Extracorporeal Life Support Organization's website (http://www.elso.med.umich.edu.).

Every attempt should be made to transport the patient to a referral center before placement on ECLS; occasionally, this is not feasible and the patient will have to begin ECLS at the referring institution. This will require the appropriate surgical equipment and supplies (including blood products) so that cannulation can take place at the bedside. The ECLS equipment weighs approximately 110 lb. It is connected to the patient by percutaneously placed cannulae in the femoral artery and vein. The battery life is only 20 min, so vehicles must be equipped with appropriate electrical inverters. Usually, the team consists of at least one ECLS technician, an ECLS physician, and one or two nurses who are familiar with ECLS.

Both ambulances and helicopters can transport patients on either IABP or ECLS. Additionally, both systems can also transport patients with left ventricular or biventricular support devices.

Biventricular Support Device

Little has been written about transporting patients using external cardiac support devices. Mestres et al. described their experience with two patients, one by ground ambulance and one by helicopter, using a paracorporeal left ventricular assist device *(35)*. The past few years have seen the development of external devices to support the failing heart. The most commonly used device is the Abiomed BVS 5000 (Abiomed, Inc, Danvers, MA), which is FDA approved for use in any cardiac condition resulting in ventricular failure. The manufacturer of the pump has recently introduced a smaller version for use in transport. The transport of a patient on the pump requires meticulous advance planning and preparation, as the patient is totally dependent on the continuous operation of the pump, and any interruption in its function can result in severe patient compromise.

The pump and its connections have many space and power requirements. Pump filling is affected by gravity, and the top of the 18-in.-long pump must be maintained level with or below the patient's left atrium. Therefore, the patient must be at least 18 in. above the floor of the vehicle. This requires a stretcher that can elevate or another means of raising the patient. The pump itself draws 280 W, so the vehicle must be equipped with an inverter capable of handling this and any other power requirements. A fully charged battery lasts only 1 h, which will probably be consumed in transporting the patient between the hospital and vehicle or vehicles. Should power fail, there is manual backup in the form of a foot pump. Regardless of the type of vehicle used in transport, preplanning is recommended to ensure that the pump can be stowed, secured,

Table 3
Early Mortality Risk

	Expected (>80%)	Very high (60–80%)	High (<60%)
Age (yr)	>80	60–80	<60
Symptom duration (h)	>12	6–12	<6
CPR	Prolonged	Short, successful	Not required
Neurologic status	Unconscious	Arousable	Conscious
Motor tone	Flaccid	Spontaneous movements	Purposeful movements
$\overline{BP}$ after pressors or IAPB (mm Hg)	<60	60–80	>80
Myocardial salvage potential by ECG	Poor	Fair	Good

Abbreviations: BP = blood pressure; CAD = coronary artery disease; CPR = cardiopulmonary resuscitation; ECG = electrocardiogram; VD = vessel disease.

and operated safely and continuously. Ideally, any team considering transport of a patient on this device should have policies and procedures in place, including a "dry run" to ensure adequate preparation for a real patient.

Ventilators

Patients in cardiogenic shock severe enough to necessitate transfer are usually intubated and require complex ventilatory parameters. In-hospital ventilators are not routinely designed for use out of the hospital and, until recently, most transport ventilators were rudimentary. Newer transport ventilators are now being introduced that are capable of more sophisticated ventilator modes. These include features such as pressure-controlled ventilation, positive end-expiratory pressure, and the ability to support inverse inspiratory : expiratory ratios. It is vitally important that transport personnel be facile with the ventilator and able to respond appropriately to changes in the patient's condition. This may necessitate including a respiratory therapist as part of the team.

CLINICAL DECISION-MAKING

The average time from chest pain onset to cardiogenic shock is 8–10 h, so cardiogenic shock is more likely to be diagnosed in the intensive care unit than in the emergency department. The results of the history and physical examination and the noninvasive evaluation with electrocardiography and echocardiography, as well as the response to initial medical interventions, should determine which patients will be candidates for transfer to a tertiary-care hospital *(36)*. Patients at high risk for death are poor candidates and should probably not be transferred (Table 3). In our experience, adverse prognostic factors include age >80 yr, symptom duration >12 h, prolonged CPR, abnormal neurological status, and mild electrocardiographic abnormalities. Good candidates are younger than 60 yr, have short symptom duration, have not required CPR and are neurologically intact, have stabilized or improved their blood pressure on vasopressors and IABP, and have a large injury current on the electrocardiogram, suggesting a large area of ischemic myocardium that can potentially be salvaged with acute reperfusion. Clinical judgment determines whether other patients should be transferred for emergency revascularization. Resources spent on preserving life are easily justifiable in this subgroup because the majority of hospital survivors have a good short-term prognosis. Conversely, expensive technology should not be employed to unnecessarily prolong life when death is inevitable.

CONCLUSION

Safety during transport depends on the quality of the ambulance or helicopter personnel and the equipment available. In published studies, patients have been selected from a much larger population presenting with ST-segment elevation or left bundle-branch block. Transfer times and distances have been relatively short; delays are likely to be longer in the real world and when extra measures are required to stabilize patients in cardiogenic shock. Nevertheless, acute transfer for primary or rescue PTCA is feasible and safe. Patients at high risk for developing cardiogenic shock should be considered for early transfer to a tertiary-care hospital with revascularization capabilities. For selected patients with cardiogenic shock, emergency transfer for coronary revascularization may be their best chance for survival.

REFERENCES

1. Serruys PW, Kay IP. Cardiogenic shock: a failure of reperfusion. Time for a strategic change? Eu Heart J 1999;20:88–89.
2. Bates ER, Topol EJ. Limitations of thrombolytic therapy for acute myocardial infarction complicated by congestive heart failure and cardiogenic shock. J Am Coll Cardiol 1991;18:1077–1084.
3. Hochman JS, Sleeper LA, Webb JG, et al. Early revascularization in acute myocardial infarction complicated by cardiogenic shock. N Engl J Med 1999;341:625–634.
4. Hochman JS, Sleeper LA, White HD, et al. One-year survival following early revascularization for cardiogenic shock. JAMA 2001;285:190–192.
5. Lee KL, Woodlief LH, Topol EJ, et al. Predictors of 30-day mortality in the era of reperfusion for acute myocardial infarction. Circulation 1995;91:1659–1668.
6. Hutter AM, Weaver WD. Task Force 2: Acute coronary syndromes: Section 2A–Prehospital issues. J Am Coll Cardiol 2000;35:846–853.
7. Menon V, Slater JN, White HD, Sleeper LA, Cocke T, Hochman JS. Acute myocardial infarction complicated by systemic hypoperfusion without hypotension: Report of the SHOCK Trial Registry. Am J Med 2000;108:374–380.
8. Hands ME, Rutherford JD, Muller JE, et al. The in-hospital development of cardiogenic shock after myocardial infarction: incidence, predictors of occurrence, outcome and prognostic factors. The MILIS Study Group. J Am Coll Cardiol 1989;14:40–46.
9. Leor J, Goldbourt U, Reicher-Reiss H, Kaplinsky E, Behar S. Cardiogenic shock complicating acute myocardial infarction in patients without heart failure on admission: incidence, risk factors, and outcome. SPRINT Study Group. Am J Med 1993;94:265–273.
10. Hasdai D, Califf RM, Thompson TD, et al. Predictors of cardiogenic shock after thrombolytic therapy for acute myocardial infarction. J Am Coll Cardiol 2000;35:136–143.
11. National Heart Attack Alert Program Coordinating Committee Access to Care Committee. Staffing and equipping emergency medical services systems: Rapid identification and treatment of acute myocardial infarction. Am J Emerg Med 1995;13:58–66.
12. Nocera A. Helicopter emergency medical services. Lancet Perspect 2000;356:S2.
13. Rodenberg H, Blumen IJ. Aeromedical transport and in-flight medical emergencies. In: Rosen P, Barkin R, eds. Emergency Medicine: Concepts and Clinical Practice. 4th ed. Mosby, St. Louis, MO, 1998, pp. 334–350.
14. Bellinger RL, Califf RM, Mark DB, et al. Helicopter transport of patients during acute myocardial infarction. Am J Cardiol 1988;61:718–722.
15. Topol EJ, Bates ER, Walton JA Jr, et al. Community hospital administration of intravenous tissue plasminogen activator in acute myocardial infarction: improved timing, thrombolytic efficacy and ventricular function. J Am Coll Cardiol 1987;10:1173–1177.

16. Goldman LE, Eisenberg MJ. Identification and management of patients with failed thrombolysis after acute myocardial infarction. Ann Intern Med 2000;132:556–565.

17. Morrison LJ, Verbeek PR, McDonald AC, Sawadsky BV, Cook DJ. Mortality and prehospital thrombolysis for acute myocardial infarction: a meta-analysis. JAMA 2000;283:2686–2692.

18. Zijlstra F, van't Hof AWJ, Liem AL, Hoorntje JCA, Suryapranata H, de Boer M-J. Transferring patients for primary angioplasty: a retrospective analysis of 104 selected high risk patients with acute myocardial infarction. Heart 1997;78:333–336.

19. Straumann E, Yoon S, Naegeli B, et al. Hospital transfer for primary coronary angioplasty in high risk patients with acute myocardial infarction. Heart 1999;82:415–419.

20. Oude Ophuis TJM, Bär FW, Vermeer F, et al. Early referral for intentional rescue PTCA after initiation of thrombolytic therapy in patients admitted to a community hospital because of a large acute myocardial infarction. Am Heart J 1999;137:846–853.

21. Vermeer F, Oude Ophuis AJM, vd Berg EJ, et al. Prospective randomised comparison between thrombolysis, rescue PTCA, and primary PTCA in patients with extensive myocardial infarction admitted to a hospital without PTCA facilities: a safety and feasibility study. Heart 1999;82:426–432.

22. Widimsky P, Groch L, Zelizko M, Aschermann M, Bednar F, Suryapranata H on behalf of the PRAGUE Study Group Investigators. Multicentre randomized trial comparing transport to primary angioplasty vs immediate thrombolysis vs combined strategy for patients with acute myocardial infarction presenting to a community hospital without a catheterization laboratory. The PRAGUE Study. Eur Heart J 2000;21:823–831.

23. Grines CL, Balestrini C, Westerhausen DR Jr, et al. A randomized trial of thrombolysis vs transfer for primary PTCA in high risk AMI patients: Results of the AIR PAMI Trial [abstract]. J Am Coll Cardiol 2000;35:376A.

24. Grines LL, Wharton TP, Balestrini C, et al. Should high-risk acute myocardial infarction patients admitted to non-surgical hospitals be transferred for primary PTCA or receive it on-site? [abstract]. Circulation 2000;102(Suppl II):II-386.

25. Anderson HR. The Danish multicenter randomized study on thrombolytic therapy versus acute coronary angioplasty in acute myocardial infarction. Presented at the XXII Congress of the European Society of Cardiology, Amsterdam, 2000.

26. Lee L, Bates E, Pitt B, Walton J, Laufer N, O'Neill W. Percutaneous transluminal coronary angioplasty improves survival in cardiogenic shock complicating acute myocardial infarction. Circulation 1988;78:1345–1351.

27. Stomel RJ, Rasak M, Bates ER. Treatment strategies for acute myocardial infarction complicated by cardiogenic shock in a community hospital. Chest 1994;105:997–1002.

28. Kovack PJ, Rasak MA, Bates ER, et al. Thrombolysis plus aortic counterpulsation: improved survival in patients who present to community hospitals with cardiogenic shock. J Am Coll Cardiol 1997;29:1454–1458.

29. Hochman JS, Buller CE, Sleeper LA, et al. Cardiogenic shock complicating acute myocardial infarction — etiologies, management and outcome: A report from the SHOCK trial registry. J Am Coll Cardiol 2000;336:1063–1070.

30. Kaplan L, Walsh D, Burney RE. Emergency aeromedical transport of patients with acute myocardial infarction. Ann Emerg Med 1987;16:55–57.

31. Gore JM, Corrao JM, Goldberg RJ, et al. Feasibility and safety of emergency interhospital transport of patients during early hours of acute myocardial infarction. Arch Intern Med 1989;149:353–355.

32. Barron HV, Malacreda R, Weaver WD. Use of helicopter transportation in acute myocardial infarction in the United States [abstract]. J Am Coll Cardiol 1998;32:269A.

33. Icenogle TB, Smith RG, Nelson R, Machamer W, Davis B. Long distance transport of cardiac patients in extremis: the mobile intensive care (MOBI) concept. Aviat Space Environ Med 1988;59:571–574.

34. Ricciardi M, Moscucci M, Zivin A, Knight BP, Bartlett RH, Bates ER. Emergency extracorporeal membrane oxygenation (ECMO) supported percutaneous coronary interventions in the fibrillating heart. Cathet Cardiovasc Diagn 1999;48:402–405.

35. Mestres CA, Sanchez-Martos A, Rodriquez-Ribo A, Davalos R, Galcera J, Fuentes M. Long distance transportation of patients with a paracorporeal left ventricular assist device. Int J Artif Organs 1998;21:425–428.

36. Bates ER, Moscucci M. Cardiogenic shock. In: Klein LW, Calvin JE, eds. Resource Utilization in Cardiac Disease. Kluwer Academic, Boston, 1999, pp. 239–250.

19 Percutaneous Mechanical Assist Devices for Severe Left Ventricular Dysfunction

Suresh R. Mulukutla, MD, John J. Pacella, MD, and Howard A. Cohen, MD

CONTENTS

INTRODUCTION

In 1968, the first clinical application of the intra-aortic balloon pump (IABP) was reported in treating patients with cardiogenic shock after acute myocardial infarction *(1)*. The IABP is only one example of a mechanical cardiac assist device. Other devices that have been developed include left ventricular assist devices (LVADs), cardiopulmonary support (CPS), the Hemopump™, percutaneous left ventricular assist devices, and the artificial heart. At present, about 100,000 IABPs are inserted every year in the United States *(2)*.

HEMODYNAMIC AND METABOLIC EFFECTS OF THE IABP

The three major aims of IABP use are to increase coronary perfusion, reduce left ventricular afterload, and increase cardiac output. There are several hemodynamic parameters that are affected by the IABP to help achieve these objectives. In a review of IABP counterpulsation, Nanas and Moulopoulos *(3)* note that counterpulsation affects several hemodynamic (Table 1) and metabolic (Table 2) parameters.

Figure 1 illustrates the several hemodynamic parameters that are affected during IABP inflation and deflation. Aortic pressure is affected directly by IABP counterpulsation. Deflation of the IABP during end diastole is an active process of drawing blood away

From: *Contemporary Cardiology: Cardiogenic Shock: Diagnosis and Treatment*
Edited by: David Hasdai et al. © Humana Press Inc., Totowa, NJ

Table 1
Hemodynamic Parameters Affected by IABP

Aortic pressure
Left ventricular end-diastolic pressure
Left ventricular work
Tension time index
Diastolic pressure time index
Ejection fraction
Cardiac output

Table 2
Metabolic Parameters Affected by IABP

Coronary blood flow
Cerebral blood flow
Renal blood flow
Myocardial oxygen supply
Myocardial oxygen consumption
Lactate production

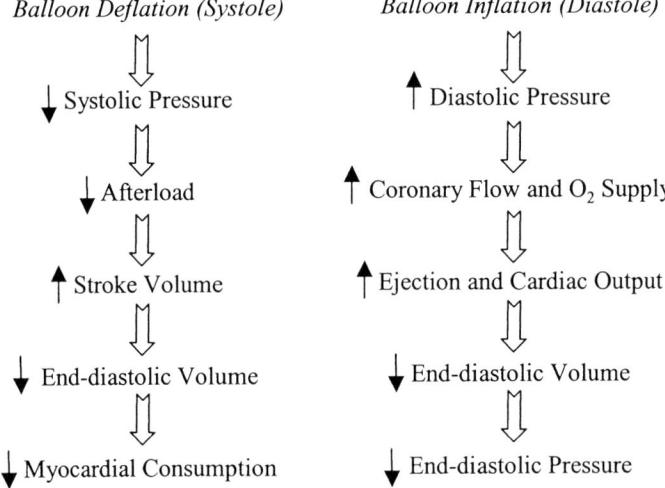

Fig. 1. Hemodynamic effects of IABP therapy.

from the central aorta and thus reduces aortic systolic pressure by 8.9–26.6% *(4)*. Left ventricular end-diastolic pressure is also reduced with IABP use by 25–40% *(5)*, and this results in an 18–50% reduction in left ventricular work *(6)*. The myocardial tension–time index is an accurate measure of total left ventricular work and is reduced by 20–40% during counterpulsation *(7)*. The diastolic pressure time index (DPTI) is the sum of diastolic aortic pressures minus left atrial pressures generated in 1 min *(3)*. It is proportional to myocardial blood flow and to the amount of oxygen available to the myocardium. With use of the IABP, there is an increase in diastolic aortic pressures (resulting from diastolic augmentation) and a decrease in left ventricular end-diastolic pressures; hence, the DPTI increases. Although there are no experimental data to suggest that IABP improves ejection fraction (EF), one would expect that with the decrease in afterload, EF might improve (provided that preload is unchanged). There are data, however, to suggest that the IABP improves cardiac output by as much as 50% (5).

With the numerous hemodynamic changes described, a number of beneficial metabolic effects have been documented. Coronary blood flow has been documented to increase anywhere from 5% to 15% in some studies (8,9). However, other investigators have found that IABP therapy does not affect coronary blood flow significantly (10). Cerebral blood flow has been shown to be increased with the use of the IABP, although renal blood flow has not been shown to increase significantly (11). Importantly, with the reduction in left ventricular end-diastolic pressures, the reduction in tension–time index, and increased DPTI, there is an increase in myocardial oxygen supply with a concomitant decrease in myocardial oxygen consumption.

INDICATIONS FOR IABP

Table 3 lists several major indications for IABP therapy. In this chapter, we will limit our discussion to only a few of these indications.

IABP in Cardiogenic Shock

In spite of the hemodynamic improvements noted already with IABP use, survival rates for patients with cardiogenic shock and treated with IABP alone have been discouraging; overall, these survival rates range from 5% to 48%, with most studies observing 20% (12–16). The wide range in survival is most likely secondary to different selection criteria, different definitions of cardiogenic shock, and different patient populations in various studies.

Because of the relatively poor survival in patients with cardiogenic shock treated with the IABP, investigators began to look at the effect of IABP therapy in patients with medically refractory heart failure but without cardiogenic shock. Hagemeijer and colleagues studied class III–IV heart-failure patients after a recent myocardial infarction and reported significant hemodynamic improvement in 80% of their patients and a 56% hospital survival rate (17). Although these results were promising, some more recent reports of similar patient populations had less favorable results with survival rates of 25–30% (18,19). One explanation for these differences may be the duration of the IABP use, with patients in the Hagemeijer study receiving IABP support for prolonged periods, some up to 24 d. Ultimately, given the relatively poor survival rates, the IABP has not developed as an independent mode of therapy for patients with cardiogenic shock; rather, it has evolved as an adjunct in the treatment of this condition.

IABP as an Adjunct to Patients Treated with Thrombolytic Therapy

Considerable data have been gathered on IABP as an adjunct to thrombolytic therapy. In one study of patients with acute MI and cardiogenic shock, those treated with IABP and thrombolysis had a significantly higher rate of hospital survival than patients treated with thrombolysis alone (20). Results of a larger, prospective study published in 2000 from the SHOCK registry also revealed the benefits of IABP therapy as an adjunct to thrombolysis/revascularization (21). In this study, patients who received

Table 3
Indications for IABP

Cardiogenic shock
   Post-acute-myocardial-infarction
   After mechanical complications of acute MI
High-risk angioplasty as prophylactic support
Unstable angina refractory to medical therapy
Bridge to cardiac surgery in patients with unstable angina
Refractory arrhythmias secondary to ischemia and/or heart failure
Acute mitral regurgitation
Perioperative low cardiac output syndrome
Bridge to cardiac transplantation
Other
   Septic shock
   High-risk patients undergoing noncardiac surgery

IABP support had a significantly lower mortality. Further, patients treated with both IABP support and thrombolytic therapy had the highest survival rates. Thus, given these results, it would appear that treatment of patients with cardiogenic shock with thrombolytic therapy and IABP support offers the best chance for survival when primary angioplasty is unavailable or not feasible.

IABP and PTCA for Acute Myocardial Infarction

Despite the theoretical benefit one would expect with IABP support in patients who are undergoing high-risk procedures, the data are somewhat conflicting. The PAMI-II trial found no significant difference in their primary combined endpoint of death, reinfarction, reocclusion of infarct-related artery (IRA), stroke, or new-onset heart failure (22). However, in another study of 1490 patients undergoing primary percutaneous transluminal angioplasty (PTCA) for acute myocardial infarction (23), IABP used before intervention was associated with fewer catheterization laboratory events in patients with cardiogenic shock (14.5% vs 35.1%, $p=0.0009$). When all "high-risk" patients were analyzed from this study, IABP use conferred a less striking, but still significant, benefit in preventing events in the catheterization laboratory (11.5% vs 21.9%, $p=0.05$). Although the data are somewhat conflicting regarding the clinical benefit in patients undergoing high-risk PTCA, IABP continues to be used frequently in this setting. The IABP support in patients undergoing percutaneous coronary intervention in the setting of acute myocardial infarction and cardiogenic shock does provide hemodynamic stability.

IABP for Postoperative Low Cardiac Output Syndrome

Among the first indications for IABP support was postcardiotomy low cardiac output syndrome. This was initially suggested by Kantrowitz's group in their seminal article from 1968 (1). Buckley et al. were among the first groups to use IABP for this clinical scenario with success (24). Although the definition of postcardiotomy low cardiac output syndrome is not standardized, for the purposes of this discussion we will use the parameters used by Rao and colleagues (25). They defined low cardiac output syndrome as a postoperative condition for which IABP or inotropic support is required to maintain a systolic blood pressure higher than 90 mm Hg or a cardiac index greater than 2.2 L/min/m^2. By this criterion, Rao diagnosed postcardiotomy low cardiac output syndrome in 9.1% of post-CABG (coronary artery bypass graft) patients. This corresponds to the prevalence found in other studies *(26–29)*.

The etiology of postcardiotomy low cardiac output syndrome is likely multifactorial, but, at its essence, this syndrome results from inadequate myocardial protection during the perioperative period. There may be multiple reasons for the lack of myocardial preservation, including recent myocardial infarction, stunned myocardium, difficulty with bypass grafting, intraoperative infarction, coronary spasm, and long periods on cardiopulmonary bypass *(30,31)*.

Factors that predispose to the development of low cardiac output syndrome include age greater than 70, left ventricular failure, NYHA functional Class III–IV, three-vessel and/or left main coronary artery disease, and redo or emergency surgery *(25,30,32)*. Several other studies have found that female gender, diabetes, and length of cardiopulmonary bypass are also risk factors for the development of low cardiac output syndrome in the postoperative period *(25,32,33)*.

The data suggest that these patients benefit greatly from IABP support. Mortality rates over 90% are reported in patients who do not receive IABP support *(34)*. However, with IABP assistance, survival rates of 40–70% are reported *(28,29,35)*. Importantly, once the need for IABP assistance is recognized, it is imperative that it be initiated quickly because mortality rises if IABP support is delayed *(36)*. Long-term survival rates are somewhat poorer. Lund et al. and Kuchar et al. reported 5-yr survival rates of 22% and 25%, respectively, in patients requiring IABP support for postcardiotomy low cardiac output syndrome *(30,37)*. Approximately 1% of cardiac surgical patients cannot be weaned from bypass in spite of inotropic and IABP support *(31)*, and in these patients ventricular assist devices (VADs) may be required.

IABP as a Bridge to Cardiac Transplantation

In the last 20 yr, cardiac transplantation has evolved into an accepted therapy for patients with end-stage heart disease. Although potentially 40,000 patients per year die of heart disease that may have been treated with cardiac transplantation *(38)*, only about 2500 donor hearts become available annually *(39)*. Of these carefully selected patients, 1-yr survival rates are 85–90% in several analyses from different institutions *(40–42)*.

The IABP has been used as a bridge to cardiac transplantation. As the number of patients eligible for transplantation has increased, however, so has the waiting period for a donor. For this reason, the IABP may be somewhat limited in its use as a bridge to transplantation; rather, devices such as VADs and the artificial heart are often preferred at certain institutions.

Nonetheless, IABPs still play a crucial role in patients awaiting cardiac transplant. Several investigators have reported success with the IABP as a bridge to cardiac transplantation *(40,41,43,44)*, and there is evidence of its efficacy in patients with ischemic cardiomyopathy as well as nonischemic cardiomyopathy *(45)*.

Survival in transplant candidates who require IABP support remains quite high. Marks and colleagues found no difference in 1-yr survival rates between patients who required mechanical support prior to cardiac transplantation and those who did not require such intervention (86% vs 88%) *(44)*. Similarly, Birovljev detected no significant difference in 1-yr or 2-yr survival rates between the two groups *(46)*. Although these studies revealed that survival rates were not worse if a patient required preoperative mechanical support, at least one study found that patients requiring mechanical support prior to transplantation had significantly poorer outcomes than patients who were not in need of mechanical assistance *(47)*. The higher mortality in this study was related to a higher rate of sepsis and a higher operative mortality in the group requiring mechanical support.

Most of the evidence suggests that IABP support is both safe and effective. Some type of mechanical circulatory assistance is required in about 9–10% of patients awaiting cardiac transplantation *(41,46,47)*, and in carefully selected patients, IABP support can provide an essential bridge as they wait for a donor organ.

CONTRAINDICATIONS TO IABP

The contraindications to IABP use include aortic insufficiency and aortic dissection. Peripheral vascular disease is a relative contraindication related to the risk of limb ischemia. In patients with documented severe focal stenosis in the iliac arteries or in the distal aorta, IABP insertion is possible without an increase in morbidity after percutaneous angioplasty of the stenosis *(48,49)*.

IABP-RELATED COMPLICATIONS

Despite the many technical advances that have helped to expand the use of intra-aortic balloon pumps, complication rates remain significant. In various studies since the introduction of the intra-aortic balloon pump, complication rates vary between 11% and 45% *(50–55)*. The more recent studies suggest that the complication rate is about 15% *(50,51)*. Major complications occur with an incidence of 4–14% and minor complications occur in 17–41% of cases *(50,51,53,56)*. Table 4 lists the some of the most common complications associated with IABP therapy.

Vascular Complications

Vascular complications account for the majority of IABP-related complications and encompass a wide range of clinical scenarios from loss of distal pulse to acute arterial thrombosis to emboli. Vascular complications can potentially result in the need for surgical therapy and even amputation. Several studies have suggested that patients at higher risk of developing IABP-related complications include female patients and those with peripheral vascular disease or diabetes *(50,54,56,57)*. In a prospective study of over 1100 patients on IABPs, Cohen and colleagues found that a history of peripheral vascular disease increases the risk of vascular complications by four times *(50)* and Gottlieb's group found that a history of peripheral vascular disease was predictive of serious vascular complications requiring surgical therapy *(54)*. Female sex has also been identified as an independent risk factor for vascular complications, with a relative risk of 2.3 *(50)*. Gottlieb suggests that the reason for the higher complication rate in women may be attributable to smaller caliber arteries. Diabetes has also been recognized as a risk factor for vascular complications *(50,58)*. Wasfie found that complications occurred in 34% of insulin-dependent diabetics, 18% of non-insulin-dependent diabetics, and 14% of nondiabetic patients *(58)*.

Catheter size and method of insertion are also factors that may increase the risk of complications. Several investigators have found that percutaneous insertion of IABPs is

Table 4
Complications Associated with IABP Use

Vascular complications
    Bleeding
    Limb ischemia
    Compartment syndrome
    Arterial dissection
    Groin hematoma
Embolic events
    Cerebrovascular accident
    Bowel infarction
    Renal infarction
    Emboli to extremities
Infection
Balloon rupture or failure
Aortic rupture
Death

associated with higher vascular complication rates than surgical insertion *(52,57,59–62)*. In patients with known peripheral vascular disease, the risk of vascular complications was 17.9% when a surgical cut-down technique was used to insert the IABP versus 38.9% when a percutaneous insertion was performed *(59)*. Pelletier's group obtained similar results with a complication rate of 11.4% associated with the surgical technique versus 30% with the percutaneous method *(62)*. Larger catheter sizes are also predictive for higher complication rates. 12 French catheters inserted percutaneously were associated with a 20.7% complication rate compared to 9.9% when 10.5 French catheters were used *(52)*. The significant decrease in vascular complications over the last 5 yr can largely be explained by the use of catheters with smaller diameters *(56)*. Retrospective studies evaluating sheathless insertion of IABPs have demonstrated a small reduction *(63)* or no reduction *(64)* in vascular complication rates.

Several studies have found that longer duration of IABP support is associated with a higher incidence of complications *(52,56,65)*. Other factors that have been implicated in higher complication rates include advanced age, hemodynamic instability, and emergency IABP insertion.

When IABP-related vascular complications occur, morbidity and mortality increase significantly. In studies by Busch and Sirbu's group, the mortality rate in patients with ischemic vascular complications was 59% *(57,66)*. Complications in these studies included acute limb arterial occlusion, compartment syndrome, arterial dissection, and groin hematoma. Of the 524 patients evaluated in this study, 26.7% experienced vascular complications requiring surgical therapy. Surgical interventions included thromboembolectomy, profundaplasties, infrainguinal bypasses, fasciotomies, and, rarely, amputations.

Other Complications

Infectious complications are also common in patients with IABPs. These include local infections, bacteremia, and sepsis. Overall, the rate of infectious complications ranges between 0% and 22% *(53–55,58,67)*. Kantrowitz's group found that the rate of infectious complications was related to the hospital location in which the device was inserted: 26% in coronary care unit, 23% in surgical intensive care unit, 17% in cardiac catheterization laboratory, and 12% in operating room *(53)*. These findings stress the importance of aseptic technique during insertion of the IABP.

Bleeding is another potentially serious complication associated with IABP use. McEnany reported major bleeding in 4% of patients studied *(68)* and this correlated with 4.6% reported by Cohen *(43)*.

Other less common complications include balloon rupture *(43)* paraplegia *(69)*, small-bowel infarction *(70)*, air embolism *(71,72)*, and acute ischemic hepatitis *(73)*. The incidence of failure to insert the IABP through the femoral artery is between 5% and 10% *(53,61,62)*.

Complications from intra-aortic balloon pump insertion, therefore, are varied and are certainly not infrequent. Fortunately, it appears that the overall complication rate is declining, probably as a result of increased experience and smaller catheters.

FUTURE DIRECTIONS

Percutaneous Cardiopulmonary Support

Counterpulsation with an intra-aortic balloon pump can help to achieve hemodynamic stability in patients with cardiogenic shock, but it is incapable of supporting a patient with complete hemodynamic collapse resulting from severe ventricular dysfunction or a patient with intractable ventricular arrhythmias. Recently, however, more complete cardiopulmonary support systems have been developed for patients with hemodynamic or potential hemodynamic collapse *(74)*. The Bard percutaneous cardiopulmonary support system (CPS) uses an 18 French arterial cannula in the descending aorta and an 18 French venous cannula in the right atrium with these cannulae connected to an external pump and membrane oxygenator to achieve full cardiopulmonary bypass (Figs. 2 and 3) *(75)*.

In 1988, Vogel first reported on the use of cardiopulmonary support using this system in patients undergoing high-risk coronary angioplasty *(76)*. In this initial report, the cannulae were inserted via surgical cut-down on the femoral artery and femoral vein. Subsequently, Shawl et al. reported on the percutaneous insertion of these cannulae for patients undergoing high-risk and emergency percutaneous intervention *(77)*. In 1990, Vogel and colleagues published the initial report from 14 centers of a national registry of elective CPS during coronary angioplasty *(78)*. Indications for this group of patients included an ejection fraction <25% or a target vessel supplying more than half of the myocardium or both. During this registry, there was a progressive change from cutdown insertion to percutaneous insertion and removal of the circulatory support cannulae. Although the angioplasty success rate was high (95%) in this group of very high-risk patients, morbidity was frequent (39%), in most cases as a result of cannulae insertion or removal. Hospital mortality was 7.6%, with half of these deaths occurring in patients with both age >75 yr and left main coronary artery stenosis. In patients without these two factors, the mortality rate was 2.6%.

Teirstein et al. reported on the use of "standby" versus "prophylactic" use of CPS in high-risk patients and found that, in most cases, high-risk angioplasty could be performed safely as long as emergency initiation of CPS was immediately available *(79)*.

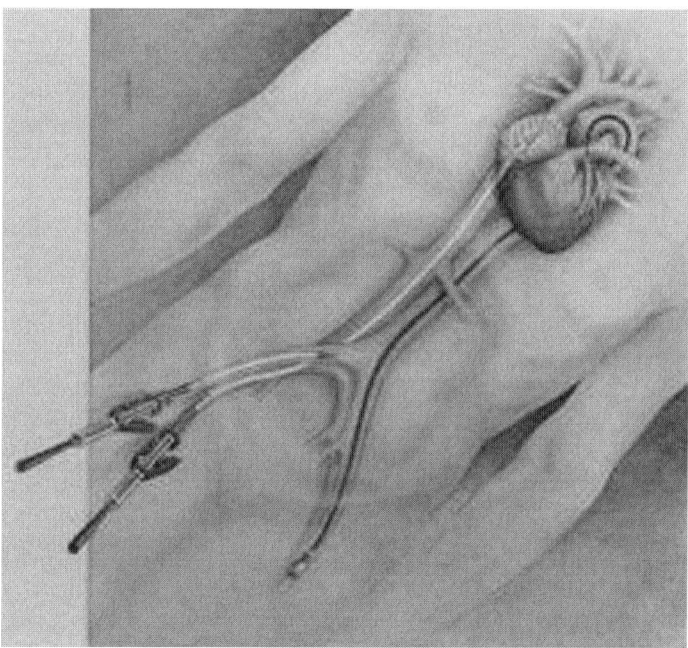

Fig. 2. Schematic representation of the appropriate position of the arterial and venous cannulae. Note placement of the tip of the venous cannula just above the junction of the inferior vena cava and right atrium. The arterial cannula is advanced until the hub is flush with the skin. Also note that a right femoral approach is shown in the diagram, whereas the left femoral approach is more commonly used in elective cases with PTCA performed from the contralateral side. Reprinted with permission from Kluwer Academic Publishers. Shawl FA, ed. Supported Complex and High Risk Coronary Angioplasty.

They concluded, however, that prophylactic CPS still appeared warranted in certain high-risk patients (Table 5).

Rapid institution of CPS allows for stabilization of patients who have cardiovascular collapse in the cardiac catheterization laboratory. Patients who have abrupt closure of a vessel may be supported until the situation is remedied either in the cardiac catheterization laboratory or in the operating room. CPS obviously does not provide myocardial blood flow beyond acutely obstructed arteries, but it allows for support of the circulation until the situation can be remedied with successful percutaneous intervention. If the cause of cardiovascular collapse cannot be rapidly corrected in the catheterization laboratory, the patient can be transferred in a stable condition to the operating room for emergency surgery. However, revascularization needs to be performed as an emergency procedure, in an effort to enhance myocardial salvage as CPS provides hemodynamic support but not distal perfusion. The duration of hemodynamic support is limited as percutaneous CPS of more than 6 h duration leads to severe hematological and pulmonary complications *(80)*.

Initiation of CPS results in a predictable hemodynamic response *(80)*. After the pump is primed with approximately 1.3 L of normosol, blood is withdrawn from the right atrium and pumped through a heat exchanger, then a membrane oxygenator, and ultimately infused into the femoral artery. There is a fall in the right atrial, pulmonary arterial, pul-

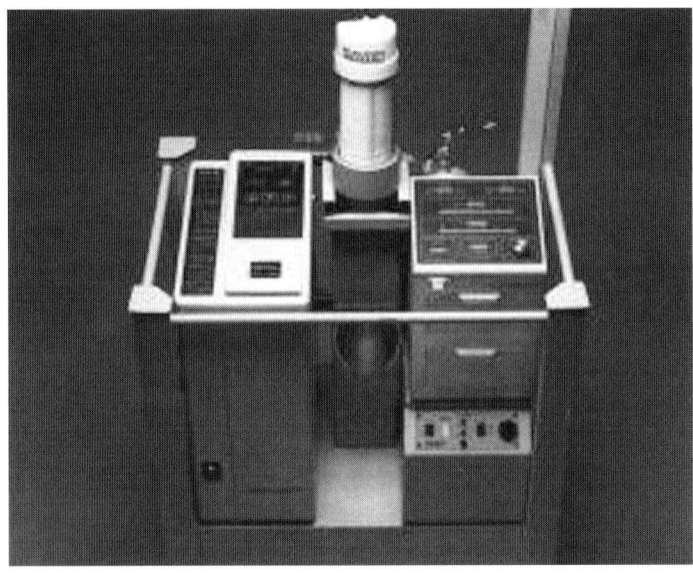

Fig. 3. Portable cardiopulmonary bypass support system. Reprinted with permission from Kluwer Academic Publishers. Shawl FA, ed. Supported Complex and High Risk Coronary Angioplasty.

Table 5
Outcome in the Subgroup of 158 Patients with a LVEF < 20%

	Prophylactic CPS (n=126)	Standby CPS (n=32)	p-Value
Procedural success	112 (90.5)	26 (81.2)	NS
Major complications			
Q-wave MI	2 (1.6)	0	NS
Emergency CABG	2 (1.6)	0	NS
Death	6 (4.8)	6 (18.8)	<0.05
Morbidity			
Femoral complications or transfusion requirement	52 (41.3)	3 (9.4)	<0.01

Source: ref. 79.

monary capillary wedge, and systemic arterial pressures. The pump provides continuous flow with maintenance of a pulsatile arterial pressure unless the circulation is being completely supported by the CPS system. Systemic anticoagulation with heparin is crucial and must be meticulously monitored to avoid thromboembolic and bleeding complications.

Although percutaneous CPS has been suggested for potential use in the setting of high-risk valvuloplasty, cardiogenic shock resulting from acute myocardial infarction, electrophysiologic testing producing hemodynamically compromising ventricular arrhythmias, hypothermia, prior to high-risk CABG, near drowning, drug overdose, and as a bridge to other mechanical assist devices or cardiac transplant, its primary use has been in the setting of abrupt vessel closure with hemodynamic collapse and refrac-

Table 6
Contraindications to the Institution of
Percutaneous Cardiopulmonary Support

Severe peripheral atherosclerotic disease
History of recent cerebral vascular accident
Pre-existing coagulopathy
Active bleeding
Untreatable or terminal disease
Suspected traumatic closed-head injury
Unwitnessed normothermic cardiac arrest
Refractory cardiac arrest of long duration
Severe aortic regurgitation

Source: Reprinted with permission from Kluwer
Academic Publishers. Shawl FA, ed. Supported Complex and High Risk Coronary Angioplasty.

tory cardiac arrest in the cardiac catheterization laboratory *(81,82)*. Contraindications to the use of CPS are listed in Table 6.

In summary, the percutaneous CPS system has been lifesaving for a small percentage of patients treated in the cardiac catheterization laboratory who have experienced hemodynamic collapse. Its use has been limited by a relatively high morbidity rate associated with vascular access as well as by the limited duration of time that the device can be employed.

Hemopump™

In 1988, Wampler and colleagues first described a retrograde, catheter-mounted left ventricular assist device intended for surgical placement via the femoral artery *(83)*. The device consists of a disposable catheter with a turbine at its tip driven by an external motor that is connected to an electrical console (Fig. 4). The disposable pumping system consists of an inlet cannula, an axial flow blood pump, and a drive cable in a polymeric sheath and a motor rotor. The sheath also serves as a conduit for purge fluid that lubricates the drive cable and hydrodynamic bearings. Purge fluid flows outward through the pump seal to prevent any blood from entering the pumping mechanism. The turbine within the catheter is driven at high speed (up to 45,000 rpm) and withdraws blood from the left ventricle and pumps it into the descending aorta. The miniature cable-driven axial flow pump is passed across the aortic valve to provide transvalvular left ventricular assistance. The catheter, available initially in size 21F, was subsequently miniaturized to 14F. Figure 5 is a diagram of the Hemopump catheter assembly. Figure 6 demonstrates the Hemopump catheter positioned in the left ventricle and the ascending aorta, the aortic arch, and descending aorta.

In 1992, Smalling and colleagues assessed the effects of ventricular unloading in a canine infarct model and concluded that the Hemopump appeared to result in significant infarct salvage compared with reperfusion alone *(84)*. In addition, the Hemopump appeared to provide superior systolic and diastolic unloading compared with intraaortic counterpulsation. In 1994, in a small pilot study, Smalling et al. reported on the use of the Hemopump in the setting of cardiogenic shock associated with acute myocardial infarction *(85)*. Hemodynamics including pulmonary capillary wedge pressure, cardiac

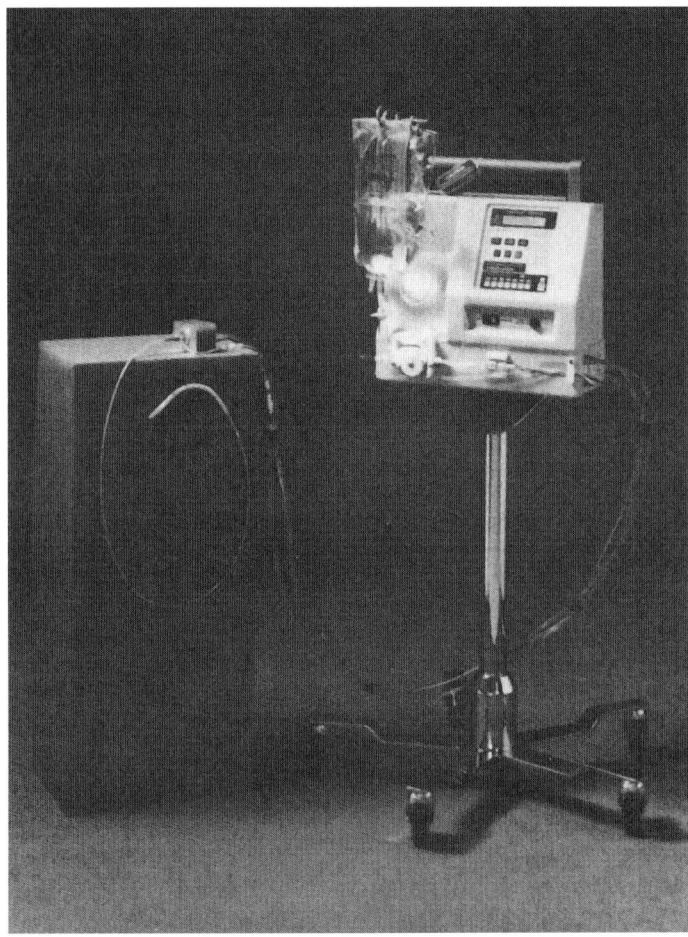

Fig. 4. Hemopump system. Reprinted with permission from Kluwer Academic Publishers. Shawl, FA, ed. Supported Complex and High Risk Coronary Angioplasty.

index, and dopamine requirements improved significantly during the first 24 h of left ventricular assistance. Four of 11 patients (36%) survived. In this small pilot trial, the authors concluded that left ventricular support with the Hemopump in patients with cardiogenic shock complicating acute myocardial infarction was feasible and that left ventricular unloading may decrease infarct expansion and improve left ventricular function over the long term.

Subsequently, Scholz et al. *(86),* in a multicenter registry, reported on the clinical experience of the Hemopump used during high-risk PTCA. The device on maximum pump speed resulted in a decrease in pulmonary artery wedge pressure from 15 ± 6 to 13 ± 6 mm Hg ($p < 0.001$). Cardiac index, mean aortic pressure, and systolic pressure did not change significantly during support. Plasma-free hemoglobin rose significantly from 4.9 ± 2.8 to 30.0 ± 21.7 mg/dL (normal range 0–10; $p < 0.001$). Serum haptoglobin did not change significantly immediately postassistance, but lactate dehydrogenase (LDH) rose significantly from 163 ± 35 to 301 ± 103 U/L ($p < 0.001$). The overall pro-

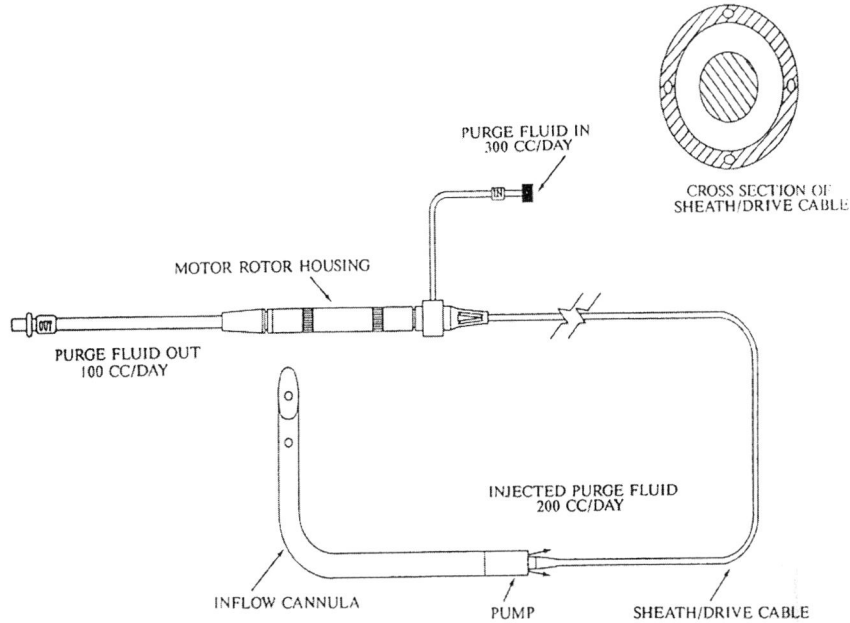

Fig. 5. Schematic of the Hemopump. Reprinted with permission from Kluwer Academic Publishers. Shawl, FA, ed. Supported Complex and High Risk Coronary Angioplasty.

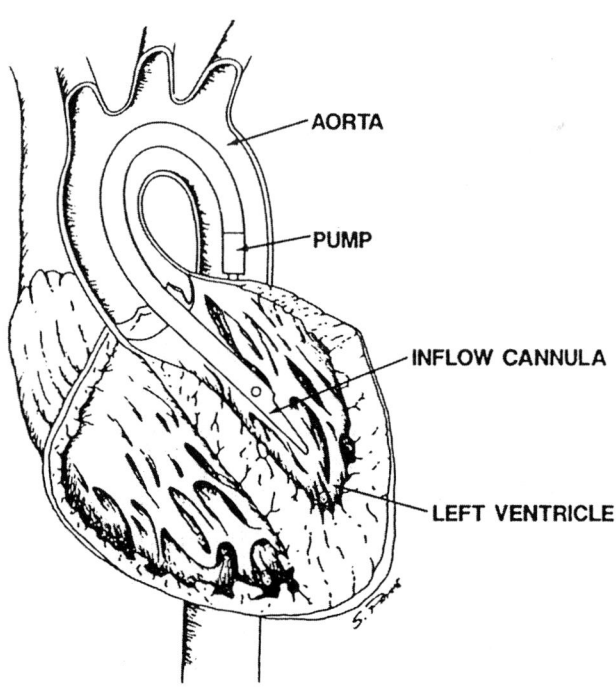

Fig. 6. Position of Hemopump in the heart. Reprinted with permission from Kluwer Academic Publishers. Shawl, FA, ed. Supported Complex and High Risk Coronary Angioplasty.

cedural mortality was 12.5% (4 of 32 patients). Two patients died of cardiogenic shock following reocclusion of the angioplasty vessel 1 and 3 h after removal of the Hemop-ump. One patient died after surgery for vascular repair of femoral artery occlusion, and one patient died 3 d after PTCA with a periprocedural cerebrovascular accident (CVA). The CVA was attributed to pre-existing severe stenosis of the middle cerebral artery and prolonged cerebral hypoperfusion during the PTCA with a marked fall in the sys-tolic aortic pressure. There was no histologic evidence of atheromatous debris or thromboembolism secondary to the device. Although the device did appear to provide hemodynamic support for many of the patients, there were significant procedure-related vascular access problems that limited the beneficial effects. In addition, the pro-cedure-related mortality of 12.5% was thought to be excessive and higher than that reported in other studies with supported high-risk PTCA. Despite these somewhat promising early results, the Hemopump never received FDA approval and further investigation was abandoned.

AB-180 Percutaneous Left Ventricular Assist Device (TandemHeart™)

The concept of ventricular assistance and unloading is particularly attractive in the setting of acute myocardial infarction with as well as without cardiogenic shock. Despite the benefits on short- and long-term mortality, reperfusion alone does not dra-matically improve global or segmental left ventricular (LV) function *(87,88)*. This para-dox of improved survival despite a lack of LV functional recovery had led to the "open artery hypothesis" with the "open artery" theoretically leading to improved LV remodel-ing, a decrease in aneurysm formation and a decrease in border zone ischemia resulting in decreased fatal arrhythmias *(89)*. Whereas, in the past, successful reperfusion follow-ing an acute MI was equated with restoration of epicardial vessel patency, there is a growing body of evidence that microvascular dysfunction and inadequate tissue perfu-sion persists despite successful opening of the epicardial vessel — the so-called "illu-sion of reperfusion" *(90,91)*. Optimal reperfusion has, therefore, been redefined to include restoration of microvascular flow as well as epicardial vessel patency *(92)*.

Several interventions have been evaluated for improving microvascular flow *(93,94)*. The intra-aortic balloon pump (IABP), for example, may be useful in supporting patients with severe LV dysfunction, but in multivariate analysis, it has not been inde-pendently associated with improved LV function or survival *(95,96)*. Animal models have demonstrated that the IABP restores epicardial blood flow but has little effect on microvascular flow in the setting of acute MI *(97)*. By contrast, the use of an LV assist device (left atrial to femoral artery bypass) in the animal model with acute MI and car-diogenic shock results in complete restoration of endocardial (microvascular) as well as epicardial flow to baseline values. In addition, the use of a left ventricular assist device (LVAD) in the setting of experimental acute MI results in a marked reduction in the extent of myocardial necrosis compared with controls *(98–100)*. The requirement for surgical placement, including a midline sternotomy, in patients with an evolving acute MI and hemodynamic instability, however, precludes the routine clinical use of a conventional LVAD *(101–104)*.

Several LVADs have been used for cardiogenic shock with acute MI. These devices are large and costly, however, and they require surgery for implantation and removal. The Jarvik 2000, the Heartmate II, and the Debakey assist device are examples of sec-ond-generation LVADs that use rotary pump technology to power blood flow. Although they are smaller and easier to insert than previous devices, they still require a thoracotomy for insertion and removal *(105)*. To date, a percutaneous system for short-term LV support is not available in the United States.

Left ventricular assist devices have been used for temporary support during acute MI. However, studies have revealed mortality rates of 75% with early implantation of LVADs *(106)*. Therefore, a strategy has evolved that delays LVAD implantation to allow for hemodynamic and end-organ stabilization.

Chen et al. *(106)* revisited the issue of early LVAD implantation in the post-MI setting, reporting on 25 patients who underwent implantation of the TCI LVAD (Thermocardiosystems, Inc.). The patients were divided into two groups: the "early cohort," who underwent device implantation less than 2 wk (average 5 d) after MI, and the "late cohort," who underwent device implantation more than 2 wk and less than 3 mo (average 23 d) after MI. In contrast to other studies, this study found a statistically significant decrease in mortality between the early and late cohorts: 26% and 40%, respectively. They also found a decreased need for right ventricular assist devices in the early group. This suggests that LV assist earlier in the MI setting has a beneficial effect on survival. However, this was a group of patients whose infarctions were already complete, rather than in the midst of an acute MI.

The concept of left heart bypass, with left atrial to femoral artery bypass, has shown promise in the treatment of acute MI. Left heart bypass (LHB) with left atrial cannulation was first reported in the early 1960s by Salisbury *(107)* and Dennis *(108)*. A method of closed-chest transseptal cannulation of the left atrium for LHB in dogs and in three patients was described in the mid-1970s *(109)*, and in 1998, three patients underwent finger-guided transseptal left atrial cannulation for LV support *(110)*. This study used a transseptal cannula placed in the left atrium and femoral artery cannulation to support patients post-cardiotomy, attaining flows of nearly 2 L/min.

The TandemHeart LVAD, currently available under an FDA-granted Investigator Device Exemption (IDE), is a simple, relatively inexpensive left atrial to femoral artery bypass system. The device consists of a small centrifugal pump with a specially designed transseptal inflow cannula and outflow conduit for percutaneous femoral artery placement. The device is powered by a DC-brushless motor and typically operates at 3000–7500 rpm. It functions as a hydrodynamic bearing with its moving surfaces suspended in a heparinized sterile water lubricant (Fig. 7). The device is connected to a controller that operates based on a back-electromagnetic force (EMF) algorithm and has several built-in safety features.

The left atrium is entered via standard transseptal technique (Fig. 8 shows the transseptal cannula after placement in the left atrium). An Inoue guidewire is used to maintain access safely in the left atrium while the intra-atrial septum is dilated with a graduated progressive dilator. The transseptal cannula, a 21F polyurethane cannula with a large end hole and 14 side holes, is then passed into the left atrium; care must be taken to be certain that all side holes are situated in the left atrium in order to avoid right-to-left shunting. The outflow cannula is inserted into the femoral artery. Less than 20 cm^3 is used to prime the pump and 60 cm^3 for the entire system. Once all air has been removed from the system and the lines are secured, the cannulae are connected to the TandemHeart using standard Tygon tubing. The power line for the device is then connected to the controller (Fig. 9), and ventricular assist may begin. With experience, the device may be inserted and left ventricular assist instituted in less than 30 min. To

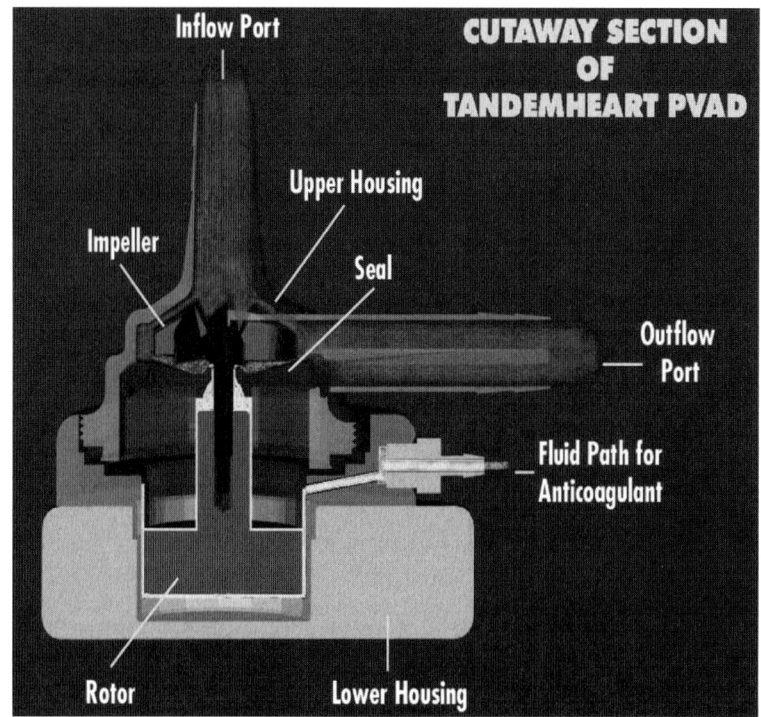

Fig. 7. Cutaway section of TandemHeart™.

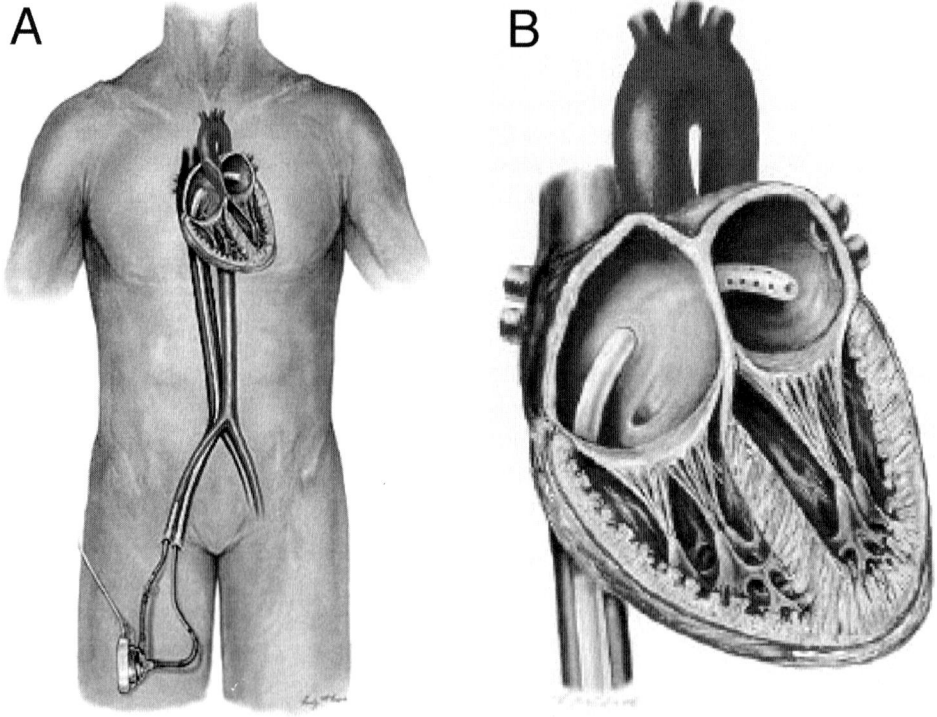

Fig. 8. (**A**) Diagram of transseptal and arterial cannulae connected to the TandemHeart. (**B**) Closeup of transseptal catheter in left atrium of the TandemHeart system.

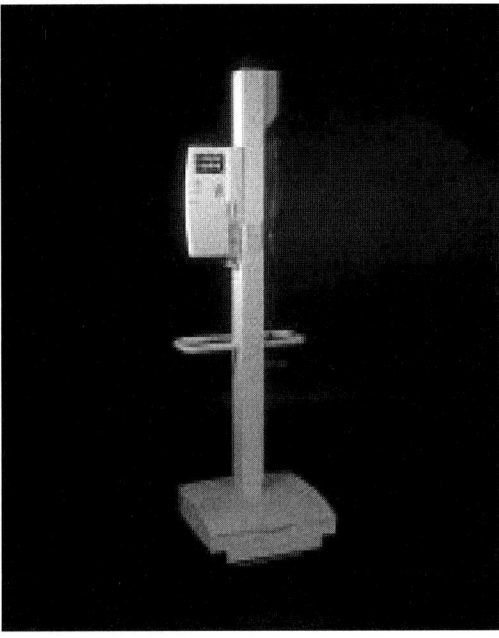

Fig. 9. TandemHeart controller.

avoid thromboembolic complications, patients must be maintained on systemic anticoagulation with heparin with the activated clotting time maintained at 200–250 s.

The TandemHeart device may be used under protocol for up to 14 d of support.
When it is decided to end its use, heparin is discontinued and the cannulae are
removed, with hemostasis achieved with direct manual pressure over the puncture sites.
The patient is left with a small iatrogenic ASD that closes gradually over the next several weeks. The ASD is no larger than that created for percutaneous balloon mitral
valvuloplasty.

Preliminary data with this device reveal that there is a significant increase in cardiac
output and blood pressure with a concomitant significant fall in pulmonary capillary
wedge, pulmonary artery, and central venous pressures. Up to 4 L/min may be provided with the device. As opposed to the CPS system, the TandemHeart may be used to
support patients in cardiogenic shock for prolonged periods of time. The device may be
useful not only in the setting of cardiogenic shock related to acute MI but also in cardiogenic shock resulting from other etiologies. Early information with this new device
demonstrates that rapid deployment is feasible in the setting of acute MI and cardiogenic shock and suggests that further trials with this device are warranted.

CONCLUSIONS

The intra-aortic balloon pump has evolved immensely over the last 30 yr. It has been
used in millions of patients. This relatively simple device has become the standard cardiac mechanical assist device, and it has been shown repeatedly to result in hemodynamic improvement. Although the indications for the IABP have expanded greatly in
recent years, cardiogenic shock remains the most significant indication for which it is

used today. Perhaps the most exciting mechanical assist devices are yet to come. The use of newer percutaneous devices remains in its infancy. As these devices become simpler and safer to deploy, their use may well increase. Although, in theory, these new assist devices, such as the TandemHeart, should be helpful, it remains to be proven whether they actually alter outcomes in patients with cardiogenic shock.

REFERENCES

1. Kantrowitz A, TjØnneland S, Freed PS, et al. Initial clinical experience with intraaortic balloon pumping in cardiogenic shock. JAMA 1968;203:135–140.
2. Kantrowitz, A. Origins of intraaortic balloon pumping. Ann Thorac Surg 1990;50:672–674.
3. Nanas JN, Moulopoulos SD. Counterpulsation: historical background, technical improvements, hemodynamic and metabolic effects. Cardiology 1994;84:156–167.
4. Talpins NL, Kripke DC, Goetz RH. Counterpulsation and intraaortic balloon pumping in cardiogenic shock. Circ Dynam Arch Surg 1968;97:991–999.
5. Kantrowitz A, Krakauer J, Zorzi G, et al. Current status of intraaortic balloon pump and initial clinical experience with aortic patch mechanical auxiliary ventricle. Transplant Proc 1971;3:1459–1471.
6. Chatterjee S, Rosensweig J. Evaluation of intraaortic balloon counterpulsation. J Thorac Cardiovasc Surg 1971;61:405–410.
7. McDonald RH Jr, Taylor RR, Cingolani HE. Measurement of myocardial developed tension and its relation to oxygen consumption. Am J Physiol 1966;211:667–673.
8. Powell WJ Jr, Daggett WM, Margo AE, et al. Effects of intraaortic balloon counterpulsation on cardiac performance, oxygen consumption, and coronary blood flow in dogs. Circ Res 1970;26:753–764.
9. Shaw J, Taylor DR, Pitt B. Effects of intraaortic balloon counterpulsation on regional coronary blood flow in experimental myocardial infarction. Am J Cardiol 1974;34:552–556.
10. Kimura A, Toyota E, Songfang L, et al. Effects of intraaortic balloon pumping on the septal arterial blood flow velocity waveform during severe left main coronary artery stenosis. J Am Coll Cardiol 1996;27:810–816.
11. Bhayana JN, Scott SM, Sethi GK, Takaro T. Effects of intraaortic balloon pumping on organ perfusion in cardiogenic shock. J Surg Res 1979;26:108–113.
12. Scheidt S, Wilner G, Mueller H, et al. Intraaortic balloon pumping in cardiogenic shock. Report of a cooperative clinical trial. N Engl J Med 1973;288:979–984.
13. Wajszczuk WJ, Krakauer J, Rubenfire M, et al. Current indications for mechanical circulatory assistance on the basis of experience with 104 patients [abstract]. Am J Cardiol 1974;33:176.
14. Kantrowitz A. The physiologic basis of in-series cardiac assistance and the clinical application of intra-aortic devices. In: Davila JC, ed. 2nd Henry Ford Hospital International Symposium on Cardiac Surgery. Appleton–Century–Crofts, New York, 1977, pp. 640–643.
15. Willerson JT, Curry GC, Watson JT, et al. Intra-aortic balloon counterpulsation in patients with cardiogenic shock, medically refractory heart failure and/or recurrent ventricular tachycardia. Am J Med 1975;58:183–191.
16. DeWood MA, Notske RN, Hensley GR, et al. Intra-aortic balloon counterpulsation with and without reperfusion for myocardial infarction shock. Circulation 1980;61:1105–1112.
17. Hagemeijer F, Larid JD, Haalebos MMP, Hugenholtz PG. Effectiveness of intraaortic balloon pumping without cardiac surgery for patients with severe heart failure secondary to a recent myocardial infarction. Am J Cardiol 1977;40:951–956.
18. Moulopoulos S, Stametelopoulos S, Petrou P. Intraaortic balloon assistance in intractable cardiogenic shock. Eur Heart J 1986;7:396–403.
19. Kuchar DL, Campbell TJ, O'Rourke MF. Long-term survival after counterpulsation for medically refractory heart failure complicating myocardial infarction and cardiac surgery. Eur Heart J 1987;8:490–502.
20. Kovack PJ, Rasak MA, Bates ER, et al. Thrombolysis plus aortic counterpulsation: improved survival in patients who present to community hospitals with cardiogenic shock. J Am Coll Cardiol 1997;29(7):1454–1458.
21. Sanborn TA, Sleeper LA, Bates ER, et al. Impact of thrombolysis, intraaortic balloon pump counterpulsation, and their combination in cardiogenic shock complicating acute myocardial infarction: a report from the SHOCK Trial Registry. J Am Coll Cardiol 2000:36(3 Suppl A):1123–1129.

22. Stone GW, Marsalese D, Brodie BR, et al. A prospective, randomized evaluation of prophylactic intraaortic balloon counterpulsation in high-risk patients with acute myocardial infarction treated with primary angioplasty. Second Primary Angioplasty in Myocardial Infarction (PAMI-II) Trial Investigators. J Am Coll Cardiol 1997;29:1459–1467.

23. Brodie BR, Stuckey TD, Hansen C, Muncy D. Intra-aortic balloon counterpulsation before primary percutaneous transluminal coronary angioplasty reduces catheterization laboratory events in high-risk patients with acute myocardial infarction. Am J Cardiol 1999;84:18–23.

24. Buckley MJ, Craven JM, Gold HK. IABP assist for cardiogenic shock after cardiopulmonary bypass. Circulation 1972;46(Suppl):II76.

25. Oldham HN Jr, Roe CR, Young WG, et al. Intraoperative detection of myocardial damage during coronary artery surgery by plasma creatine phosphokinase isoenzyme analysis. Surgery 1973;74:917–925.

26. Rao V, Ivanov J, Weisel R, et al. Predictors of low cardiac output syndrome after coronary artery bypass. J Thorac Cardiovasc Surg 1996;112:38–51.

27. The Warm Heart Investigators. Normothermic versus hypothermic cardiac surgery: a randomized trial of 1732 coronary bypass patients. Lancet 1994;343:559–563.

28. McGee NG, Zillgitt SL, Trono R, et al. Retrospective analyses of the need for mechanical circulatory support (intraaortic balloon pump/abdominal left ventricular assist device or partial artificial heart) after cardiopulmonary bypass. A 44 month study of 14,168 patients. Am J Cardiol 1980;46:135–142.

29. Norman JC, Cooley DA, Igo SR, et al. Prognostic indices for survival during postcardiotomy intra-aortic balloon pumping. Methods of scoring and classification, with implications for left ventricular assist device utilization. J Thorac Cardiovasc Surg 1977;74:709–720.

30. Lund O, Johansen G, Allermand H, et al. Intraaortic balloon pumping in the treatment of low cardiac output following open heart surgery—immediate results and long-term prognosis. Thorac Cardiovasc Surg 1988;36:332–337.

31. Campbell CD, Tolitano DJ, Weber KT, et al. Mechanical support for postcardiotomy heart failure. J Cardiac Surg 1988;3:181–191.

32. Kurki TS, Kataja M. Preoperative prediction of postoperative morbidity in coronary artery bypass grafting. Ann Thorac Surg 1996;61:1740–1745.

33. Royster RL. Myocardial dysfunction following cardiopulmonary bypass: recovery patterns, predictors of inotropic need, theoretical concepts of inotropic administration. J Cardiothorac Vasc Anesth 1993;7:19–25.

34. Najafi H, Henson D, Dye WS, et al. Left ventricular hemorrhagic necrosis. Ann Thorac Surg 1969;7:550–561.

35. Hedenmark J, Ahn H, Henze A, et al. Intra-aortic balloon counterpulsation with special reference to determinants of survival. Scand J Thorac Cardiovasc Surg 1989;23:57–62.

36. Bolooki H, William W, Thurer RJ, et al. Clinical and hemodynamic criteria for use of intraaortic balloon pump in patients requiring cardiac surgery. J Thorac Cardiovasc 1976;72:756–758.

37. Kuchar DL, Campbell TJ, O'Rourke MF. Long-term survival after counterpulsation for medically refractory heart failure complicating myocardial infarction and cardiac surgery. Eur Heart J 1987;8:490–502.

38. Kottke TE, Pesch DG, Frye RL. The potential contribution of cardiac replacement to the control of cardiovascular disease: a population based estimate. Arch Surg 1990;125:1148–1151.

39. Hosenpud JD, Bennett LE, Keck BM, et al. The Registry of the International Society for Heart and Lung Transplantation: fourteenth official report—1997. J Heart Lung Transplant 1997;16:691–712.

40. Carrier M, White M, Pelletier G, et al. Ten-year follow-up of critically ill patients undergoing heart transplantation. J Heart Lung Transplant 2000;19:439–443.

41. Marks JD, Karwande SV, Richenbacher WE, et al. Perioperative mechanical circulatory support for transplantation. J Heart Lung Transplant 1992;11:117–128.

42. Kaye MP. The registry of the International Society for Heart Transplantation: fourth official report—1987. J Heart Transplant 1987;6:64–67.

43. Hardesty RL, Griffith BP, Trento A, et al. Mortally ill patients and excellent survival following cardiac transplantation. Ann Thorac Surg 1986;41:126–129.

44. O'Connell JB, Renlunnd DG, Robinson JA, et al. Effect of preoperative hemodynamic support on survival after cardiac transplantation. Circulation 1988;78(Suppl III):78–82.

45. Rosenbaum AM, Murali S, Uretsky BF. Intra-aortic balloon counterpulsation as a "bridge" to cardiac transplantation. Effects in nonischemic and ischemic cardiomyopathy. Chest 1994;106:1683–1688.

46. Birovljev S, Radovancevic B, Burnett CM, et al. Heart transplantation after mechanical circulatory support: four years' experience. J Heart Lung Transplant 1992;11:240–245.

47. Carrier M, White M, Pelletier G, et al. Ten-year follow-up of critically ill patients undergoing heart transplantation. J Heart Lung Transplant 2000;19:439–443.

48. Lewis BE, Sumida C, Hwang MH, Loeb HS. New approach to management of intraaortic balloon pumps in patients with peripheral vascular disease: case reports of four patients requiring urgent IABP insertion. Cathet Cardiovasc Diagn 1992;26:295–299.

49. Coyler WR Jr, Moore JA, Buket MW, Cooper CJ. Intraaortic balloon pump insertion after percutaneous revascularization in patients with severe peripheral vascular disease. Cathet Cardiovasc Diagn 1997;42:1–6.

50. Cohen M, Dawson MS, Kopistansky C, McBride R. Sex and other predictors of intra-aortic balloon counterpulsation-related complications: prospective study of 1119 consecutive patients. Am Heart J 2000;139:282–287.

51. Cook L, Pillar B, McCord G, Josephson R. Intra-aortic balloon pump complications: a five-year retrospective study of 283 patients. Heart Lung 1999;28:195–202.

52. Scholz KH, Ragab S, von zur Muhlen F, et al. Complication of intra-aortic balloon counterpulsation. The role of catheter size and duration of support in a multivariate analysis of risk. Eur Heart J 1998;19:458–465.

53. Kantrowitz A, Wasfie T, Freed PS, et al. Intraaortic balloon pumping 1967 through 1982: analysis of complications in 733 patients. Am J Cardiol 1986;57:976–983.

54. Gottlieb SO, Brinker JA, Borkon AM, et al. Identification of patients at high risk for complications of intraaortic balloon counterpulsation: a multivariate risk factor analysis. Am J Cardiol 1984;53:1135–1139.

55. Lefemine AA, Kosowsky B, Madoff I, et al. Results and complications of intraaortic balloon pumping in surgical and medical patients. Am J Cardiol 1977;40:416–420.

56. Arafa OE, Pedersen TH, Svennevig JL, et al. Vascular complications of the intraaortic balloon pump in patients undergoing open heart operations: 15-year experience. Ann Thorac Surg 1999;67:645–651.

57. Busch T, Sirbu H, Zenker D, Dalichau H. Vascular complications related to intraaortic balloon counterpulsation: an analysis of ten years' experience. Thorac Cardiovasc Surg 1997;45:55–59.

58. Wasfie T, Freed PS, Rubenfire M, et al. Risk associated with intraaortic balloon pumping in patients with and without diabetes mellitus. Am J Cardiol 1988;61:558–562.

59. Miller JS, Dodson TF, Salam AA, Smith RB III. Vascular complications following intra-aortic balloon pump insertion. Am Surg 1992:58:232–238.

60. Curtis JJ, Bolan M, Bliss D, et al. Intra-aortic balloon cardiac assist: complication rates for the surgical and percutaneous insertion techniques. Am Surg 1988;54:142–147.

61. Goldberg MG, Rubenfire M, Kantrowitz A, et al. Intraaortic balloon pump insertion: a randomized study comparing percutaneous and surgical techniques. J Am Coll Cardiol 1987;9:515–523.

62. Pelletier LC, Pomar JL, Bosch X, et al. Complications of circulatory assistance with intra-aortic balloon pumping: a comparison of surgical and percutaneous techniques. J Heart Transplant 1986;5:138–142.

63. Tatar H, Cicek S, Demirkilic U, et al. Vascular complications of intraaortic balloon pumping: unsheathed versus sheathed insertion. Ann Thorac Surg 1993;55:1518–1521.

64. Gol MK, Bayazit M, Emir M, et al. Vascular complications related to percutaneous insertion of intraaortic balloon pumps. Ann Thorac Surg 1994;58:1476–1480.

65. Manord JD, Garrard CL, Mehra MR, et al. Implications for the vascular surgeon with prolonged (3 to 89 days) intraaortic balloon pump counterpulsation. J Vasc Surg 1997;26:511–515.

66. Sirbu H, Busch T, Aleksic I, et al. Ischaemic complications with intraaortic balloon counter-pulsation: Incidence and management. Cardiovasc Surg 2000;8:66–71.

67. Beckman CB, Geha AS, Hammond GL, Baue AE. Results and complications of intraaortic balloon counterpulsation. Ann Thorac Surg 1977;24:550–559.

68. McEnany MT, KayHR, Buckley MJ, et al. Clinical experience with intraaortic balloon pump support in 728 patients. Circulation. 1978;58(Suppl I):124–132.

69. Seifert PE, Silverman NA. Late paraplegia resulting from intra-aortic balloon pump. Ann Thorac Surg 1986;41:700.

70. Jamolowski CR, Poirier RL. Small bowel infarction complicating intra-aortic balloon counterpulsation via the ascending aorta. J Thorac Cardiovasc Surg 1980;79:735–737.

71. Tomatis L, Nemiroff M, Riahi M, et al. Massive air embolism due to rupture of pulsatile assist device: Successful treatment in the hyperbaric chamber. Ann Thorac Surg 1981;32:604–608.

72. Haykal HA, Wang AM. CT diagnosis of delayed cerebral air embolism following intraaortic balloon pump catheter insertion. Comput Radiol 1986;10:307–309.

73. Shin H, Yozu R, Sumida T, Kawada S. Acute ischemic hepatic failure resulting from intraaortic balloon pump malposition. Eur J Cardiothorac Surg 2000;17:492–494.

74. Figulla HR. Circulatory support devices in clinical cardiology. Cardiology 1994;84:149–155.

75. Shawl F. Percutaneous cardiopulmonary bypass support: technique, indications and complications. In: Shawl FA, ed. Supported Complex and High Risk Coronary Angioplasty. Kluwer Academic, Boston, 1991 pp. 65–100.

76. Vogel RA, Tommaso CL, Gundry SR. Initial experience with coronary angioplasty and aortic valvuloplasty using elective semi-percutaneous cardiopulmonary support. Am J Cardiol 1988;62:811–813.

77. Shawl FA, Domanski MJ, Punja S. Percutaneous cardiopulmonary bypass support in high risk patients undergoing percutaneous transluminal coronary angioplasty. Am J Cardiol 1989;64:1258–1263.

78. Vogel RA, Shawl FA, Tommaso CL, et al. Initial report of the National Registry of Elective Cardiopulmonary Bypass Supported Coronary Angioplasty. J Am Coll Cardiol 1990;15:23–29.

79. Teirstein PS, Vogel RA, Dorros G, et al. Prophylactic versus standby cardiopulmonary support for high risk percutaneous transluminal coronary angioplasty. J Am Coll Cardiol 1993;21:590–596.

80. Ronan JA, Shawl FA. Echocardiographic and hemodynamic changes during percutaneous cardiopulmonary bypass. In: Shawl FA, ed. Supported Complex and High Risk Coronary Angioplasty. Kluwer Academic, Boston, 1991. pp. 57–63.

81. Shawl FA, Domanski MJ, Hernandez TJ, et al. Emergency percutaneous cardiopulmonary bypass with cardiogenic shock from acute myocardial infarction. Am J Cardiol 1989;64:967–970.

82. Shawl FA, Domanski MJ, Wish MH, et al. Emergency cardiopulmonary bypass support in patients with cardiac arrest in the catheterization laboratory. Cathet Cardiovasc Diagn 1990;19:8–12.

83. Wampler RJ, Moise JC, Frazier OH, et al. In vivo evaluation of a peripheral vascular access axial flow blood pump. Trans ASAIO 1988;34:450–455.

84. Smalling RW, Cassidy DB, Barrett R, et al. Improved regional myocardial blood flow, left ventricular unloading, and infarct slavage using an axial-flow, transvalvular left ventricular assist device. A comparison with intraaortic balloon counterpulsation and reperfusion alone in a canine infarction model. Circulation 1992;85:1152–1159.

85. Smalling RW, Sweeney M, Lachterman B, et al. Transvalvular left ventricular assistance in cardiogenic shock secondary to acute myocardial infarction — evidence for recovery from near fatal myocardial stunning. J Am Coll Cardiol 1994;23:637–644.

86. Scholz KH, Figulla Jr, Schweda F, et al. Mechanical left ventricular unloading during high risk coronary angioplasty — first use of a new percutaneous left ventricular assist device. Cathet Cardiovasc Diagn 1994;31:61–65.

87. Christian TF, Schwartz RS, Gibbons RJ. Determinants of infarct size in reperfusion therapy for acute myocardial infarction. Circulation 1992;86:81–90.

88. Miller TD, Christian TF, Hopfenspirger MR, et al. Infarct size after acute myocardial infarction measured by quantitative tomographic ^{99m}Tc sestamibi imaging predicts subsequent mortality. Circulation 1995;92:334–341.

89. Braunwald E. Myocardial reperfusion, limitation of infarct size, reduction of left ventricular dysfunction, and improved survival: should the paradigm be expanded? Circulation 1989;79:441–444.

90. Kloner RA, Ganote CE, Jennings RB. The "no-reflow" phenomenon after temporary occlusion in the dog. J Clin Invest 1974;54:1496–1508.

91. Lincoff AM, Topol EJ. "Illusion of reperfusion": does anyone achieve optimal reperfusion during acute myocardial infarction? Circulation 1993;88:1361–1374.

92. Roe MT, Ohman EM, Maas AC, et al. Shifting the open-artery hypothesis downstream: the quest for optimal reperfusion. J Am Coll Cardiol 2001;37:9–18.

93. Lincoff AM, Popma JJ, Ellis SG, et al. Percutaneous support devices for high risk or complicated coronary angioplasty. J Am Coll Cardiol 1991;17:770–780.

94. Vogel JH, Ruiz CE, Jahnke EJ, et al. Percutaneous (nonsurgical) supported angioplasty in unprotected left main disease and severe left ventricular dysfunction. Clin Cardiol 1989;12:297–300.

95. Stone GW, Marsalese D, Brodie BR, et al. A prospective, randomized evaluation of prophylactic intraaortic ballon counterpulsation in high risk patients with acute myocardial infarction treated with primary angioplasty. Second Primary Angioplasty in Myocardial Infarction (PAMI-II) Trial Investigators. J Am Coll Cardiol 1997;29:1459–1467.

96. Berger PB, Holmes DR Jr, Stebbins AL, et al. Impact of an aggressive invasive catheterization and revascularization strategy on mortality in patients with cardiogenic shock in the Global Utilization of Streptokinase and Tissue Plasminogen Activator for Occluded Coronary Arteries (GUSTO-1) trial. Circulation 1997;96:122–127.

97. Hata M, Shiono M, Orime Y, et al. Coronary microcirculation during left heart bypass with a centrifugal pump. Artif Organs 1996;20:678–680.
 98. Catinella FP, Cunningham JN, Glassman E, et al. Left atrium-to-femoral artery bypass: effectiveness in reduction of acute experimental myocardial infarction. J Thorac Cardiovasc Surg 1983;86:887–896.
 99. Grossi EA, Krieger KH, Cunningham JN, et al. Time course of effective interventional left heart assist for limitation of evolving myocardial infarction. J Thorac Cardiovasc Surg 1986;91:624–629.
100. Laschinger JC, Grossi EA, Cunningham JN, et al. Adjunctive left ventricular unloading during myocardial reperfusion plays a major role in minimizing myocardial infarct size. J Thorac Cardiovasc Surg 1985;90:80–85.
101. Frazier OH, Rose EA, Macmanus Q, et al. Multicenter clinical evaluation of the HeartMate 1000 IP left ventricular assist device. Ann Thorac Surg 1992;53:1080–1090.
102. Vetter HO, Kaulbach HG, Schmitz C, et al. Experience with the Novacor left ventricular assist system as a bridge to cardiac transplantation, including the new wearable system. J Thorac Cardiovasc Surg 1995;109:74–80.
103. Farrar DJ, Hill JD. Univentricular and biventricular Thoratec VAD support as a bridge to transplantation. Ann Thorac Surg 1993;55:276–282.
104. Marelli D, Laks H, Amsel B, et al. Temporary mechanical support with the BVS 5000 assist device during treatment of acute myocarditis. J Cardiac Surg 1997;12:55–59.
105. Westaby S, Katsumata T, Houel R, et al. Jarvik 2000: potential for bridge to myocardial recovery. Circulation 1998;98:1568–1574.
106. Chen JM, DeRose JJ, Slater JP. Improved survival rates support LVAD implantation early after myocardial infarction. J Am Coll Cardiol 1999;33:1903–1908.
107. Salisbury PF. Comparison of two types of mechanical assistance in experimental heart failure. Circ Res 1960;8:431.
108. Dennis C. Left atrial cannulation without thoractomy for total left heart bypass. Acta Chir, Scand 1962;123:267–279.
109. Glassman E, Engelman RM, Boyd AD, et al. A method of closed-chest cannulation of the left atrium for left atrial-femoral artery bypass. J Thorac Cardiovasc Surg 1975;69:283–290.
110. Pavie A, Leger P, Nzomvuama A, et al. Left centrifugal pump cardiac assist with transseptal percutaneous left atrial cannula. Artif Organs 1998;22:502–507.

20 Mechanical Alternatives to the Human Heart

Jacob Lavee, MD

So Oz brought a pair of tinsmith's shears and cut a small, square hole in the left side of the Tin Woodman's breast. Then, going to a chest of drawers, he took out a pretty heart, made entirely of silk and stuffed with some sawdust.

Isn't it a beauty? He asked.

L. Frank Baum, The Wizard of Oz

INTRODUCTION

Heart failure afflicts close to 1% of the adult population in the United States, is a contributing factor in over 250,000 deaths annually, is the primary diagnosis for more than 900,000 hospitalizations per year, and commands total treatment costs that approach $38 billion annually or nearly 4% of total health care costs. Despite the availability of heart transplantation as the preferred surgical treatment for end-stage heart disease, this mode of therapy is limited and clearly insufficient to meet the increasing demands for donor organs. Figures available from the United Network for Organ Sharing for 1999 report that although 4152 patients were listed for heart transplantation, only 2180 received a donor organ, a situation that is mirrored all over the globe. Even if the availability of donor hearts increases, it is unlikely that donor availability will keep pace with the escalating prevalence of end-stage heart failure, underscoring the crucial need for alternatives to cardiac allotransplantation. This chapter will attempt to summarize the current status of available mechanical alternatives to the human heart covering their indications for use, performance, and results. To complete the picture, devices that are under investigation will be described.

From: *Contemporary Cardiology: Cardiogenic Shock: Diagnosis and Treatment*
Edited by: David Hasdai et al. © Humana Press Inc., Totowa, NJ

INDICATIONS

There are currently three major indications for mechanical assistance to the failing heart: (1) bridge to myocardial or hemodynamic recovery; (2) bridge to cardiac transplantation; (3) destination therapy: permanent devices as an alternative to transplantation.

Severe cardiogenic shock from a potentially reversible cardiac insult can be successfully bridged to myocardial recovery by an assist device. Specific diagnoses for this category include acute viral cardiomyopathy, postpartum cardiomyopathy, postcardiotomy syndromes, anterior wall myocardial infarction (with revascularization), and reperfusion injury in cardiac allografts. The goal of an implanted assist system is decompression of the injured myocardium, allowing cardiac recovery and remodeling while providing physiologic support. Studies have shown that support with an assist device may decrease myocyte necrosis and apoptosis, decrease myocytolysis, and improve myocyte contractility *(1)*. These beneficial changes in the biology of the failing myocardium have been accompanied by favorable changes in the left ventricle geometry, left ventricular wall thickness, and volume. Normalization of ventricular structure does not necessarily mean that ventricular function is normalized, however. Following successful recovery of the heart the assist device may be weaned and subsequently explanted, although there are no guidelines as to the right timing and clinical features for a successful recovery.

Bridging cardiac transplant candidates to heart transplantation is currently the most common indication for implantation of an assist device. Candidates for transplant for whom no donor organ is immediately available and who continue to deteriorate despite aggressive pharmacologic support can benefit from implantation of an assist device. Such a device can sustain them, sometimes for months or even years, until a donor heart becomes available. The assist device is explanted at the time of transplantation.

The third, and currently still investigational, indication for assist system is as an alternative to cardiac transplantation. The recently published multicenter REMATCH trial (Randomized Evaluation of Mechanical Assist Treatment for Congestive Heart failure) compared outcomes for 68 nontransplant candidates in New York Heart Association Class IV heart failure supported with Thoratec Corporation's (formerly Thermo Cardiosystems Inc.) HeartMate vented electric left ventricular assist system (VE LVAS) to 61 similar patients who received optimal medical management *(2)*. The rates of survival at one year were 52% in the device group and 25% in the medical-therapy group ($p = 0.002$), and the rates at two years were 23% and 8% ($p = 0.09$), respectively. Although the frequency of serious adverse events in the device group was 2.35 times that in the medical-therapy group, the quality of life was significantly improved at one year in the device group. Based on the REMATCH trial results the Thoratec Corporation has filed a PreMarket Approval Supplement with the FDA seeking approval to expand the intended use of its HeartMate VE LVAS to include long-term support for heart failure patients on optimal medical management who are not eligible for heart transplants.

CURRENT SYSTEMS

The currently approved mechanical alternatives to the human heart can be categorized as paracorporeal assist systems, intracorporeal assist systems, or total artificial hearts.

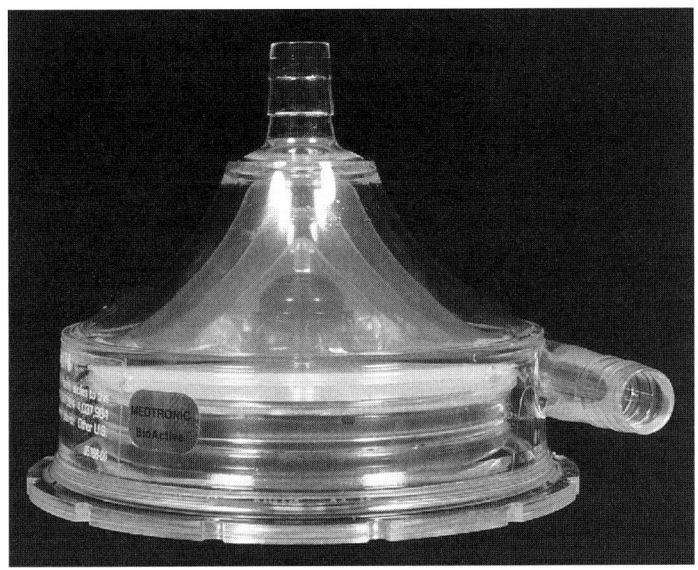

Fig. 1. The Bio-Medicus Bio-Pump centrifugal pump head (Medtronic Bio-Medicus, Inc., Eden Praire, MN).

Paracorporeal Assist Systems

Currently there are four paracorporeal assist systems approved for use:

1. Centrifugal pumps
2. ABMIOMED BVS 5000 (Abiomed, Danvers, MA)
3. Thoratec Ventricular Assist Device (Thoratec Corporation, Pleasanton, CA)
4. The Berlin Heart (Berlin Heart AG, Berlin, Germany)

CENTRIFUGAL PUMPS

Of the available cardiac assist devices, centrifugal pumps are most commonly used *(3)* because they are relatively simple to operate, require no special training, and are inexpensive compared with other devices. In centrifugal pumps, blood enters the pump axially from an inlet tube and is caught up between vanes or stages and whirled outward. Rotation of the impellers or stages causes the velocity of the blood to change while it moves toward the periphery of the pump. As the blood exits through the outlet tube, pressure is increased. Centrifugal pumps can provide high flow rates with low pressure rises. Most centrifugal pumps have only one moving part and, hence, can be manufactured inexpensively.

Several centrifugal pumps are available: The Bio-Medicus Bio-Pump (Medtronic Bio-Medicus, Inc., Eden Praire, MN) (Fig. 1), the Sarns Centrifugal System (Terumo Cardiovascular Systems, Ann Arbor, MI) (Fig. 2), the Lifestream centrifugal pump (Lifestream International, Haverhill, MA) (Fig. 3), and the Nikkiso centrifugal pump (Nikkiso Co., Ltd., Shizuoka, Japan). All use the impellers technique, varying only in the number of impellers, except the Medtronic Bio-Pump, which consists of two concentric cones made to impart a circular motion to incoming blood by viscous drag and constrained vortex principles. Each system consists of a disposable pump coupled to a motorized pump drive unit containing monitors and blood flow controls. In vitro and in

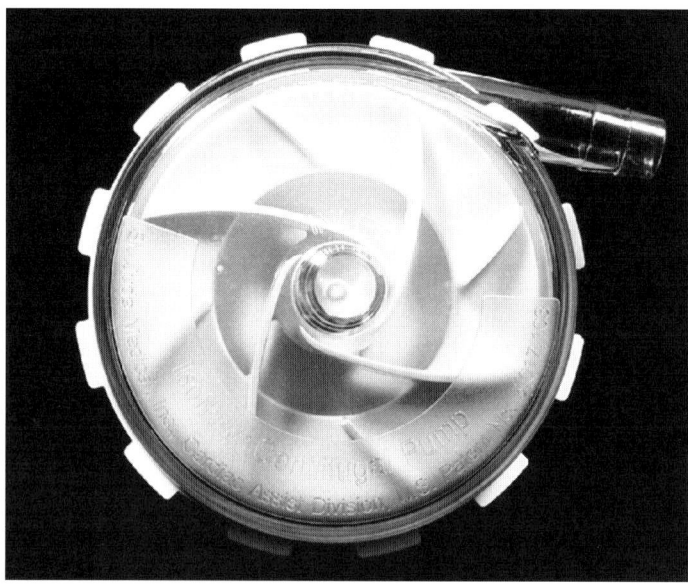

Fig. 2. The Sarns centrifugal pump head (Terumo Cardiovascular Systems, Ann Arbor, MI).

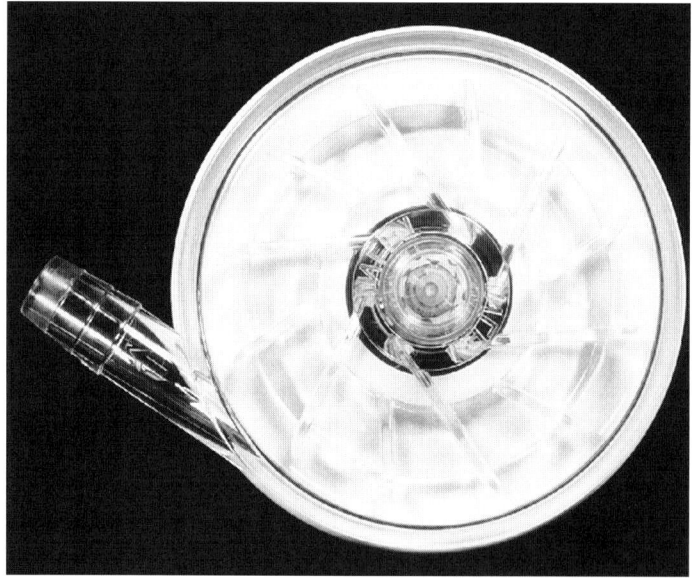

Fig. 3. The Lifestream centrifugal pump head (Lifestream International, Haverhill, MA).

vivo testing, which compared mechanical function, hematological effects (specifically hemolysis), and incidence of thromboembolism, revealed no compelling features that would dictate clear superiority of one centrifugal pump over another *(4)*.

Implantation techniques for centrifugal pumps, although simple, require great attention to detail to avoid bleeding, which is the most frequent complication. For left-heart

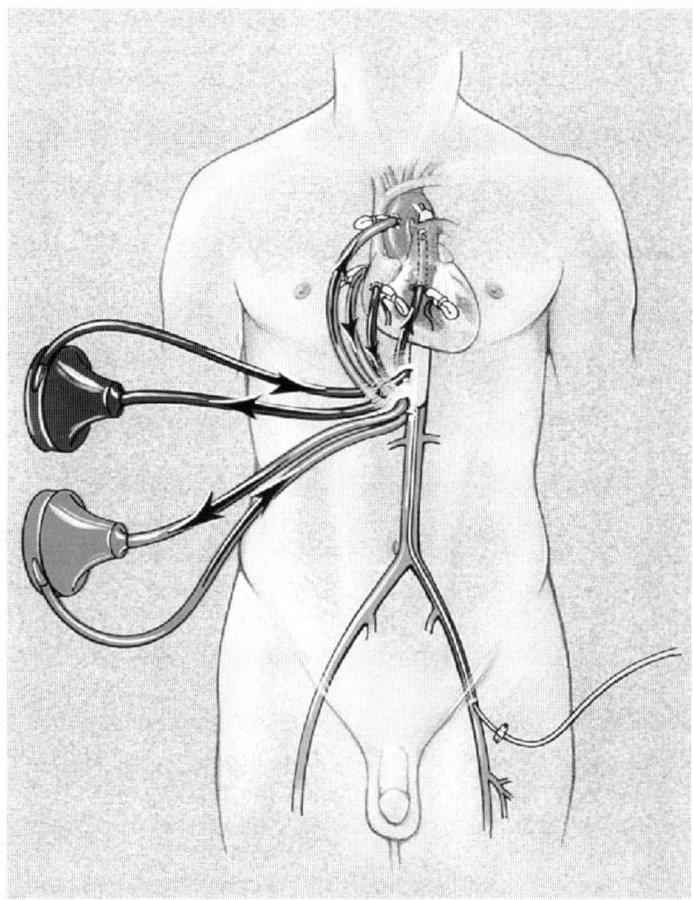

Fig. 4. Patient with a Bio-Medicus centrifugal biventricular assist device and intra-aortic balloon pump. Reproduced with permission from Noon GP, Lafuente JA, Irwin S. Acute and temporary ventricular support with bioMedicus centrifugal pump. Ann Thorac Surg 1999;68:650–654.

bypass, several cannulation sites are available: the junction of the left atrium and the superior pulmonary vein, between the superior and inferior pulmonary veins, at the left atrial appendage or dome, and at the left ventricular apex. Blood from the centrifugal pump can be returned via the ascending aorta, the aortic arch, the subclavian artery, or the femoral artery. For right-heart bypass, the right atrium can be cannulated at the appendage or at the junction of the inferior vena cava. Blood can be returned directly to the pulmonary artery or via the right ventricular outflow tract (Fig. 4).

Whichever site is selected, it is important to avoid movement at the cannulation site postoperatively to prevent bleeding. Therefore, cannulae are usually exited from the median sternotomy incision or inferior to the left or right costal margin and are secured to the skin with heavy silk sutures. The sternum is usually left open, and if the skin cannot be closed, a transparent silicone sheeting is sutured to the edges and covered by an iodophor adhesive drape.

All centrifugal pumps require anticoagulation medication for prevention of thromboembolism, one of the major hazards of these devices. If used for postcardiotomy failure, following complete reversal of heparin with protamine in the operating room, a heparin drip is begun to maintain the partial thromboplastin time between 40 and 60 s.

Centrifugal pumps were designed for short-term support. Although there has been a report of implantation for 18 d without malfunction *(5)*, these pumps usually require replacement within a median of 48 h for left ventricular assist and 83 h for right ventricular assist because the seal is disrupted within the pump head, allowing fluid to accumulate in the magnet chamber *(5)*. Patients supported with centrifugal pumps remain bedridden, usually sedated and ventilated.

The most common current indication for centrifugal pumps is postcardiotomy ventricular failure *(3,6)*. They have also been successfully used as a bridge to heart transplantation *(7)*, although because of the scarcity of donors and long waiting times, they are rarely chosen for this purpose if other devices are available. An additional indication for their use is as a short-term bridge device to one of the long-term pulsatile electric or air-driven mechanical assist devices—the so-called bridge-to-bridge indication. In this setting, centrifugal pumps may allow time to assess the patient's neurologic status and the function of other organs to determine if the patient is a candidate for cardiac transplantation. If a long-term device is not available, the patient can be maintained on the centrifugal pump while being transferred to a referral hospital.

Any comparison of clinical outcomes of centrifugal pump assistance for postcardiotomy ventricular failure from different institutions is flawed because of varying hemodynamic indications and timing of the device application. In general, 20–25% of patients who would have been perioperative fatalities can be salvaged with the centrifugal mechanical assistance *(6–8)*. Patients who survive postcardiotomy mechanical assist ultimately do reasonably well, with 82% of hospital survivors alive at 2 yr, 86% of them in NYHA class I or II *(3)*.

THE ABIOMED BVS 5000

The ABIOMED BVS 5000 is a paracorporeal pulsatile ventricular assist device capable of providing short-term left, right, or biventricular support. The device is a dual-chamber pump contained in a hard polycarbonate housing. The upper (atrial) chamber is a passive, gravity-filled reservoir and the lower (ventricular) chamber is the pumping chamber (Fig. 5). Each chamber contains a smooth polyurethane bladder. The lower pumping chamber is isolated by two polyurethane trileaflet valves, which ensure unidirectional blood flow. A compressed air driveline connects the console with the ventricular chamber. Blood drains by gravity from the atria into the upper chamber of the device, which is located on the side of the bed (Fig. 6). During pump systole, compressed air enters the device's ventricular chamber, causing the bladder to collapse and return its blood volume to the patient. During diastole, air is vented through the console allowing the ventricular bladder to fill (Fig. 5).

The BVS 5000 console is an automated, self-regulating, pulsatile support device, which operates asynchronously relative to the native heart rhythm. The console adjusts the external pump beat rate as well as the duration of diastole and systole to compensate for changes in preload and afterload. The console senses bladder filling and returns blood to the patient whenever the ventricle is full. The BVS maintains a constant stroke volume (80 mL) and can provide a maximal output of 6 L/min. A single console can operate and adjust one or two blood pumps independently.

Left-heart assistance by the BVS 5000 is achieved by cannulating the left atrium, or preferably the left ventricular apex, for inflow, and anastomosing the Dacron graft of

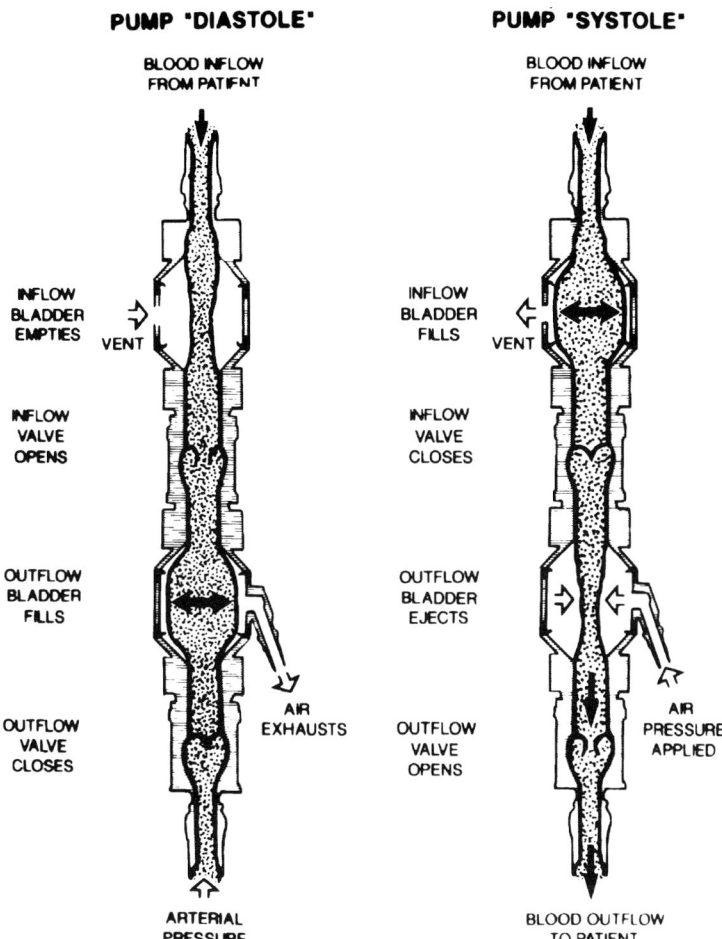

PUMP "DIASTOLE"

BLOOD INFLOW
FROM PATIENT

INFLOW
BLADDER
EMPTIES
VENT

INFLOW
VALVE
OPENS

OUTFLOW
BLADDER
FILLS

OUTFLOW
VALVE
CLOSES

AIR
EXHAUSTS

ARTERIAL
PRESSURE

PUMP "SYSTOLE"

BLOOD INFLOW
FROM PATIENT

INFLOW
BLADDER
FILLS
VENT

INFLOW
VALVE
CLOSES

OUTFLOW
BLADDER
EJECTS

OUTFLOW
VALVE
OPENS

AIR
PRESSURE
APPLIED

BLOOD OUTFLOW
TO PATIENT

Fig. 5. Schematic illustration of the ABIOMED BVS 5000 blood pump during pump systole and diastole. Reprinted with permission from ABIOMED Inc., Danvers, MA.

the outflow cannula to the anterior aspect of the ascending aorta. Right-heart assistance is achieved by cannulating the right atrium through the mid right atrial wall for inflow and anastomosing the outflow cannula to the pulmonary artery. All cannulae are externalized subcostally. Once the patient is off cardiopulmonary bypass and BVS support has been initiated, heparin is completely reversed by protamine, but reinstated later on a full anticoagulation protocol to prevent thromboembolism.

Postcardiotomy low cardiac output is the most common indication for the BVS 5000 support, comprising approximately 63% in ABIOMED's worldwide registry, which currently includes more than 3000 cases. Other forms of heart failure have also been successfully supported to recovery, including acute myocardial infarction with cardiogenic shock *(9)* and acute myocarditis *(10)*. If recovery does not occur, the BVS 5000 may be used to bridge to transplant or to another device for long-term support. It is the most commonly used device for temporary right-heart assistance when right-heart failure follows donor heart transplantation or insertion of an intracorporeal left ventricular assist device.

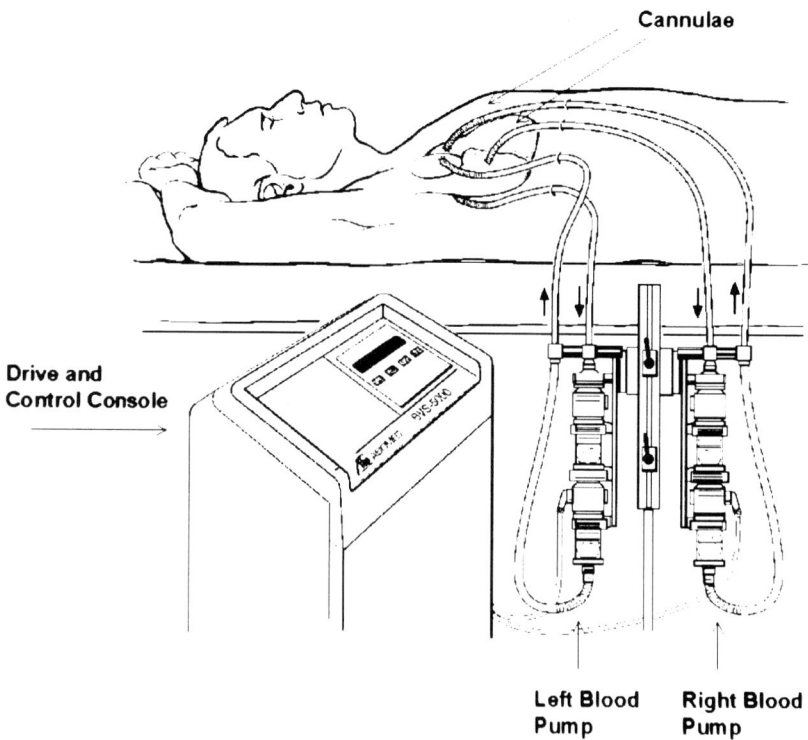

Fig. 6. ABIOMED BVS 5000 system. Reprinted with permission from ABIOMED Inc., Danvers, MA.

The ABIOMED BVS 5000 is used for a short period, with most patients being supported for 5–8 d. Patients mobility is limited and most remain bedridden.

According to the worldwide voluntary registry maintained by ABIOMED, survival is related to the indication and the type of support. Postcardiotomy patients have a 31% discharge rate compared with a 40% rate for patients with cardiomyopathy and a 33% rate for patients with acute myocardial infarction. Recipients of univentricular support have generally fared better than patients requiring biventricular support. As with all other devices, the best determinant of survival was early insertion of the device. When the device was inserted within 3 h of the decision to implant, the survival was 60%, versus 20% when device insertion was delayed. In addition, if the decision is made within 3 h, the likelihood that a left ventricular assist device will be sufficient is greater than when the decision is delayed. Complications have been most common in postcardiotomy patients. This is the result of the lengthy cardiopulmonary bypass time before the device is inserted. Cardiomyopathy patients have experienced less bleeding and other complications than postcardiotomy patients.

THE THORATEC VENTRICULAR ASSIST DEVICE

The Thoratec ventricular assist device (VAD) is the only system capable of providing long-term biventricular support, with more than 1300 patients being supported so far.

The Thoratec VAD blood pump is positioned paracorporeally on the patient's abdomen with cannulae piercing the skin below the costal margin, crossing the diaphragm, and

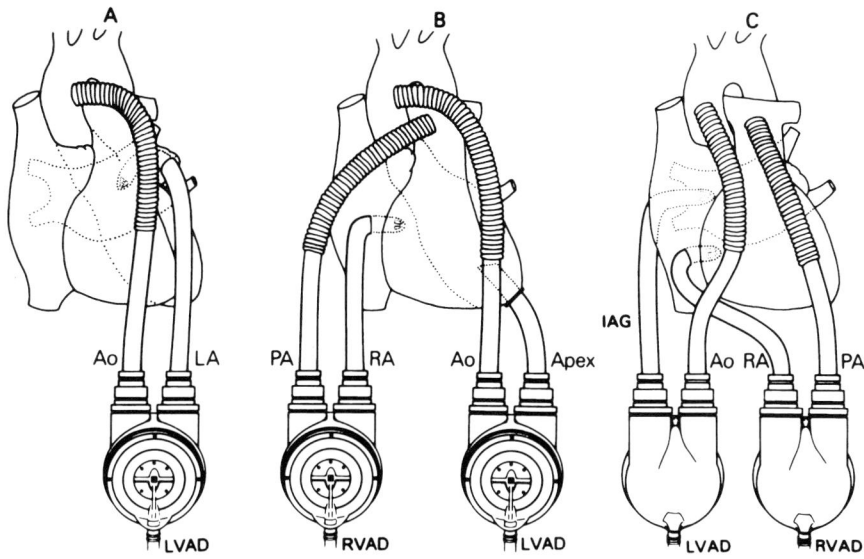

Fig. 7. Schematic illustration of the Thoratec biventricular assist device connections. Reprinted with permission from Thoratec Laboratories, Pleasanton, CA.

entering the mediastinum, where they are connected to the heart and great vessels (Fig. 7). The pump connects via a pneumatic driveline to a dual-drive console that controls and monitors the pump. The pump is made of a flexible blood sac contained within a rigid outer casing (Fig. 8). The console provides alternating positive and negative air pressures that activate the blood sac. Monostrut tilting Delrin disk mechanical valves located in the inflow and outflow ports ensure unidirectional blood flow through the device.

Left- and/or right-heart support is possible with the Thoratec VAD. The console is usually run in the volume (or fill-to-empty) mode in which the pump operates on a fixed stroke volume with a variable pump rate, producing a variable pump output. Increased pump filling causes an increase in pump rate, which results in a higher pump output.

Left-heart support with the Thoratec VAD is achieved by anastomosing the outflow cannula Dacron graft to the ascending aorta and cannulating the left atrium (dome, appendage, or interatrial groove) or left ventricular apex for inflow (Fig. 7). Right-heart support is achieved by anastomosing the outflow cannula Dacron graft to the main pulmonary artery and cannulating the right atrium for inflow (Fig. 7). After all cannulae have been brought out through the skin in the anterior abdominal wall, the blood pumps are connected to them, and following de-airing maneuvers, the console begins operating gradually as the patient is weaned off cardiopulmonary bypass. The drive console must be carefully managed to adjust diastolic vacuum, systolic duration, and driveline pressure so that pump output is optimal. Patients on the Thoratec VAD require anticoagulation therapy with warfarin.

Although the Thoratec VAD is currently the only device capable of providing long-term biventricular support, its major limitation is the restricted mobility and independence it imposes on the patient. Patients supported with the Thoratec VAD can walk throughout the hospital, but they usually cannot leave it because of the size of the con-

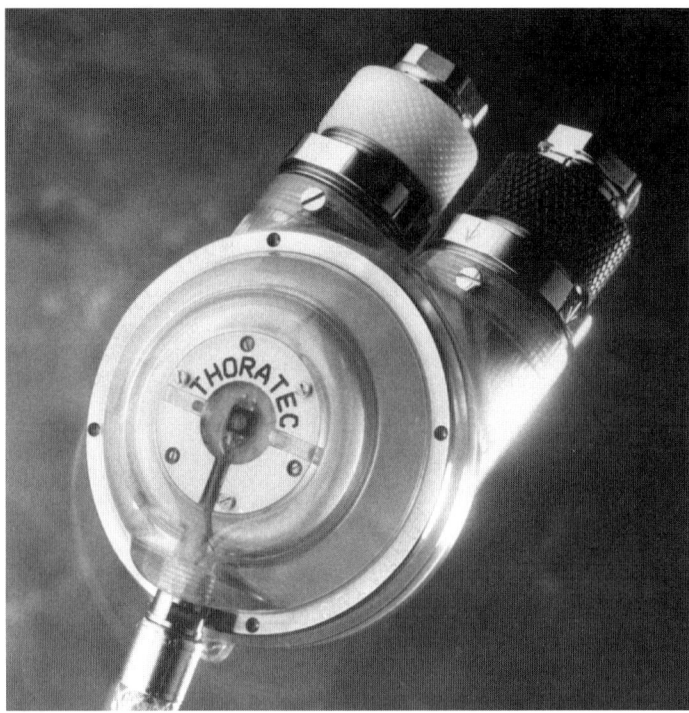

Fig. 8. The Thoratec VAD blood pump. Reprinted with permission from Thoratec Laboratories, Pleasanton, CA.

sole. Thoratec has recently developed a compact and lightweight (9.1 kg) battery or line-operated biventricular pneumatic drive unit designed to promote greater mobility and self-care. It is intended to allow the patient to exercise easily and move freely around the hospital grounds, and eventually to be discharged *(11)*. This device provides three portability options: hand-carrying the driver, using a shoulder strap, or using a small custom trolley.

The Thoratec VAD, as all other currently available VAD systems, carries the risk of infection because of the need for connecting the device transcutaneously. Compared with intracorporeal electric devices, which are precluded in small patients, the Thoratec VAD has been used in adult as well as some adolescent patients with a body surface area as low as 0.73 m². An intracorporeal version of the device is now being developed *(12)*.

The current indications for use of the Thoratec VAD are as a bridge to cardiac transplantation or as a temporary support for native heart recovery. Most patients can be successfully bridged to transplantation with an LVAD and pharmacologic support of the right ventricle. It is often not possible to predict preoperatively which patients will require biventricular assist devices. However, patients with clinically severe right-heart failure, cardiogenic shock with end-organ failure *(13,14)*, elevated pulmonary vascular resistance, and intractable ventricular arrhythmias should be considered for biventricular support. The final decision to use biventricular support can be made intraoperatively after insertion of the LVAD. The Thoratec VAD is sometimes used as a hybrid system

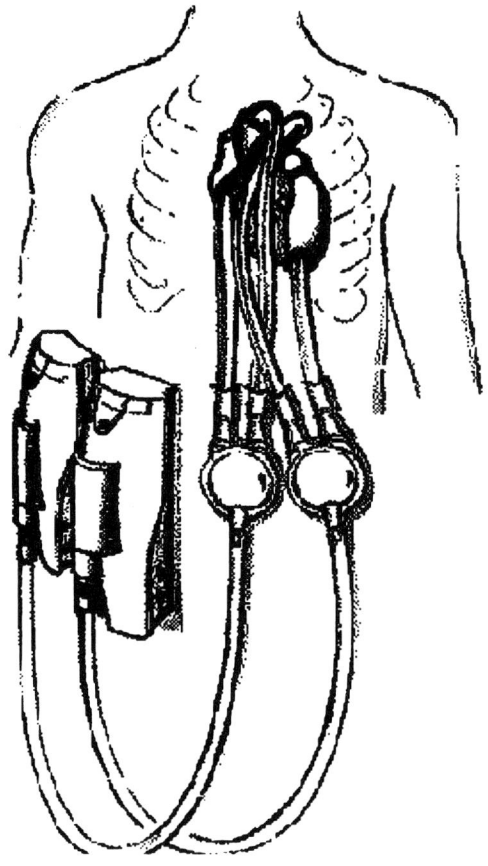

Fig. 9. The Berlin Heart biventricular assist device.

when inserted as an RVAD following right ventricular failure after implantation of an intracorporeal LVAD.

In a multicenter review *(15),* the most common complications following Thoratec VAD insertion were bleeding (42%), renal failure (36%), infection (36%), hepatic failure (24%), hemolysis (19%), respiratory failure (17%), multiorgan failure (16%), nonthromboembolic neurologic events (14%), and embolic neurologic events (8%). Another large multicenter study *(16)* showed survival to transplantation of 74% of LVAD patients and 58% of biventricular patients, with a hospital discharge rate of 89% and 81%, respectively. The Thoratec voluntary registry indicates that, as of May 2000, 60% of the 828 patients bridged to transplant underwent transplantation, with a post-transplant survival rate of 86% *(17).* Survival rates following implantation of the Thoratec VAD for postcardiotomy cardiogenic shock or other forms of cardiogenic shock are lower, ranging between 30% and 47% *(14,17).* The longest duration of support with a Thoratec LVAD has been for 515 d *(17).*

THE BERLIN HEART

The Berlin Heart assist device solves the problem of support for small children. The Berlin Heart is built very similar to the Thoratec VAD but is available in small sizes, making it a particularly suitable paracorporeal device for the pediatric population. This device is not available for use in the United States.

The Berlin Heart is a univentricular or biventricular air-driven device, with a unique three-layered flexible polyurethane blood pump membrane encased within a semirigid transparent polyurethane housing (Fig. 9). The three membranes are separated from one another with a graphite powder lubricant to minimize friction. The innermost membrane, which is the only one that comes in contact with blood, is smooth and heparin coated. The Berlin Heart blood pumps are available in 80-, 60-, 30-, 25-, and 12-mL sizes. The adult-size pumps are supplied with monoleaflet tilting disk valves (Sorin Biomedica, Turin, Italy) in the inflow and outflow sides, whereas the pediatric-size pumps are supplied with heparin-coated polyurethane trileaflet valves, marked by flat construction, which provides optimal washout behind the leaflets.

A variety of steel-reinforced silicone cannulae, available also in small diameters, enable the paracorporeal blood pump to be connected to the heart and great vessels (Fig. 9). The blood pump is operated by a variety of stationary or wearable electro-pneumatic drive units, each containing redundant drive units for safety. All drive units are equipped with rechargeable batteries to provide for patient's mobility.

The Berlin Heart implantation techniques are identical to those of the Thoratec VAD. Recently, as a left ventricular apical cannula became available, the device was implanted in several patients who had undergone previous cardiac surgery. To avoid a repeat sternotomy, the device was implanted by a left lateral thoracotomy using femo-rofemoral bypass, with the outflow graft anastomosed to the descending aorta *(18)*. Adult patients assisted by the Berlin Heart are kept on warfarin, aspirin, and dipyri-damole; pediatric patients are kept on intravenous heparin.

The largest experience with the Berlin Heart VAD has been accumulated at the Deutsches Herzzentrum Berlin *(19)*. By February 1999, the device had been implanted in 346 patients, including 34 children under the age of 16 yr. A biventricular support mode was chosen for 81%, isolated left ventricular support for 17%, and isolated right ventricular support for 2%. The main indications for support were bridge to transplant (59%), postcardiotomy heart failure (15%), and posttransplantation cardiac dysfunc-tion (9%). The overall mean duration of support was 63 d, and the current longest sup-port period was 525 d on biventricular assistance. Of the adult patients bridged to transplant, 52% underwent transplantation and 74% of those were discharged. Of the 34 children assisted with the Berlin Heart (aged between 6 d and 16 yr, mean 7.5 yr), 19 (56%) were taken off the device either after complete cardiac recovery or at the time of transplantation. Of the 14 transplanted children, 10 were discharged.

Intracorporeal Assist Systems

Currently there are two approved intracorporeal assist systems:

1. The HeartMate LVAD (Thoratec Corporation, formerly Thermo Cardiosystems Inc., Woburn, MA)
2. The Novacor LVAD (WorldHeart, Ottawa, Ontario, Canada)

The HeartMate LVAD

The HeartMate LVAD is an implantable pulsatile blood pump that is available in pneumatically driven (implantable pneumatic, or IP) or electrically powered (vented electric, or VE) (Fig. 10) models. More than 2300 devices have been implanted since

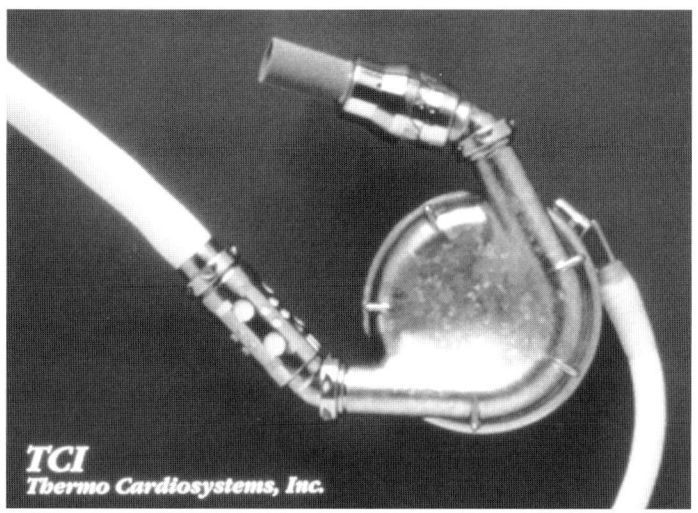

Fig. 10. The HeartMate vented electric (VE) left ventricular assist device. Reprinted with permission from Thermo Cardiosystems, Inc., Wobourn, MA.

1986, establishing its current position as one of the major cornerstones in long-term, often out-of-hospital, left ventricular assistance.

Both models of the HeartMate are fabricated from sintered titanium and house a flexible, textured, polyurethane diaphragm bound to a rigid pusher-plate. In the IP model, the pusher-plate is activated pneumatically from a portable external console; in the VE model, the pusher-plate is activated by a low-speed torque motor that drives a pair of nested helical cams. A single, two-channeled, velour-covered driveline extends from the implanted LVAD, through the skin, to the external environment (Fig. 11). In the IP model, one of the channels contains an electric cable conveying performance data to the bedside console, whereas the other transfers the air. In the VE model, one of the driveline channels contains the electric cable from the portable battery pack to the motor, whereas the other acts as an air vent, allowing air transfer in and out of the motor chamber to maintain it near-atmospheric conditions.

A unique property of the HeartMate is the design of the blood-contacting portions. The titanium housing incorporates titanium microspheres and the flexible diaphragm is covered with textured polyurethane, both promoting the adherence of cellular blood elements and the formation of a pseudointimal layer, leading to an exceptionally low thromboembolic risk *(20)*. Both models of the HeartMate are equipped with inflow and outflow porcine xenograft valves. Both models can generate a maximum stroke volume of 85 mL and a maximum pump output of 11 L/min. They are usually operated in an automatic mode, in which the eject cycle begins only after the pump is at least 90% filled. The VE model, with its wearable two-battery pack, provides patients with 6–8 h of untethered activity.

Most HeartMate LVADs were implanted in a preperitoneal pocket behind the left rectus abdominis posterior sheath. Some centers prefer the intra-abdominal placement, although internal organ erosions, bowel obstruction, and intra-abdominal adhesions have made this approach less favorable. Following preparation of the

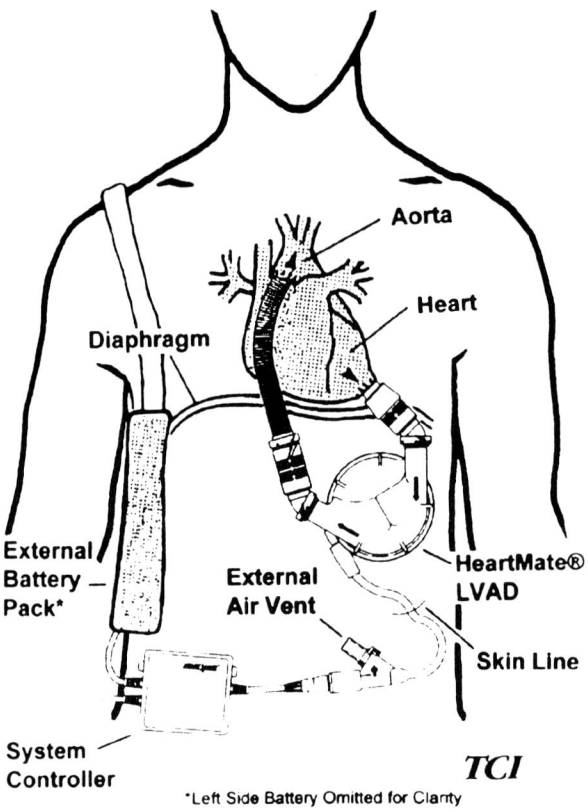

Fig. 11. Schematic illustration of the implanted HeartMate VE LVAS. Reprinted with permission from Thermo Cardiosystems, Inc., Wobourn, MA.

preperitoneal pocket, the patient is placed on cardiopulmonary bypass and an apical silicone cuff is sewn to the left ventricular apex, which has been cored out by a circular coring knife. The LVAD is brought into its pocket, tunneling its driveline subcutaneously to exit in the right mid- to upper-quadrant area. The pump inflow cannula is then brought through the diaphragm and inserted through the apical cuff. The outflow Dacron graft is anastomosed to the right lateral surface of the ascending aorta, and following meticulous de-airing maneuvers, the outfow graft is screwed to the pump outflow port (Fig. 11). As the cardiopulmonary bypass is weaned, the device is activated first in a slow fixed mode, to be replaced by the automatic mode when the hemodynamic status stabilizes.

Patients assisted by the HeartMate LVAD are maintained on aspirin alone, with no need for anticoagulation. Patients implanted with the HeartMate VE experience a significant improvement in quality of life during LVAD support, as many of them are discharged from the hospital while on the device and can return to their families and their work or school activities (Fig. 12).

The HeartMate LVAD is usually used as a bridge to transplantation. As such, any contraindication to transplantation negates candidacy for this device. Incidence of right-heart failure and the need for temporary RVAD assistance following HeartMate

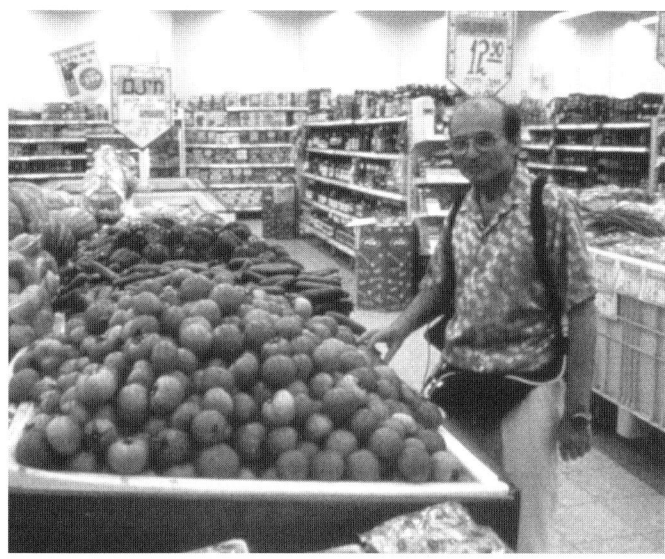

Fig. 12. Our first HeartMate VE LVAS recipient, bridged to heart transplantation for 350 d, spent more than 300 d at home, leading normal daily activities.

LVAD implantation have been greatly reduced since the introduction of routine inhaled nitric oxide *(21)*. Preoperative low pulmonary artery pressure and low right ventricular stroke work index have been shown to be significant risk factors for RVAD use *(22)*. The following predictive factors have been shown to be associated with perioperative mortality: oliguria (urine output <30 mL), elevated central venous pressure (>16 mm Hg), need for mechanical ventilation, elevated prothrombin time (>16 s), and prior mediastinal operation *(23)*.

According to the last reported data from the Thermo Cardiosystems Worldwide Registry on September 2000, 65% of the 2265 patients implanted with the HeartMate IP or VE survived implantation, 63% underwent transplantation, and 2% recovered native heart function and had the device explanted. Infections, the Achilles' heel of all devices, have always been one of the major causes of failure with this device *(24,25)*. More than 250 patients were supported with the device for over 6 mo, and more than 60 patients were supported for over 1 yr. Some patients were supported for over 2 yr, which sparked interest in the device as an alternative to transplantation, leading to the aforementioned REMATCH trial *(2)*.

THE NOVACOR LVAD

The Novacor LVAD was the first electrically powered implantable assist device; since its first human use at the Stanford University Medical Center in 1984, more than 1000 patients have been supported by it worldwide.

The Novacor LVAD blood pump (Fig. 13) is made of a smooth polyurethane sac activated by a pulsed solenoid energy converter motor, which activates two identical pivoted pusher-plates. Inflow and outflow porcine valves maintain unidirectional blood flow through knitted, gelatin-sealed Vascutek inflow and outflow grafts. A percuta-

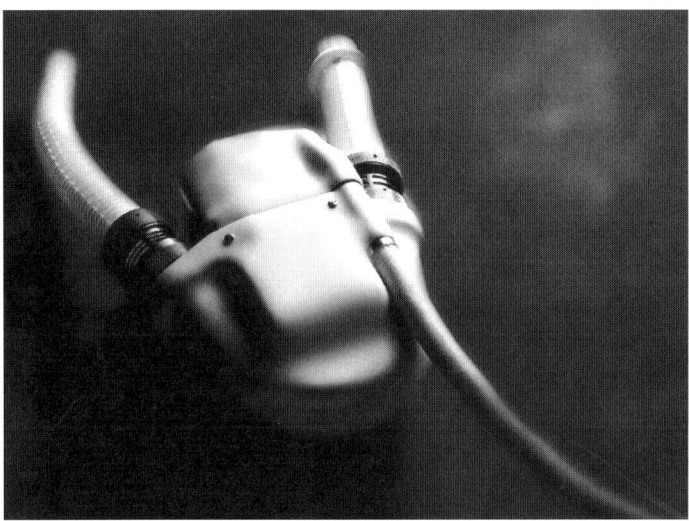

Fig. 13. The Novacor left ventricular assist device. Reprinted with permission from WorldHeart Corporation, Ottawa, Ontario, Canada.

neous vent tube, containing power and control leads, connects the internalized blood pump to an extracorporeal electronic control and wearable batteries.

Implantation technique of the Novacor LVAD is very similar to that of the Heart-Mate (Fig. 14), with the pump usually implanted in a preperitoneal pocket behind the left rectus muscle. The device's vent tube is tunneled subcutaneously and exits midway between the right costal margin and the anterosuperior iliac crest. The need for temporary RVAD assistance following implantation of the Novacor LVAD has been reduced to less than 6% since the introduction of inhaled nitric oxide *(21)*. Patients assisted by the Novacor LVAD are usually maintained on warfarin and aspirin. Novacor-assisted patients can be discharged from the hospital and can return home to normal daily activities, allowing for a better quality of life while awaiting transplantation.

The recent results of the global experience with the Novacor LVAD, comprising 1040 implants, show that the device was used as a bridge to transplant in 93.4% of the patients, as a bridge to recovery in 4.3%, and as an alternative to transplant in 2.3%. Half of the patients were supported for more than 6 mo, with mean duration of 254 d. The longest support was for over 4 yr, the longest time that any recipient has lived with continuous support from a heart assist device.

A high incidence of embolic stroke, ranging between 21% with the previously used woven, unsupported Cooley grafts, and 12% with the newer knitted, gelatin-sealed, supported Vascutek grafts, has always been one of the major disadvantages of the Novacor LVAD *(26,27)*. In contrast, an excellent reliability record, with only 0.8% pump replacements, has been one of its virtues.

In a US multicenter bridge-to-transplant study including 156 Novacor LVAD recipients, 73% were successfully bridged to transplant *(26)*. In a single center (Deutches Herzzentrum in Berlin) experience with the Novacor LVAD as a bridge to recovery for 23 patients, stable cardiac recovery occurred in 13 patients for 3–49 mo. Three patients

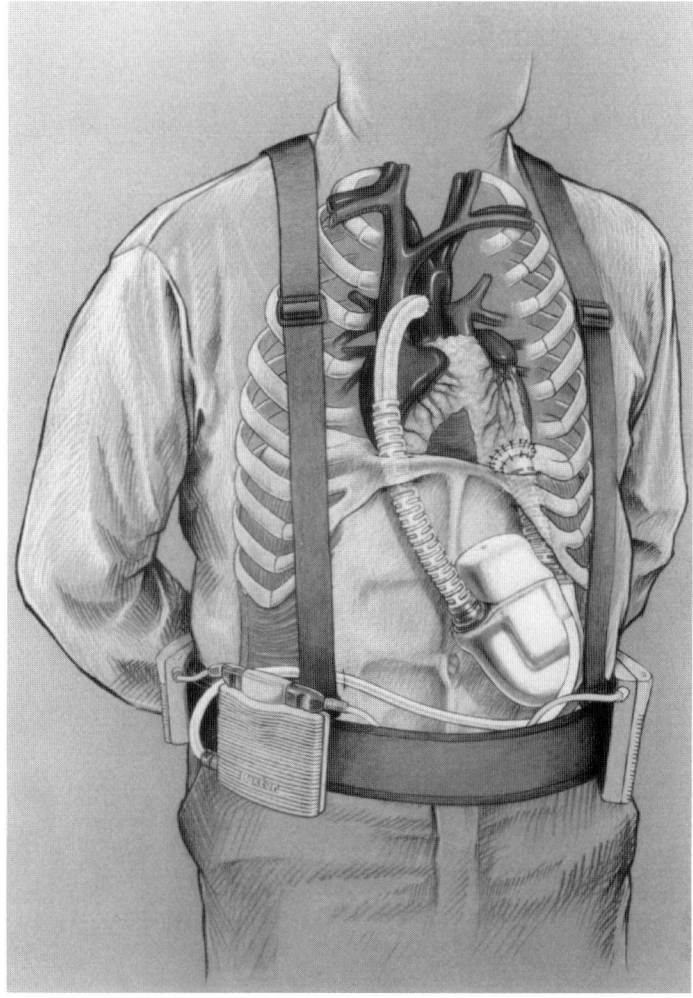

Fig. 14. Schematic illustration of the implanted Novacor LVAS. Reprinted with permission from WorldHeart Corporation, Ottawa, Ontario, Canada.

died of noncardiac causes within a period of 4 mo and 3 d after removal of the assist device. Seven patients had recurrent cardiac failure after 4–24 mo; transplantation was performed in six of them and 1 died while on the waiting list *(28)*. As yet, there are insufficient data to determine the viability of this form of therapy.

The CardioWest Total Artificial Heart

The total artificial heart (TAH) was first used at the University of Utah in 1982 as the Jarvik-7 TAH *(29),* followed for several years as the Symbion TAH; its use was halted in 1991 following loss of its investigational device exemption because of a high incidence of morbidity and mortality. Since 1993, a new investigational device exemption study was begun at the University Medical Center in Tucson, Arizona with the Cardio West TAH (Cardio West Technologies, Inc.), and a multicenter trial was undertaken.

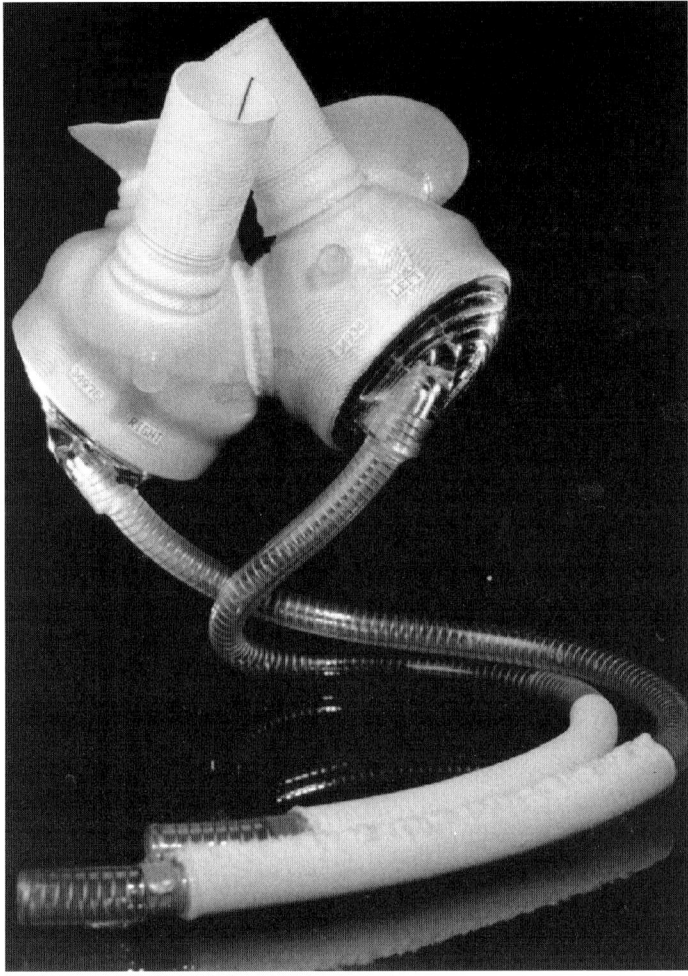

Fig. 15. CardioWest total artificial heart. Reproduced from ref. *30* with permission.

The CardioWest TAH (Fig. 15) is a pneumatic biventricular pump that is implanted in the orthotopic position. It consists of two ventricles connected to the native atria and great vessels. A velour-covered air driveline passes from each of the ventricles transcutaneously to a large console that pulses pressurized air and monitors pump function (Fig. 16). Each ventricle consists of a spherical polyurethane chamber, half of it immobile, anchored to the chamber rigid wall and half of it a mobile four-layered diaphragm. Pulses of air pressure from the console push the diaphragm and, thus, blood is ejected from the chamber. Vacuum added to the device in diastole improves ventricular filling at low venous pressures. Medtronic–Hall mechanical valves located at the inflow and outflow of each chamber provide for unidirectional blood flow. Specialized cuffs anastomosed to the native atria allow for quick connection of the ventricles, whereas Dacron outflow grafts connect to the great vessels. The maximal blood volume of each of the chambers is 70 mL, and the cardiac output is generally between 6 and 8 L/min.

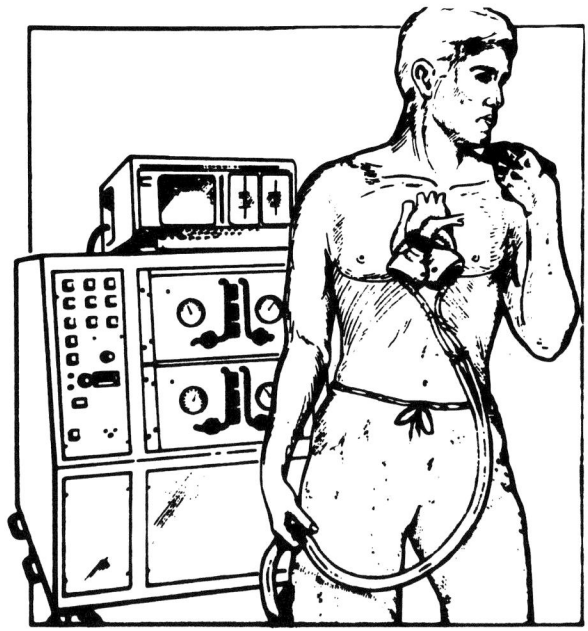

Fig. 16. Schematic illustration of a CardioWest total artificial heart recipient. Reproduced from ref. *30* with permission.

Because of the considerable size of the implanted CardioWest TAH, adherence to stringent fitting criteria must be followed in order to prevent bad outcomes. Patients with a body surface area less than 1.7 m², thin chests, or cardiothoracic ratio less than 0.5 are at increased risk of inferior vena cava or left pulmonary vein compression.

Implantation starts with a total cardiectomy, leaving behind maximal length of the great vessels and the two atria, which are cut at the atrioventricular groove *(30)*. The atrial quick connector cuffs are anastomosed to each of the two native atria, followed by end-to-end anastomosis of the two outflow grafts to the aorta and pulmonary artery. Next, the atrial connector of the left ventricle is snapped onto the left atrial quick connector, the ventricle is filled with saline, and the aortic connection is made. A similar approach is made with the right ventricle. After de-airing, console pumping is started and the patient is rapidly weaned off cardiopulmonary bypass. The device's two air drivelines are tunneled to the left epigastrium.

Patients on the Cardio West TAH are maintained on warfarin, aspirin, dipyridamole, and pentoxyphylline (Trental). These patients need to be permanently tethered to a large console, which makes out-of-hospital existence impractical; walking within the confines of the hospital is possible for short periods with battery power and air tanks.

Current indication for use of the CardioWest TAH is as a bridge to transplant in patients with rapid decompensation involving biventricular failure unresponsive to maximal medical therapy *(13,31)*.

A US national trial of the CardioWest TAH *(31)* showed that of 27 patients supported for an average of 52 d (range 12–186 d), 93% underwent heart transplantation and 89% were discharged home. The most common source of morbidity was infection in 90% of the patients, but in only 10% was it considered serious. No fatal neurologic events occurred, although nonserious neurologic events included nine transient ischemic attacks, three seizures, two episodes of impaired state of consciousness, one retinal hemorrhage, one retinal embolus, and one cerebrovascular accident. Internationally, there have been 175 implants with a 65% transplantation rate and 88% discharge rate for transplanted patients *(32)*.

FUTURE DEVICES

A survey of the existing mechanical alternatives to the human heart would not be complete without a short glimpse at alternatives that are in the pipeline, some of which are undergoing preliminary clinical investigation. One or more of the following devices will probably dominate the future of mechanical heart assistance or even permanent replacement:

1. Axial flow pumps
2. The LionHeart left ventricular assist system (Arrow International Inc., Reading, PA)
3. Penn State University total artificial heart (Abiomed, Danvers, MA)
4. The AbioCor total artificial heart (Abiomed, Danvers, MA)
5. The HeartSaver ventricular assist device (WorldHeart Corp., Ottawa, Ontario, Canada)

Axial Flow Pumps

The cumulative experience with the various pulsatile systems has highlighted their lack of long-term durability resulting from the need for moving flexible diaphragms and unidirectional valves. Hence, research has focused on producing axial nonpulsatile flow devices that would contain a single moving part and be valveless and, therefore, be potentially more durable and suitable for chronic ventricular assistance. Long-term support with axial flow pumps in various animal models has failed to demonstrate significant clinical, biochemical, or microscopic end-organ damage for up to 6 mo of nonpulsatile support *(33,34)*.

Three axial blood flow pumps are currently undergoing preliminary clinical investigation:

1. Jarvik 2000 Ventricular Assist System (Jarvik Heart, Inc., New York, NY)
2. HeartMate II Left Ventricular Assist System (Thoratec Corporation, Woburn, MA)
3. The MicroMed-DeBakey Ventricular Assist Device (MicroMed Technology, Inc., Houston, TX)

THE JARVIK 2000 VAD

This is an axial flow pump, measuring 2.5 cm in diameter and 5.5 cm in length and weighing 90 g (Fig. 17). The pump's only moving part is the impeller, which is housed in a titanium casing and is supported by ceramic bearings that are immersed in the bloodstream. The impeller is activated at a fixed rate of 8000–12,000 rpm by an electromagnetic field across the motor air gap through which the blood flows, delivering a blood flow of 3–8 L/min, depending on the systemic vascular resistance. The device is implanted, through a left thoracotomy, inside the left ventricle via its apex, with the outflow Dacron graft anastomosed to the descending aorta (Fig. 18). Power is supplied through a small cable, which passes from the device to the apex of the chest, then through the neck to a titanium pedestal screwed into the skull behind the mastoid

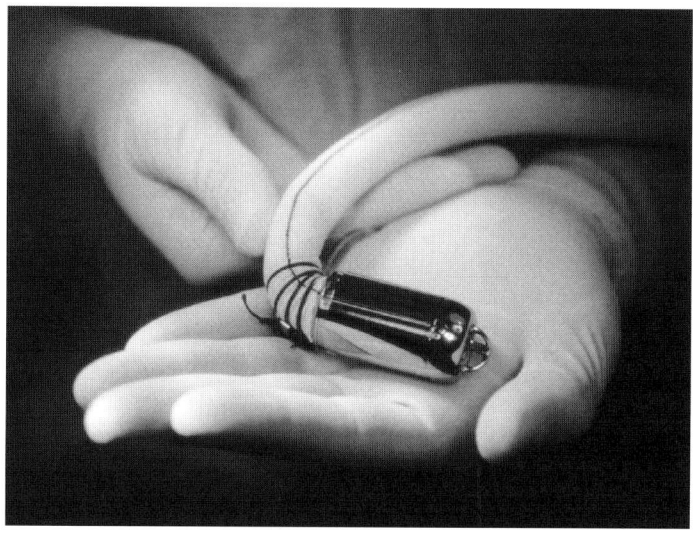

Fig. 17. The Jarvik 2000 ventricular assist device.

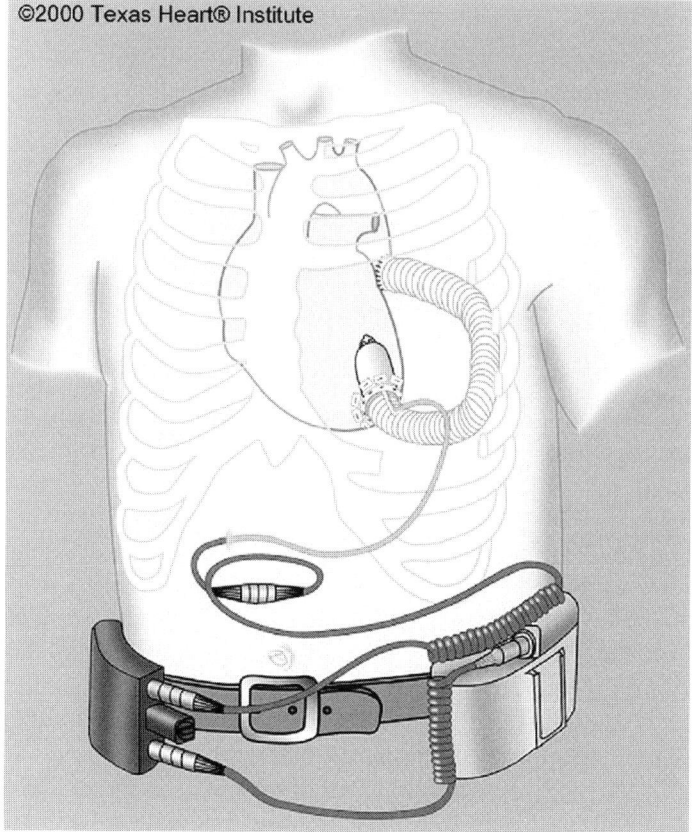

Fig. 18. Schematic illustration of the implanted Jarvik 2000 VAD.

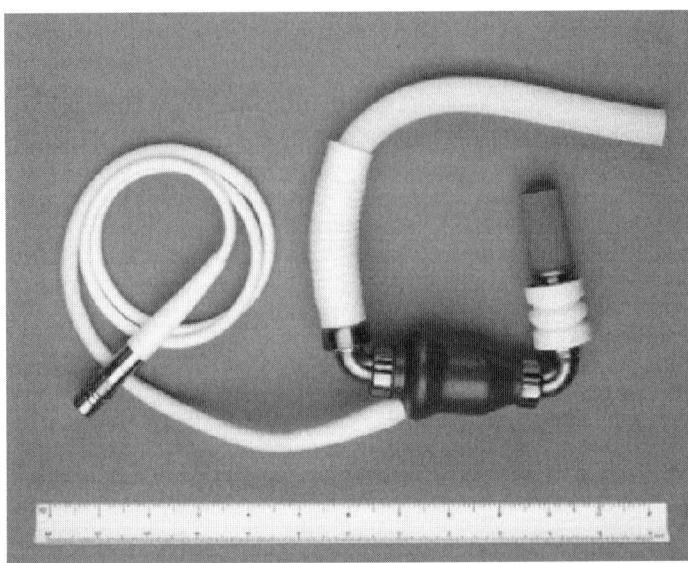

Fig. 19. The HeartMate II left ventricular assist system. Reprinted with permission from Thermo Cardiosystems, Inc., Woburn, MA.

process. This percutaneous pedestal transmits the cable to an external portable controller and battery, both of which are worn unobtrusively on the patient's belt or waistcoat.

Fourteen human implantations of the Jarvik 2000 VAD have been performed so far, in 10 patients at the Texas Heart Institute as a bridge to transplantation and in four patients in Europe as a permanent device. The first implantation took place on April 2000, and involved a 52-yr-old female in whom the device was successfully implanted for 79 d as a bridge to transplantation *(35)*. Seven of the 10 bridged patients were transplanted and six of them were discharged home. The longest duration on the device so far has been for 214 d. On June 2000, at the Oxford Heart Center, a 61-yr-old man with end-stage congestive heart failure due to idiopathic dilated cardiomyopathy received the device as an alternative to heart transplantation, and was discharged home *(36)*. One additional patient who received the Jarvik 2000 VAD as an alternative to transplantation was also discharged home, one patient died, and one is waiting to be discharged.

THE HEARTMATE II LVAS

This device, developed jointly by Nimbus Inc. and the University of Pittsburgh *(37)*, is an electromagnetically driven, axial flow, rotary blood pump. Measuring 2.5 cm in diameter and 4 cm in length and weighing 370 g (Fig. 19), this titanium device incorporates a high-speed rotor whose integral vanes create a blood vortex that accelerates the blood using axial and centrifugal force (Fig. 20). Operating at up to 12,000 rpm, the device is capable of producing over 10 L/min flow.

One feature of the pump is that a decrease in pressure difference between the pump inlet and outlet results in a significant increase in flow. Thus, at any set speed of the pump, small pulsations from the left ventricle will be magnified, amplifying pulsatile blood flow. The textured surface of the sintered titanium technology used in the Heart-

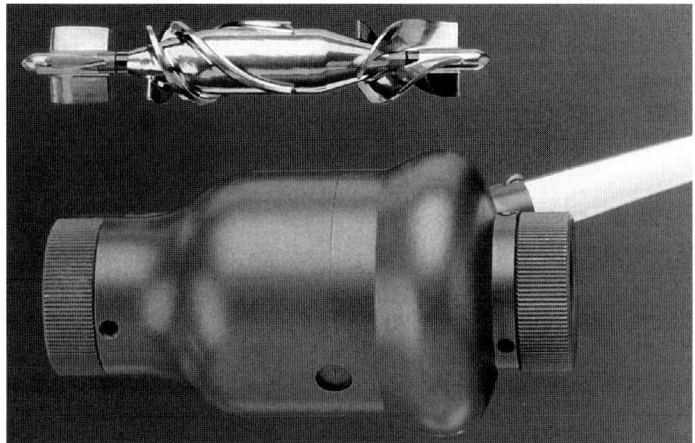

Fig. 20. The HeartMate II LVAS and its rotor. Reprinted with permission from Thermo Cardiosystems, Inc., Wobourn, MA.

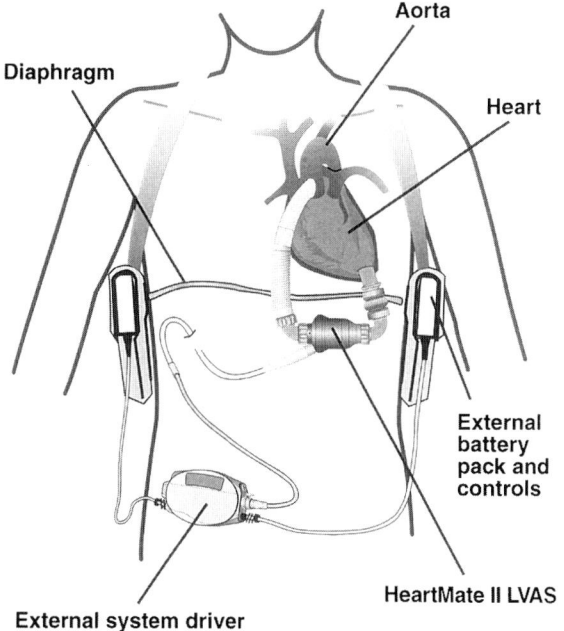

Fig. 21. Schematic illustration of the implanted HeartMate II LVAS. Reprinted with permission from Thermo Cardiosystems, Inc., Woburn, MA.

Mate I devices to reduce thromboembolic risk is also used in all blood-contacting surfaces of the HeartMate II.

The device is implanted in a small preperitoneal pocket, draining blood from the left ventricular apex via a rigid inlet cannula and ejecting into the aortic root via an outflow graft (Fig. 21). The power and control of the pump are delivered through a thin electrical cable that exits the skin on the right abdomen and connects to wearable batteries and system driver (Fig. 21). An animal-tested transcutaneous energy transmission sys-

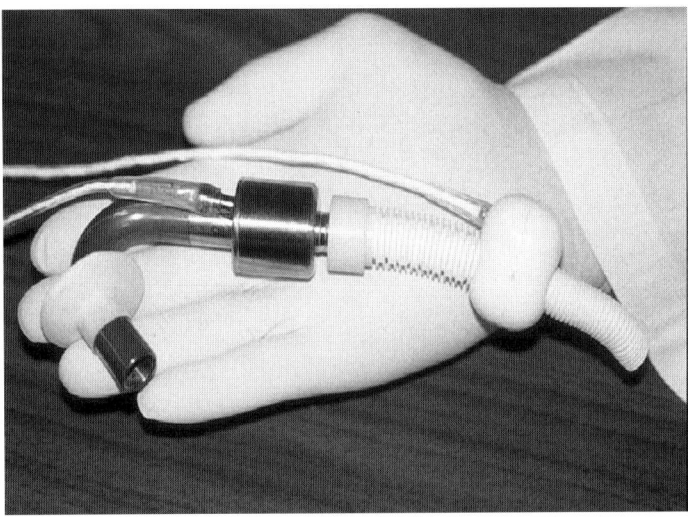

Fig. 22. The Micromed-DeBakey ventricular assist device. Reprinted with permission from MicroMed Technology, Inc., Houston, TX.

tem will eliminate, in the future, the current need to perforate the skin and thus minimize the risk of infection.

We performed the first human implant of the HeartMate II LVAS at the Sheba Medical Center in Israel on July 2000 *(37)*. This implant marked the start of a multinational study aimed at evaluating the efficacy and safety of the device in patients at risk of imminent death from refractory end-stage heart failure. A 64-yr-old man suffering from end-stage heart failure resulting from ischemic cardiomyopathy was implanted with the device because a prostate malignancy precluded heart transplantation. The device functioned flawlessly for 4 d before the patient succumbed to irreversible pulmonary hypertension causing severe right-heart failure. Five more patients were since implanted in Europe. Two implantations of the device at the Heart and Diabetes Center in Bad Oeynhausen, Germany, were also unsuccessful and terminated with the patients death due to multiorgan failure or sudden cardiac arrest, one patient was transplanted after 33 d, one patient, implanted by Prof. Magdi Yacoub at the Harefield Hospital in England, recoverd the use of his natural heart after 156 d of support on the device, and the sixth patient is still ongoing.

The MicroMed-DeBakey VAD

This is an axial flow pump measuring 3.5 cm in diameter, 7.6 cm in length, and weighing 93 g (Fig. 22). An electromagnetic motor stator drives the six-bladed impeller, which is housed within a titanium tube, at speeds of 7500–12,500 rpm. An inflow cannula connects the device to the left ventricular apex and a flow probe-fitted Dacron outflow graft connects the pump to the ascending aorta (Fig. 23). The electric cable, which traverses the skin at the right lower abdomen, connects the pump to an external wearable controller, which provides energy to the device from the clinical data acquisition system (CDAS) or batteries (Fig. 23). The CDAS receives measurements of pump speed, flow,

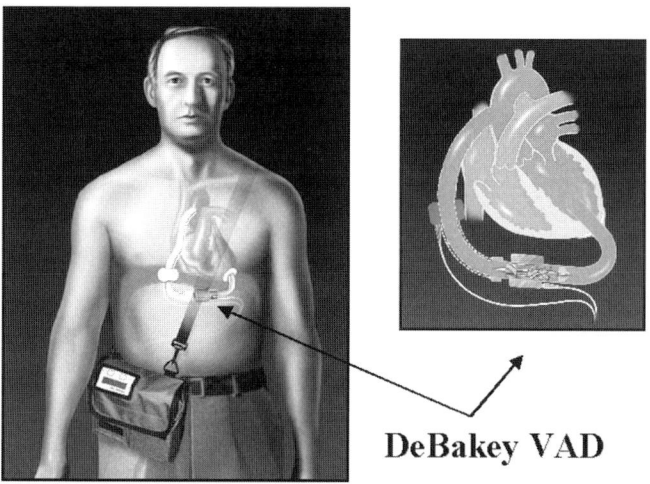

DeBakey VAD

Fig. 23. Schematic illustration of the implanted Micromed-DeBakey VAD. Reprinted with permission from MicroMed Technology, Inc., Houston, TX.

power, and current signals from the controller and is also used to adjust the pump speed while the patient is in the hospital. The MicroMed-DeBakey VAD is implanted in a preperitoneal abdominal pocket via a mid-sternotomy incision.

As reported by Noon et al. *(38)*, one of the device's coinventors, as of September 2000, 51 patients have been implanted with the MicroMed-DeBakey VAD in 12 European centers and at the Methodist Hospital in Houston, Texas. All implants were done as a bridge to transplantation. Fourteen patients have undergone successful transplantations. The principal complication has been late bleeding, with most events occurring more than 5 d after the implantation. Some incidences of hemolysis have also been observed, but there have been no device-related infections. In a small number of patients, a pump thrombus or embolus has affected pump function, requiring pump exchange or outflow graft ligation to prevent regurgitant flow.

LionHeart LVAS

The LionHeart completely implanted LVAS, developed at the Pennsylvania State College of Medicine, is designed for use as long-term destination therapy for patients with progressive, irreversible, end-stage congestive heart failure for which heart transplantation is not an option *(39)*. It is not intended as a bridge to transplant or as a bridge to recovery of ventricular function. The electrically powered blood pump is implanted in the preperitoneal space beneath the left costal margin (Fig. 24). The blood pump features a motor, a pusher-plate mechanism, a smooth blood sac, and two tilting disk valves for unidirectional flow. The blood pump is connected to the native circulation via a left ventricular apical inlet and an aortic outlet cannula.

Percutaneous drivelines and external tethers can be eliminated by a transcutaneous energy transmission system implanted under the anterior chest wall, which delivers power by induction from wearable batteries (Fig. 24). Rechargeable implanted batter-

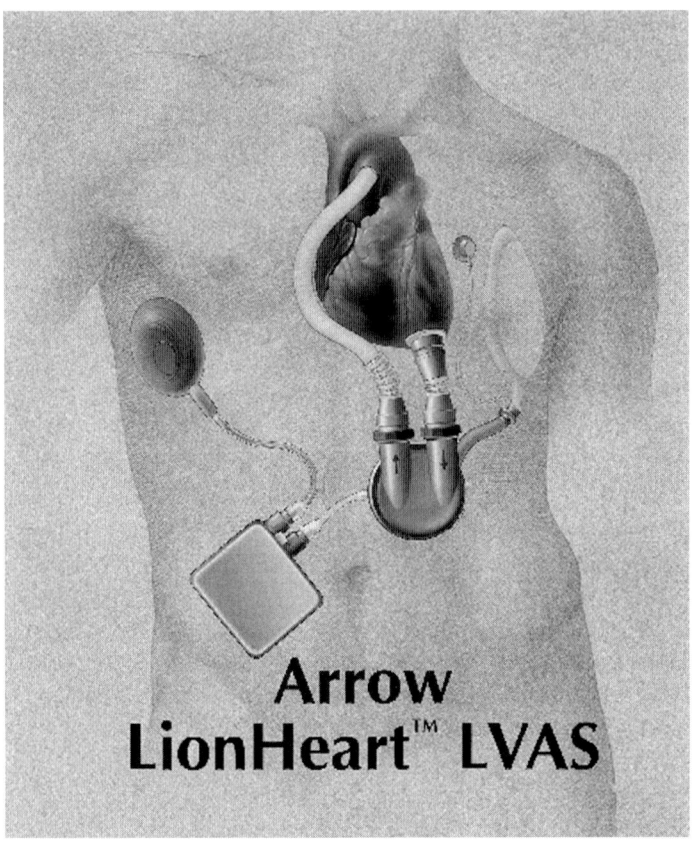

Fig. 24. The LionHeart fully implantable left ventricular assist system. Reprinted with permission from Arrow International, Inc., Reading, PA.

ies allow patients to be untethered for approximately 20 min. An implantable motor controller is placed under the anterior abdominal wall in the preperitoneal space, beneath the right costal margin. Finally, a compliance chamber, approachable by an access port, serves as a gas-volume accumulator, providing gas to evacuated chambers of the blood pump during its operation and eliminating the need for a vent tube. The compliance chamber is placed in the left pleural space and is periodically charged with room air via the access port, which is passed through the intercostal space and located in the subcutaneous tissue over the left anterior chest wall (Fig. 24).

The first human implant of the LionHeart LVAS occurred in October 1999 at the Heart and Diabetes Center in Bad Oeynhausen, Germany. This patient had a stroke early on, but has recovered and is living at home with the device continuing to function as expected. As of January 2001, 10 patients had been implanted with the device as part of an ongoing European clinical investigation to demonstrate the safety and performance of the device. Six patients have died of multiorgan failure and four are at home. There has been no significant pump or controller dysfunction (personal communication, Benjamin C. Sun, MD, Pennsylvania State University).

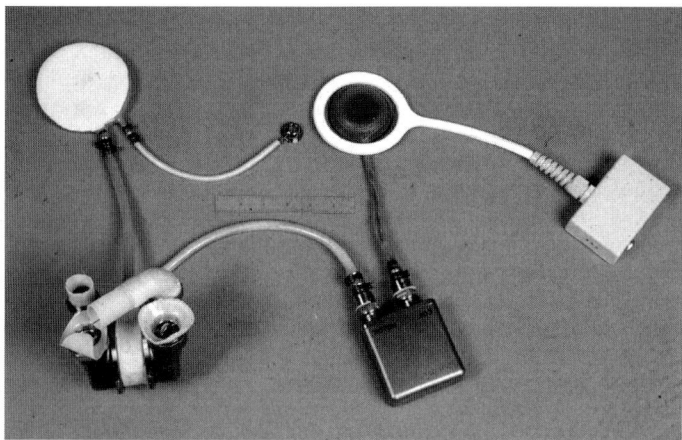

Fig. 25. The Penn State University total artificial heart. Reprinted with permission from Abiomed, Danvers, MA.

Pennsylvania State University Total Artificial Heart (BeneCor)

The Pennsylvania State University (PSU) TAH is an electrically driven pump with no percutaneous connections. The pump's titanium casing encloses two polyurethane blood sacs separated by a central energy converter, including a motor, which activates a roller screw with pusher-plates at either end. Mechanical compression of the blood sacs against the rigid housing is induced by the pusher-plates and results in alternate emptying of the blood sacs. Unidirectional blood flow is maintained by Delrin monostrut valves located at the inlet and outlet connectors of each pumping chamber. The remaining device components include an implantable controller, rechargeable batteries, and telemetry hardware, all encased in a single electronics canister, as well as an implantable compliance chamber (Fig. 25). Power is supplied by a transcutaneous transmission of energy from externally wearable batteries. The implanted batteries can provide up to 45 min of totally untethered activity. The PSU TAH is implanted in an orthotopic position following total cardiectomy, which leaves behind the native atria and the great vessels. Animal implants and durability studies are ongoing, with clinical implants planned to commence in 2002 *(40)*.

AbioCor Total Artificial Heart

The AbioCor TAH is a fully implantable device, intended to serve as an alternative to heart transplantation, consisting of two blood sacs encased within a titanium housing, separated by an electric motor that drives the centrifugal pumping system *(41)* (Fig. 26). The blood sacs, as well as the four unidirectional valves incorporated in the device, are made of Angioflex, a proprietary polyurethane material. An internal controller regulates power delivered to the prosthetic heart. Without penetrating the skin, an external unit transmits power to the internal unit using transcutaneous energy transmission. A rechargeable internal battery will allow the patient to be completely free of the external power transmission unit for 30 min. The system is designed to increase or decrease its pump rate in response to the body's needs. The first human implant of the AbioCor TAH took place on July 2, 2001 at the Jewish Hospital in

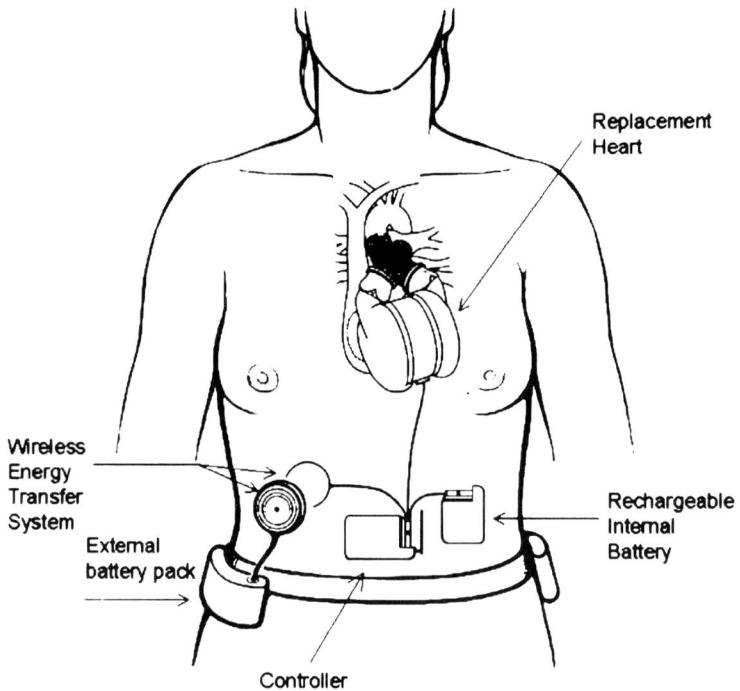

Replacement
Heart

Wireless
Energy
Transfer
System

External
battery pack

Rechargeable
Internal
Battery

Controller

Fig. 26. The AbioCor fully implantable total artificial heart. Reprinted with permission from Abiomed, Danvers, MA.

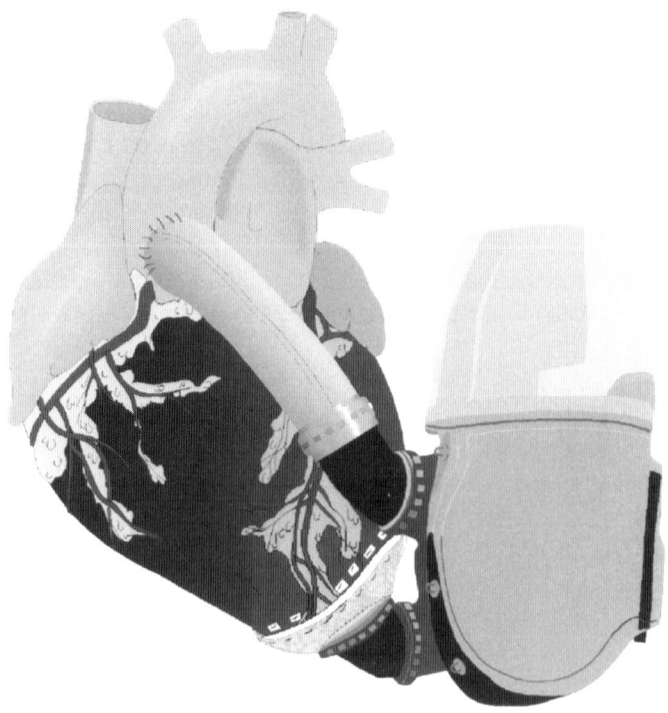

Fig. 27. The HeartSaver fully implantable ventricular assist device. Reprinted with permission from WorldHeart Corporation, Ottawa, Ontario, Canada.

Louisville, Kentucky. The patient, a 59-yr-old male, who has been rapidly deteriorating from severe end-stage ischemic heart disease, was implanted with the TAH after being considered as unsuitable for heart transplantation. The highly publicized patient who has been living with the AbioCor TAH making good progress overall and enjoying a relatively high quality of life, making frequent trips outside the hospital and beginning to improve his ability to eat, has suffered a major stroke 135 d after the implantation. Five months after the implantation the patient died of complications due to gastrointestinal bleeding. So far five more patients were implanted with the AbioCor TAH. One of them died intra-operatively secondary to uncontrolled bleeding due to coagulopathy, and the other four are reported to make good progress although still hospitalized.

HeartSaver VAD

The HeartSaver VAD, developed at the University of Ottawa Heart Institute, is a unique heart-assist device that will be fully implantable in the left hemithorax for long-term use. The device's key features include the incorporation of the controller and the hydraulic fluid volume displacement chamber into the implanted unit, which also includes the blood chamber and the electrohydraulic axial flow pump (Fig. 27). The device will be remotely powered, monitored, and controlled using transcutaneous energy transfer and biotelemetry technologies. The device has a unique shape that follows the contour of the chest wall and connects via short conduits, equipped with porcine valves, to the apex of the left ventricle and to the ascending aorta. Following successful long-term in vitro and in vivo studies in calves *(42),* the initial clinical use of the HeartSaver VAD is planned for 2001.

CONCLUSION

Since 1963, when the first intrathoracic LVAD was implanted in a patient *(43),* major technological advances have been made in the field of mechanical alternatives to the failing heart by the combined efforts of the medical and industrial communities. Although heart transplantation is the preferred choice for patients with end-stage cardiomyopathy, the supply of human donor hearts will continue to fall far short of the demand. With xenotransplantation not yet established as a safe and suitable solution for human use, there is a definite need for long-term mechanical circulatory support. As smaller and more durable cardiac-assist devices and total artificial hearts become available, and as the potential for thromboembolism and the need for percutaneous drive-lines decrease, the number of patients who will benefit from permanent circulatory support will increase considerably.

L. Frank Baum predicted this future in *The Wizard of Oz* when he wrote:

Wizard of Oz:
As for you, my galvanized friend—you want a heart!
You don't know how lucky you are not to have one.
Hearts will never be practical until they can be made unbreakable.

Tin Man:
  But I – I still want one.

REFERENCES

1. Mann DL, Willerson JT. Left ventricular assist devices and the failing heart. A bridge to recovery, a permanent assist device, or a bridge too far? [editorial]. Circulation 1998;98:2367–2369.
2. Rose EA, Gelijns AC, Moskowitz AJ, et al. Long term use of a left ventricular assist device for end-stage heart failure. N Engl J Med 2001;345:1435–1443.
3. Pae WE, Miller CA, Matthews Y, et al. Ventricular assist devices for postcardiotomy cardiogenic shock. J Thorac Cardiovasc Surg 1992;104:541–553.
4. Curtis JJ. Centrifugal mechanical assist for postcardiotomy ventricular failure. Semin Thorac Cardiovasc Surg 1994;6:140–141.
5. Curtis JJ, Boley TM, Walls JT, et al. Frequency of seal disruption with the Sarns centrifugal pump in postcardiotomy assist. Artif Organs 1994;18:235–237.
6. Noon GP, Ball JW, Papaconstantinou HT. Clinical experience with the BioMedicus centrifugal ventricular support in 172 patients. Artif Organs 1995;19:756–760.
7. Mehta SM, Aufiero TX, Pae WE, et al. Combined registry for the clinical use of mechanical ventricular assist pumps and the total artificial heart in conjuction with heart transplantation: sixth official report—1994. J Heart Lung Transplant 1995;14:585–593.
8. Joyce LD, Kaiser JC, Frasier L, et al. Experience with generally accepted centrifugal pumps. Ann Thorac Surg 1996;61:287–290.
9. Grossman DS, Levy N, Sears N (1999). Temporary ventricular assist using the ABIOMED system as a new option for cardiogenic shock due to myocardial infarction. Heart Failure Summit IV.
10. Chen JM, Spanier TB, Gonzalez JJ, et al. Improved survival in patients with acute myocarditis using external pulsatile mechanical ventricular assistance. J Heart Lung Transplant 1999;18:351–357.
11. Farrar DJ, Korfer R, E1-Banayosy A, et al. First clinical use of the Thoratec TLC-II Portable VAD Driver in ambulatory and patient discharge settings. ASAIO J 1998;44:35A.
12. Farrar DJ, Reichenbach SH, Rossi SA, et al. Development of intracorporeal Thoratec ventricular assist device for univentricular or biventricular support. ASAIO J 2000;46:351–353.
13. Hendry PJ, Masters RG, Mussivand TV, et al. Circulatory support for cardiogenic shock due to acute myocardial infarction: a Canadian experience. Can J Cardiol 1999;15:1090–1094.
14. Korfer R, El-Banayosy A, Arusoglu L, et al. Single center experience with the Thoratec ventricular assist device. J Thorac Cardiovasc Surg 2000;119:596–600.
15. Farrar DJ, Hill JD. Univentricular and biventricular Thoratec ventricular assist device support as bridge to transplantation. Ann Thorac Surg 1993;55:276–283.
16. Farrar DJ, Hill JD, Pennington DG, et al. Preoperative and postoperative postoperative comparison of patients with univentricular and biventricular support with the Thoratec ventricular assist device as a bridge to cardiac transplantation. J Thorac Cardiovasc Surg 1997;113:202–209.
17. Farrar DJ. The thoratec ventricular assist device: a paracorporeal pump for treating acute and chronic heart failure. Semin Thorac Cardiovasc Surg 2000;12(3):243–250.
18. Pasic M, Bergs S, Hennig E, et al. Simplified technique for implantation of a left ventricular assist system after previous cardiac operations. Ann Thorac Surg 1999;67:562–564.
19. Loebe M, Kaufmann F, Hetzer R. The Berlin Heart. In: Goldstein DJ, Oz MC, eds. Cardiac Assist Devices. Futura, Armonk, NY, 2000, pp. 275–287.
20. Rose EA, Levin HR, Oz MC, et al. Artificial circulatory support with textured interior surfaces: a counterintuitive approach to minimizing thromboembolism. Circulation 1994;90(Suppl II):II87–I191.
21. Argenziano DJ, Choudhri A, Moazami N, et al. Randomized, double-blind trial of inhaled nitric oxide in LVAD recipients with pulmonary hypertension. Ann Thorac Surg 1998;65:340–345.
22. Fukamachi K, McCarthy PM, Smedira NG, et al. Preoperative risk factors foe right ventricular failure after implantable left ventricular assist device insertion. Ann Thorac Surg 1999;68:2181–2184.
23. Oz MC, Goldstein DJ, Pepino P, et al. Screening scale predicts patients successfully receiving long term implantable left ventricular assist devices. Circulation 1995;92(Suppl II):II-169–II-173.
24. Holman WL, Skinner JL, Waites KB, et al. Infection during circulatory support with ventricular assist devices. Ann Thorac Surg 1999;68:711–716.
25. El-Banayosy A, Arusoglu L, Kizner L, et al. Novacor left ventricular assist system versus Heartmate vented electric left ventricular assist system as a long-term mechanical circulatory support device in bridging patients: a prospective study. J Thorac Cardiovasc Surg 2000;119:581–587.
26. Kormos RL, Ramasamy N, Sit S, et al. Bridge to transplant experience with the Novacor left ventricular assist system: results of a multicenter US study [abstract]. J Heart Lung Transplant 1999;18:163.

27. Portner PM, Jansen PGM, Oyer PE, et al. Improved outcomes with an implantable left ventriculat assist system: a multicenter study. Ann Thorac Surg 2001:71:205–209.

28. Hetzer R, Mueller JH, Weng YG, et al. Midterm follow-up of patients who underwent removal of a left ventricular assist device after cardiac recovery from end-stage dilated cardiomyopathy. J Thorac Cardiovasc Surg 2000;120:843–855.

29. Devries WC, Anderson JH, Joyce LD, et al. Clinical use of the total artificial heart. N Engl J Med 1984;310:273–278.

30. Arabia FA, Copeland JG, Smith RG, et al. Implantation technique for the CardioWest total artificial heart. Ann Thorac Surg 1999;68:698–704.

31. Copeland JG, Arabia FA, Banchy ME, et al. The CardioWest total artificial heart bridge to transplantation: 1993 to 1996 national trial. Ann Thorac Surg 1998;66:1662–1669.

32. Arabia FA, Copeland JG, Smith RG, et al. International experience transplantation. with the CardioWest total artificial heart as a bridge to heart transplantation. Eur J Cardiothorac Surg 1997;11(Suppl):S5–S10.

33. Sezai A, Shiono M, orime Y, et al. Renal and cellular metabolism during left ventricular assisted circulation: comparison study of pulsatile and nonpulsatile assists. Artif Organs 1997;21:830–835.

34. Tominga R, Smith WA, Massielo A, et al. Chronic nonpulsatile blood flow I. Cerebral autoregulation in chronic nonpulsatile biventricular bypass: carotid blood flow response to hypercapnia. J Thorac Cardiovasc Surg 1994;108:907–912.

35. Frazier OH, Myers TJ, Jarvik RK, et al. Research and development of an implantable, axial-flow left ventricular assist device: the Jarvik 2000 Heart. Ann Thorac Surg 2001;71:S125–S132.

36. Westaby S, Banning AP, Jarvik R, et al. First permanent implant of the Jarvik 2000 Heart. Lancet 2000;356:900–903.

37. Griffith BP, Kormos RL, Borovetz HS, et al. HeartMate II left ventricular assist system: from concept to first clinical use. Ann Thorac Surg 2001;71:S116–S120.

38. Noon GP, Morley DL, Irwin S, et al. Clinical experience with the MicroMed DeBakey ventricular assist device. Ann Thorac Surg 2001;71:S133–S138.

39. Mehta SM, Pae WE, Rosenberg G, et al. The LionHeart LVD-2000: a completely implanted left ventricular assist device for chronic circulatory support. Ann Thorac Surg 2001;71:S156–S161.

40. Hoenicke EM, Strange RG, Weiss WJ, et al. Modifications in surgical implantation of the Penn State Electric Total Artificial Heart. Ann Thorac Surg 2001;71:S150–S150.

41. Dowling RD, Etoch SW, Stevens KA, et al. Current status of the AbioCor implantable replacement heart. Ann Thorac Surg 2001;71:S147–S149.

42. Mussivand T, Hendry PJ, Masters RG, et al. Progress with the HeartSaver ventricular assist device. Ann Thorac Surg 1999;68:785–789.

43. Hall CW, Liotta D, Henly WS, et al. Development of artificial intrathoracic circulatory pumps. Am J Surg 1964;108:685–692.

21 Treatment of Cardiogenic Shock
Future Perspective

Jonathan Leor, MD,
Israel M. Barbash, MD,
Alexander Battler, MD,
and Robert A. Kloner, MD, PhD

CONTENTS

INTRODUCTION

During the past few years, powerful technological advancement in molecular and cellular biology has provided hope for the future treatment of irreversible myocardial damage. One of the most fascinating goals of myocardial infarction and heart-failure therapy is myocardial regeneration: molecular and cellular manipulation leading to regeneration of new contractile tissue to replace scar tissue. This myocardial regeneration strategy may improve viability and enhance contractility of the heart that has suffered a large infarction. Furthermore, it may be possible to apply this strategy to critically ill patients with cardiogenic shock who are dependent on a left ventricular assist device (LVAD).

The aim of this chapter is to review selected topics that cover recent developments and opportunities in the research of myocardial regeneration that may be relevant to survivors of cardiogenic shock. We shall focus on the potential of and obstacles to cell transplantation as a future therapy for myocardial regeneration. In addition, we shall critically outline tissue and genetic engineering as a prospective future strategy.

From: *Contemporary Cardiology: Cardiogenic Shock: Diagnosis and Treatment*
Edited by: David Hasdai et al. © Humana Press Inc., Totowa, NJ

THE LIMITATIONS OF CURRENT TREATMENT

Following myocardial infarction, the heart cannot regenerate because cardiac myocytes cannot replicate significantly after injury *(1)* and because no muscle stem cells exist in the myocardium. The inability of mature cardiac myocytes to undergo significant cell division, although questioned and debated *(2–5),* contributes to progressive damage following myocardial infarction. As a result, patients who suffer large myocardial infarctions have significantly compromised cardiac function.

Despite significant advances in management and outcome of patients with cardiogenic shock, the prognosis remains poor *(6–8),* with many patients not receiving appropriate treatment or receiving it too late *(9).* For those patients remaining in shock, mortality may be as high as 90% *(6–8).* Patients who survive the first days experience severe and irreversible myocardial damage. This damage is progressive and such patients are prone to develop left ventricular dilatation, infarct expansion, cardiac deterioration, advanced heart failure, and life-threatening arrhythmias. With the advance of interventional cardiology and revascularization strategies, the number of survivors from cardiogenic shock will increase and concomitantly the number of patients with heart failure will rise.

The problem of how to treat the thousands of patients per year worldwide who survive an extensive myocardial infarction and develop advanced heart failure despite optimal medical therapy has not been resolved. Failure to prevent morbidity associated with heart failure places an enormous burden on patients, their families, and community. Heart donor supply is declining, increasing the gap between supply and demand for heart replacement therapies *(10).* Left ventricular assist devices may provide a temporary therapeutic option for patients with pump failure, but, at best, they serve as only a bridge to transplantation and do not provide definitive therapy. As a result, there has been great interest in alternative therapeutic strategies to reverse this common and deadly disease.

Cell Transplantation

A possible strategy to restore heart function after myocardial injury is to replace the damaged with healthy tissue. Cell transplantation is a promising approach that offers the creation of new functional tissue to replace lost or failing myocardium *(11–13).* The implanted cells may have the potential for growth, self-repair, and remodeling. It has been hypothesized that embryonic cardiomyocyte transplantation could result in the formation of alternative cardiac tissue that could replace the scar tissue and improve cardiac function after extensive myocardial infarction (MI). This technology could also be used for the delivery of therapeutic recombinant proteins to the heart, thereby providing an alternative strategy for gene therapy *(12,13).*

In the past few years, cell transplantation biology has advanced considerably. Fetal myocytes *(14–18),* bone marrow cells *(19,20),* skeletal myocytes *(21–24),* and intraventricular septal cells *(25,26)* have all been transplanted into the hearts of animal models. Although embryonic cells may be the best candidates, they are not readily available for ethical reasons. Transplantation of other cell types has produced significant success, but this, too, has its limitations. It is encouraging to note that cells derived from mature animals appear to have broader differentiation potential than thought previously. The surprising ability of adult animal cells to develop into various types of tissue — a process that was once thought to be unique to embryonic stem cells — is already being reported for cells derived from bone marrow *(20,27–29)*, liver *(30)*, and mouse brain tissue *(31)*.

Cardiomyocyte Transplantation

In their breakthrough experiment, Soonpaa and associates *(14)* showed that fetal cardiomyocytes can be transplanted and integrated within the normal myocardium of mice. This group also reported on the formation of stable fetal cardiomyocyte grafts in the myocardium of dystrophic mice and dogs *(32)*. Other studies showed that fetal or neonatal cardiomyocytes can be engrafted into infarcted, cryoinjured, or cardiomyo-pathic hearts and survive *(15–18,33–35)*. Cell transplantation was associated with smaller infarcts *(34)* and improved heart function as assessed by echocardiography *(35,36)* or ex vivo hemodynamic studies on excised hearts *(33,37)*. The transplanted cells formed sarcomeres and junctions between each other *(17)*. In addition, the development of cardiac tissue was associated with increased angiogenesis *(34)*. However, several months after transplantation, the transplanted tissue decreased in size, probably secondary to rejection *(17,34)*.

The biology by which cardiomyocyte transplantation has improved heart function is unclear. Possible mechanisms include direct contribution of the transplanted myocytes to contractility, attenuation of infarct expansion by the elastic properties of transplanted cardiomyocytes, or angiogenesis induced by growth factors secreted from the embryonic cells resulting in improved collateral flow *(13)*.

Problems and Limitations: Despite encouraging results, the strategy of fetal or neonatal cardiomyocyte transplantation is limited, as fetal or neonatal cardiomyocytes have little growth potential in vitro and they are relatively sensitive to ischemic injury. In a few studies, the implanted cells kept their embryonic phenotype *(16,38)* and remained isolated from the host myocardium by scar tissue *(16,17,38)*. These islands of cells could be an electrophysiologic substrate for life-threatening arrhythmias. In addition, fetal cell transplantation creates an ethical dilemma and could be restricted by a donor shortage and immune rejection of the engrafted cells. Several alternative approaches have been developed to overcome these limitations.

Alternative Source of Cells

AUTOLOGOUS SKELETAL MYOBLASTS

Each mature skeletal myofiber bears a few satellite cells. These myogenic cells are activated following skeletal injury, enter the mitotic cycle, and fuse with each other and with injured myofibers, thereby restoring continuity and skeletal muscle function. Skeletal myoblasts have many desirable properties as donor cells, including the ability to be amplified in an undifferentiated state in vitro and to remain viable in ischemic tissue. Continued proliferation in vivo may be an advantage when engrafting into an injured heart, because the input of a smaller number of cells could give rise to a larger graft *(21,22,39)*. In addition, skeletal myoblasts are autologous cells, obviating the need for immune suppression. Several groups have investigated the hypothesis that following transplantation into the heart, satellite myogenic skeletal muscle cells might undergo transdifferentiation into functioning cardiac-like myocytes. This has been demonstrated during cardiomyoplasty, in which the skeletal muscle latissmus dorsi is preconditioned with repeated electrical stimulation and converts from fast to slow (cardiac-like) twitch fibers *(40)*. Promising recent data have shown that skeletal myoblasts engrafted into cryoinjured hearts have successfully seeded damaged tissue and formed nascent myotubes in rats, dogs, and rabbits *(21–24,41,42)*. The myotubes differentiated into mature myofibers and later converted to "cardiaclike" fibers *(22)*. The engrafted cells improved cardiac function in cryoinjured rabbit hearts when compared with nonengrafted controls *(20)*. In another study, skeletal myoblasts were as effective as fetal cardiomyocytes for improving postinfarction left ventricular function in a rat model of myocardial infarction *(42)*. Given our capacity to amplify primary myoblasts from humans, the potential use of skeletal grafts for treating heart disease has generated enthusiasm and hope as an alternative for heart transplantation.

Most recently, Menasche and colleagues *(43)* have reported, for the first time, the successful transplantation of autologous human skeletal myoblasts into the scar tissue of a patient with severe ischemic left ventricular (LV) dysfunction during coronary artery bypass grafting of remote myocardial areas. Five months later, the investigators identified contraction and viability in the grafted scar on echocardiography and positron emission tomography (PET). This encouraging observation requires validation by additional randomized controlled trials *(43)*.

Problems and Limitations: The use of autologous myogenic cells may be restricted by low recovery of satellite cells from muscle biopsies of elderly patients, resulting in difficulty in obtaining a reasonable number of cells. The ability of engrafted myoblasts to integrate within the host myocardium has been questioned and debated. Reinecke et al. *(44)* reported that cultured rat skeletal myoblasts expressed N-cadherin and connexin43, major adhesion and gap-junction proteins of the intercalated disk, yet both proteins were markedly downregulated after differentiation into mature myotubes. Also, differentiated skeletal muscle grafts in injured hearts had no detectable N-cadherin or connexin43; hence, electromechanical coupling is not likely to occur after in vivo grafting *(44)*. These findings have raised concern regarding the prospects of myoblast-based therapy in the repair of infarcted myocardium.

Transplantation of satellite cells that are able to proliferate in vivo has both advantages and disadvantages: excess proliferation may cause grafts to distort the ventricular wall and possibly impair contractility and relaxation. Thus, cardiac repair strategies may need to incorporate methods to control graft cell proliferation *(39)*.

Stem-Cell–Derived Myocytes

Stem cells are a unique population of cells characterized by their pluripotency (i.e., the ability to differentiate into multiple cell lineage). Basically, there are two potential sources for stem cells: embryonic-derived stem cells *(45)* and bone-marrow-derived mesenchymal stem cells *(46)*. Stem cells are unlimited in number because they have self-regenerating capacity and can be expanded in vitro. After expansion, these pluripotent cells can be directed to differentiate into cardiomyogenic lineage by various techniques *(47–49)*. For these reasons, stem-cell-based therapy for cardiac muscle regeneration has been under intense research and progress during the last decade.

Embryonic Stem Cells

Recently, Thomson et al. *(45)* succeeded in isolating embryonic stem cells from a 140-cell blastocyst of human embryo and established a stable cell line that was found to be totipotent. The major advantages, therefore, of embryonic stem cells are that they are totipotent (i.e., can differentiate into all three embryonic layers) and that these cells can be maintained and expanded in vitro without limitation.

The first study in which embryonic stem cells were used as a source for transplantation into the myocardium was performed by Klug et al. *(50)*. This group generated pure cultures of cardiomyogenic cells that were differentiated in vitro from murine embryonic stem cells by transfection with a vector, carrying both a cardiac myosin heavy-chain promotor and sequences encoding aminoglycoside phosphotransferase for selection of differentiated cells with G418. The differentiated cells developed myofibers and gap junctions between adjacent cells and showed synchronous contractile activity in vitro for a long period of time (up to 11 mo). The differentiated cells were transplanted into the myocardium of adult dystrophic mice and were shown to integrate and survive in the myocardium for 7 wk. This study proved, for the first time, the ability to direct an unlimited number of embryonic stem cells into cardiomyogenic cell lineage and to use them for myocardial regeneration. The breakthrough of establishing an embryonic stem cell line *(50)* has opened up new frontiers in the research for *in utero* cues that direct embryonic cells to differentiate into mature cardiomyocytes.

The finding that human embryonic stem-cell-derived cardiomyocytes displayed structural and functional properties of early-stage cardiomyocytes may enhance the prospects of cell therapy and tissue engineering for heart disease *(47)*.

Limitations and Problems: The use of embryonic stem cells does not overcome one of the major obstacles of using allogeneic cells (i.e., the need for immunosuppression). In addition, there is an ongoing controversy regarding the ethical justification of using human embryos for such purposes.

Mesenchymal Stem Cells

Another potential source for a cell reservoir is bone-marrow-derived mesenchymal stem cells *(46)*. The bone marrow contains cells that possess the properties of stem cells (i.e., pluripotency), in addition to blood-forming progenitors *(28,51)*. These cells are referred to as mesenchymal stem cells.

Mesenchymal stem cells are theoretically the ultimate cell source for cardiac muscle regeneration, as they are pluripotent and can be expanded in vitro *(52)*. Because they reside in the bone marrow of all patients they can be obtained by a bedside procedure of bone marrow aspiration, expanded in vitro with or without differentiation, and retransplanted to the patient, thus eliminating the need for immunosuppression *(20)*.

Makino et al. *(49)* treated murine mesenchymal stem cells with 5-azacytidine and, after repeated screening of spontaneously beating cells, isolated a cardiomyogenic cell line. 5-Azacytidine causes hypomethylation of specific genes and possibly activates the myogenic master gene *MyoD,* thus converting mesenchymal stem cells into myoblasts *(48,49)*. The authors verified the characteristics of the cardiomyogenic cell line with electron microscopy analysis and immunologic staining, directed at specific contractile proteins (e.g., myosin heavy chain). Despite these encouraging results, however, it is not clear whether this conversion technique is actually efficient and whether the long-term effects of 5-azacytidine treatment, known to have mitogenic properties, are recognized. Tomita and his colleagues *(19)* have shown that the transplantation of 5-azacytidine-treated mesenchymal stem cells into scar tissue has decreased the scar area, limited left ventricular dilatation, and increased regional angiogenesis, as compared to transplantation of mesenchymal stem cells not treated with 5-azacytidine or to culture medium only.

Most recently, Orlic et al. *(27)* reported, for the first time, that a subpopulation of bone marrow stem cells are capable of generating myocardium in vivo. They sorted lineage-negative bone marrow cells from transgenic mice, expressing enhanced green fluorescent protein by fluorescence-activated cell sorting on the basis of c-kit expression. Shortly after coronary ligation, cells were injected into the contracting wall bordering the infarct. They observed that newly formed myocardium occupied 68% of the infarcted portion of the ventricle 9 d after bone marrow cell transplantation. The developing tissue comprised proliferating myocytes and vascular structures. These findings provide a preliminary indication of the wide variety of possibilities in the use of mesenchymal stem cells in cardiac muscle regeneration *(28,29,51,53,54)*.

An additional remarkable property has now been added to the already impressive potential of stem cells: the power to help heal a damaged heart by inducing new capillary formation in the remaining viable myocardial tissue, thereby increasing survival and restoring heart function. Several studies imply that a specific subset of bone-marrow-derived angioblasts, expressing endothelial precursor markers, is responsible for neovascularization and angiogenesis *(55–58)*. Kocher et al. *(59)* demonstrated that an intravenous injection of human bone marrow donor cells to the infarcted myocardium of athymic rat recipients resulted in a significant increase in neovascularization of postinfarction myocardial tissue, attenuation of cardiomyocyte apoptosis, and LV remodeling. Building on previous observations that autologous bone-marrow-derived mesenchymal stem cells injected directly into the damaged rodent heart improved cardiac function *(19)*, the investigators confirmed the healing properties of a different subpopulation of human bone marrow cells that lack mesenchymal stem cell markers.

Limitations and Problems: Many issues still need to be clarified. The presence of stem cells in the heart itself has not yet been established. Several researchers *(27,28)* have reported finding stem cells for cardiomyocytes in other parts of the body, such as in bone marrow, but no such claim has yet won worldwide acceptance. The next critical step is to establish a method of inducing stem cell development into fully differentiated cardiomyocytes in large enough numbers for transplantation. Because of its mitogenic properties, 5-azacytidine treatment is unlikely to be applied in clinical practice. Finally, although the intravenous injection protocol of endothelial progenitor cells is a significant improvement over transthoracic delivery, obtaining adequate autologous cells from a myocardial infarction patient in time to prevent postinfarction remodeling may be difficult. Furthermore, the safety and efficacy of the intravenous administration of mesenchymal stem cells has been questioned *(60)*.

Therapeutic Cloning

Transfer of a somatic cell nucleus into a donor oocyte from which the nucleus has been removed could be used to clone mammalian species *(61)*. The oocyte containing the replaced nucleus carries the genetic information of the donor. This technique was used to clone Dolly the sheep *(62)*. Blastocysts can be developed in vitro from such manipulated oocytes, and embryonic stem cells that are genetically matched to the donor can be derived from the inner cell mass of the blastocysts—a procedure that takes several months.

Such a procedure for generating cardiac cells from embryonic stem cells could be developed (a supply of oocytes could be provided from fertility clinics) to produce an alternative approach for myocardial regeneration. Stem cells are isolated from the resulting clone and then differentiated in vitro into genetically matched cardiomyocytes for transplantation *(61)*. The major advantage of this cloning technology is, of course, that the embryonic stem cells would generate cardiomyocytes with a patient's own genetic information, thus avoiding allogeneic host-versus-graft reactions.

Limitations and Problems: Currently, the concept of therapeutic cloning is limited by ethical dilemma and regulatory restrictions. Therapeutic cloning has certain risks, such as the introduction of genetic mutations in vitro during cell expansion and differentiation. With advanced medicine and biological technology, this powerful technique might be approved for creating autologous cell replacement tissues for transplantation. In order to realize the full potential of therapeutic cloning, it is essential to understand how to reconstitute more complex tissue and organs in vitro *(61)*.

Tissue Engineering

Tissue engineering is a rapidly emerging interdisciplinary field that applies the principles and knowledge of biology, medicine, materials science, and engineering to the development of biocompatible substitutes for the restoration, maintenance, and improvement of human tissue functions *(63)*. Unlike blood or bone marrow tissues, which can be regenerated by intravenous injection of cells, regeneration of most anatomical tissues requires a template scaffolding. This scaffold temporarily provides the biomechanical structural characteristics for the seeded cells until they produce their own extracellular matrix, which ultimately provides the structural integrity and biomechanical profile for the replacement tissue.

The potential additional advantage of this tissue engineering over the isolated cell transplantation approach is improved control of the tissue formation process, of the graft shape and size, and of the ability to determine the consistency of the graft (e.g., number of cardiomyocytes to the ratio of other cells) *(64)*.

Recent advances in methods of cardiomyocyte isolation and three-dimensional culture *(64–68)* show promise and will contribute to cardiac tissue engineering in vitro. Most recently, we reported *(69)* on the successful seeding of fetal cardiomyocytes into scaffolds composed of alginate sponges. Following implantation of the cellular constructs into the infarcted myocardium of rat, some of the cells appeared to differentiate into mature myocardial fibers. The implanted grafts were supplied by intensive neovascularization. The biografts prevented LV dilatation and deterioration of heart function after infarction.

The mechanism behind this beneficial effect was unclear. A direct contribution of the biograft to contractility is unlikely because only a relatively small fraction of the biograft was composed of myocardial tissue. Attenuation of infarct expansion by virtue of the elastic properties of bioartificial grafts is possible. Restraining the expansion of the left ventricle by a mesh placed over the infarcted myocardium preserves LV geometry and resting function in a sheep model of myocardial infarction. Angiogenesis induced by growth factors secreted from the embryonic cells, resulting in improved collateral flow and augmentation of contractility, is also a possible mechanism. Finally, a nonspecific immune response against the implanted biograft followed by cytokine release could enhance scar formation and cardiac function.

The success of these pioneering experiments provides potential methods for tissue engineering into myocardial infarction. The bioengineered tissue could be used for local gene delivery *(69)* and surgical repair of the infarcted myocardium or of congenital cardiac defects.

Limitations and Problems: For tissue engineering technology to be effective in humans, however, it is critical that the number of myofibers in the graft increase and that the cells differentiate and organize in a systemic manner,

THE FUTURE

Rejuvenated Cells

The inability of mature cardiac myocytes to undergo significant cell division, although questioned and debated *(2–5)*, contributes to progressive damage following myocardial infarction. An alternative approach to increase the number of viable myocytes is to control the cell-cycle regulatory molecules *(70,71)*. Terminal differentiation of cardiac myocytes occurs at or shortly after birth in most mammals and is characterized by transition from hyperplastic growth (cell division) to hypertrophic growth (an increase in cell size) *(72)*. Therefore, the ability to control the growth of cardiac myocytes in the myocardium may result in reinitiating DNA synthesis and cell division, thus controlling the repair of damaged myocardium.

The mechanism of cell-cycle withdrawal in cardiomyocytes is complicated and poorly understood. In general, the cell cycle is controlled at various cell-cycle checkpoints by cyclins, cyclin-dependent kinases (cdks), and cdk inhibitors *(70,71,73,74)*. In cardiomyocytes, however, the regulation of the cell-cycle process is not well characterized. Several groups have shown that overexpression of cell-cycle regulators induces DNA synthesis in cardiomyocytes *(75–78)*. Transgenic models expressing high levels of c-*myc* mRNA resulted in a two-fold increase in the number of cardiomyocytes in the fetus *(79,80)*. Furthermore, Soonpaa et al. *(81)* reported that over-expression of cyclin D1 promotes cardiomyocyte DNA synthesis and multinucleation. These studies indicate that altered levels of cell-cycle regulators can increase DNA synthesis and possibly increase cardiomyocyte numbers. This strategy might be applied both in vitro and in vivo.

Limitations and Problems: Uncontrolled proliferation of cardiomyocytes can lead to tumor formation that will deform the left ventricular geometry and lead to arrhythmias, conduction defects, pump dysfunction, and death. Thus, the success of this strategy depends on tight control of cell proliferation.

Genetic Engineering

Gene therapy offers new therapeutic options for the infarcted myocardium *(13)*. The ability to introduce recombinant transgenes that encode therapeutic proteins into the infarcted myocardium may stimulate new vessel formation, accelerate healing, and enhance myocardial performance. One of the most fascinating goals in the field of gene therapy for myocardial infarction and heart failure is genetic modulation *in situ* or ex vivo, leading to regeneration of new contractile tissue. One possible approach to muscle regeneration is to convert fibroblasts in the healing heart lesions to muscle cells. At present, there is insufficient knowledge regarding cardiac muscle determination and differentiation to induce cells to form myocardium. In skeletal muscle, however, the muscle-specific *MyoD* family of transcription factors is able to prompt the skeletal muscle differentiation program in a variety of cells including fibroblasts *(82–84)*. The efficiency of this process is directly related to the lineage relationship with myoblasts and is highest in fibroblasts *(82–84)*. Transformation of cardiac fibroblasts in scar tissue of a myocardial infarction into skeletal myocytes could add to myocardial contractility.

Murry et al. *(83)* reported successful *in situ* transduction with *MyoD* gene transfer using a rat model of myocardial cryoinjury. One week after cryoinjury, they injected adenovirus encoding the *MyoD* gene into myocardial granulation tissue. Rats were treated with cyclosporine to suppress the adenoviral immune response. One week after gene transfer, cells that expressed both myogenin and embryonic skeletal myosin heavy chain were identified. In several hearts, they observed structures resembling multinucleated myotubes.

Most recently, Lattanzi et al. *(82)* showed that an adenoviral vector expressing *MyoD* can induce massive myogenic conversion of human and murine primary fibroblasts in culture. Primary human fibroblasts were expanded in culture, converted to myogenesis by adeno-delivered *MyoD,* and injected into regenerating muscles of severe combined immunodeficiency/beige (scid/bg) recipient mice, where they formed apparently normal fibers at an efficiency comparable to that of myogenic satellite cells. The use of genetically modified autologous myogenic cells should avoid most of the immunological problems associated with the allogeneic approach and also offer an abundant resource for cell transplantation. If these promising results in a model of muscular disease can be replicated in a model of myocardial infarction and heart failure, it may prove a feasible alternative for cell transplantation and ex vivo gene therapy.

Limitations and Problems. One of the most important difficulties in in vivo gene therapy is the low transfection efficiency and immune reaction in target tissue *(85,86)*. Both efficiency and safety need to be improved with the development of better gene-delivery methods and expression vectors. Genetic engineering has certain risks, such as the introduction of genetic mutations. Major chromosomal abnormalities and other somatic mutations could remain silent within the genome until after the time of transplantation, possibly leading to abnormal cell growth and differentiation and to the development of cancer. Further development in gene therapy vectors is needed to improve safety, immunological tolerance, and expression of the transgene before this strategy can be applied in the clinical practice.

Molecular Myoplasty

Heart failure is an attractive candidate for gene therapy, as several targets have been identified as either functionally impaired or defective *(87)*. Studies using animal models and failing human hearts have identified several abnormalities that affect excitation–contraction coupling *(88,89)*. In particular, changes at the level of sarcolemmal/sarcoplasmic reticulum Ca^{2+} transport and contractile proteins are thought to contribute to depressed contractile function. Cardiomyocytes from failing animal and human hearts reveal abnormal Ca^{2+} homeostasis, such as reduced sarcoplasmic reticulum (SR) Ca^{2+} release, elevated diastolic Ca^{2+}, and reduced rate of Ca^{2+} removal *(87)*. There is strong evidence that reduced expression or activity of the SR Ca^{2+} ATPase (SERCA) and increased expression of Na^+–Ca^{2+} exchanger are key changes contributing to alterations in calcium homeostasis in the failing heart *(87–89)*. Abnormalities in calcium cycling may be responsible for attenuating the frequency potentiation of contractile force in the failing human heart *(87–89)*. SR Ca^{2+} ATPase plays a dominant role in removing cytosolic Ca^{2+} and is the main mechanism for restoring SR Ca^{2+} load. Therefore, a possible strategy to improve systolic and diastolic function of the failing heart may be stimulation of SR Ca^{2+} ATPase activity either by increasing pump expression or inhibiting phospholamban interaction, a modulator of SR pump function. This should increase SR Ca^{2+} transport and SR Ca^{2+} load (89).

Xenotransplantation

Porcine cells have been suggested as a virtually unlimited supply of cells for transplantation (90). However, two major hurdles remain before xenotransplantation can enter the clinic (91). The first is the technical issue of being able to overcome the human immune response that leads to rejection of transplanted organs/cells from other species. The second concerns the potential risk of inadvertent transfer of animal viruses present in the xenotransplant capable of infecting the human recipient (92). The threat from viruses is a particularly contentious topic because it poses a risk not only to those individuals who receive xenotransplants but also to healthy individuals who come into contact, either directly or indirectly, with the xenotransplant recipient. Until these serious problems have been resolved, xenotransplantation will remain an academic approach.

TIMING AND MODE OF DELIVERY

The optimal time for cell delivery is uncertain. A patient in cardiogenic shock dependent on LVAD requires prompt treatment. In a mouse model of myocardial infarction (27), mesenchymal stem cell injection into the border of the infarcted myocardium several hours after coronary occlusion resulted in enhanced healing and heart function within 9 d. If these exciting results could be reproduced in a clinical setting, they would provide an efficient tool for self-healing of the human heart.

However, the relevance of these experimental conditions to humans is difficult to assess. Previous reports have indicated that several hours of acute ischemia would induce a cascade of proteolytic enzyme activation and inflammation leading to tissue destruction and possibly death of the engrafted cells (93,94). Furthermore, the production and preparation of autologous cells for transplantation may take several weeks or even months. Obtaining sufficient autologous cells from a patient in time to prevent postinfarction remodeling could be difficult. The solution, therefore, for the majority of patients in urgent need of cell transplantation, may stem from a reservoir of donor cells or tissue. This approach, however, would require immunosupression. For stable patients supported by LVAD, adequate time exists to produce and amplify autologous mesenchymal stem or satellite cells. It is possible that in the distant future, with the advancement of therapeutic cloning and tissue engineering techniques, each patient will have a bank of autologous stem cells and tissue ready for transplantation to replace damaged organs.

The cells could be delivered via intramyocardial injection during coronary artery bypass grafting (CABG) or by using a catheter-based transendocardial injection system. Left ventricular electromechanical mapping could be used to distinguish among infarcted, ischemic, and normal myocardium (95). Biografts or artificial tissue would need open heart surgery and could be implanted during CABG. Although the protocol of stem cell intravenous injection is a significant improvement over transthoracic delivery, it is not yet clear whether cytokine activation of a patient's bone marrow cells alone would be enough or whether concentration of endothelial precursors ex vivo will be a necessary intermediary step.

SUMMARY AND IMPLICATIONS

During the last few years, we have witnessed incredible progress and achievements in experimental strategies for myocardial regeneration, particularly in cell transplantation. These innovations hold promise for treating or preventing end-stage heart failure.

For patients in refractory shock complicating acute MI, various LVADs are now available and may provide an effective bridging option. In light of the success with LVAD bridge therapy for transplantation in patients with chronic heart failure, improved survival could be achieved in patients with MI in cardiogenic shock with LVAD bridge therapy to recovery or transplantation (96).

The concept of cellular cardiomyoplasty and tissue repair after myocardial injury promises a revolutionary approach for myocardial regeneration. These strategies still face significant difficulties before they can develop into clinically therapeutic tools.

A major barrier for cell transplantation is generation of a sufficient number of suitable cells. Strategies aimed at limiting the process of cell necrosis or apoptosis would need to be developed (12,93). Other issues that warrant further, in-depth investigation are cell integration and function, and the development of methodologies to control donor cell growth and differentiation. By enhancing the proliferative capacity of the donor cells, we might obtain larger grafts (12).

Tissue engineering offers the possibility of organizing cells into three-dimensional myocardial "patches" that could be used to repair the damaged portions of the heart. Creating more complex vital organs, such as the entire heart, is a much greater challenge, requiring the assembly of different cell types and materials in great combinations and complexity. Our knowledge of the molecular pathways of tissue growth and differentiation are limited, and we still have a long way to go before we can understand and control the process well enough to channel in vitro differentiation of human embryonic stem cells into all the various cell replacement types.

Where the clinical applications of these exciting investigations will lead remains to be demonstrated, but the research potential is enormous. Myocardial regeneration and tissue repair are now in sight and, if successful, will have a dramatic impact on the practice of cardiovascular medicine, becoming increasingly important as the number of heart-failure patients increases.

ACKNOWLEDGMENTS

This work was supported by grant Nos. 95-00294/1 and 98-414 from the United States–Israel Binational Science Foundation and a grant from the Israel Science Foundation.

Dr. Kloner is supported by a grant from the National Heart, Lung and Blood Institute (HL 61488).

REFERENCES

1. Soonpaa MH, Field LJ. Assessment of cardiomyocyte DNA synthesis in normal and injured adult mouse hearts. Am J Physiol 1997;272:H220–H226.
2. Beltrami AP, Urbanek K, Kajstura J, et al. Evidence that human cardiac myocytes divide after myocardial infarction. N Engl J Med 2001;344:1750–1757.
3. Rosenthal N. High hopes for the heart. N Engl J Med 2001;344:1785–1787.
4. Kajstura J, Leri A, Finato N, Di Loreto C, Beltrami CA, Anversa P. Myocyte proliferation in end-stage cardiac failure in humans. Proc Natl Acad Sci USA 1998;95:8801–8805.

5. Anversa P, Kajstura J. Ventricular myocytes are not terminally differentiated in the adult mammalian heart. Circ Res 1998;83:1–14.

6. Barbash IM, Ilia R, Gilutz H, Boyko V, Battler A, Leor J. Cardiogenic shock: single center experience with and without on-site catheterization facilities. Cardiology 2000;93:87–92.

7. Goldberg RJ, Samad NA, Yarzebski J, Gurwitz J, Bigelow C, Gore JM. Temporal trends in cardiogenic shock complicating acute myocardial infarction. N Engl J Med 1999;340:1162–1168.

8. Menon V, Hochman JS, Stebbins A, et al. Lack of progress incardiogenic shock: lessons from the GUSTO trials. Eur Heart J 2000;21:1928–1936.

9. Barbash IM, Behar S, Battler A, et al. Management and outcome of cardiogenic shock complicating acute myocardial infarction in hospitals with and without on-site catheterization facilities. Heart 2001;86:145–149

10. Hosenpud JD, Bennett LE, Keck BM, Fiol B, Boucek MM, Novick RJ. The Registry of the International Society for Heart and Lung Transplantation: sixteenth official report—1999. J Heart Lung Transplant 1999;18:611–626.

11. Kessler PD, Byrne BJ. Myoblast cell grafting into heart muscle: cellular biology and potential applications. Annu Rev Physiol 1999;61:219–242.

12. Reinlib L, Field L. Cell transplantation as future therapy for cardiovascular disease? A workshop of the National Heart, Lung, and Blood Institute. Circulation 2000;101:E182–E187.

13. Leor J, Prentice H, Sartorelli V, et al. Gene transfer and cell transplant: an experimental approach to repair a "broken heart." Cardiovasc Res 1997;35:431–441.

14. Soonpaa MH, Koh GY, Klug MG, Field LJ. Formation of nascent intercalated disks between grafted fetal cardiomyocytes and host myocardium. Science 1994;264:98–101.

15. Scorsin M, Marotte F, Sabri A, et al. Can grafted cardiomyocytes colonize peri-infarct myocardial areas? Circulation 1996;94(Suppl II):II-337–II-340.

16. Leor J, Patterson M, Quinones MJ, Kedes LH, Kloner RA. Transplantation of fetal myocardial tissue into the infarcted myocardium of rat. A potential method for repair of infarcted myocardium? Circulation 1996;94(Suppl II):II-332–II-336.

17. Reinecke H, Zhang M, Bartosek T, Murry CE. Survival, integration, and differentiation of cardiomyocyte grafts: a study in normal and injured rat hearts [In Process Citation]. Circulation 1999;100:193–202.

18. Li RK, Mickle DA, Weisel RD, Zhang J, Mohabeer MK. In vivo survival and function of transplanted rat cardiomyocytes. Circ Res 1996;78:283–288.

19. Tomita S, Li RK, Weisel RD, et al. Autologous transplantation of bone marrow cells improves damaged heart function. Circulation 1999;100(Suppl II):II-247–II-256.

20. Wang JS, Shum-Tim D, Galipeau J, Chedrawy E, Eliopoulos N, Chiu RC. Marrow stromal cells for cellular cardiomyoplasty: feasibility and potential clinical advantages. J Thorac Cardiovasc Surg 2000;120:999–1005.

21. Chiu RC. Card cell transplantation: the autologous skeletal myoblast implantation for myocardial regeneration. Adv Cardiac Surg 1999;11:69–98.

22. Murry CE, Wiseman RW, Schwartz SM, Hauschka SD. Skeletal myoblast transplantation for repair of myocardial necrosis. J Clin Invest 1996;98:2512–2523.

23. Pouzet B, Vilquin JT, Hagege AA, et al. Intramyocardial transplantation of autologous myoblasts: can tissue processing be optimized? Circulation 2000;102(Suppl III):III-210–III-2105.

24. Taylor DA, Atkins BZ, Hungspreugs P, et al. Regenerating functional myocardium: improved performance after skeletal myoblast transplantation [published erratum appears in Nature Med 1998;4(10):1200]. Nature Med 1998;4:929–933.

25. Li RK, Weisel RD, Mickle DA, et al. Autologous porcine heart cell transplantation improved heart function after a myocardial infarction. J Thorac Cardiovasc Surg 2000;119:62–68.

26. Sakai T, Li RK, Weisel RD, et al. Autologous heart cell transplantation improves cardiac function after myocardial injury. Ann Thorac Surg 1999;68:2074–2080; discussion 2080–2081.

27. Orlic D, Kajstura J, Chimenti S, et al. Bone marrow cells regenerate infarcted myocardium. Nature 2001;410:701–705.

28. Liechty KW, MacKenzie TC, Shaaban AF, et al. Human mesenchymal stem cells engraft and demonstrate site-specific differentiation after in utero transplantation in sheep. Nat Med 2000;6:1282–1286.

29. Jackson KA, Majka SM, Wang H, et al. Regeneration of ischemic cardiac muscle and vascular endothelium by adult stem cells. J Clin Invest 2001;107:1395–1402.

30. Malouf NN, Coleman WB, Grisham JW, et al. Adult-derived stem cells from the liver become myocytes in the heart in vivo. Am J Pathol 2001;158:1929–1935.

31. Clarke DL, Johansson CB, Wilbertz J, et al. Generalized potential of adult neural stem cells. Science 2000;288:1660–1663.

32. Koh GY, Soonpaa MH, Klug MG, et al. Stable fetal cardiomyocyte grafts in the hearts of dystrophic mice and dogs. J Clin Invest 1995;96:2034–2042.

33. Li RK, Jia ZQ, Weisel RD, et al. Cardiomyocyte transplantation improves heart function. Ann Thorac Surg 1996;62:654–660; discussion 660–661.

34. Li RK, Mickle DA, Weisel RD, et al. Natural history of fetal rat cardiomyocytes transplanted into adult rat myocardial scar tissue. Circulation 1997;96:II-179–II-186; discussion 186–187.

35. Scorsin M, Hagege AA, Marotte F, et al. Does transplantation of cardiomyocytes improve function of infarcted myocardium? Circulation 1997;96:II-188–II-193.

36. Scorsin M, Hagege AA, Dolizy I, et al. Can cellular transplantation improve function in doxorubicin-induced heart failure? Circulation 1998;98:II-151–II-155; discussion II-155–II-156.

37. Sakai T, Li RK, Weisel RD, et al. Fetal cell transplantation: a comparison of three cell types. J Thorac Cardiovasc Surg 1999;118:715–724.

38. Etzion S, Barbash IM, et al. Influence of embryonic cardiomyocyte transplantation on the progression of heart failure in a rat model of extensive myocardial infarction. J Mol Cell Cardiol 2001;33:1321–1320.

39. Reinecke H, Murry CE. Transmural replacement of myocardium after skeletal myoblast grafting into the heart. Too much of a good thing? Cardiovasc Pathol 2000;9:337–344.

40. Hooper TL, Stephenson LW. Cardiomyoplasty for end-stage heart failure. Surg Annu 1993;25:157–173.

41. Robinson SW, Cho PW, Levitsky HI, et al. Arterial delivery of genetically labelled skeletal myoblasts to the murine heart: long-term survival and phenotypic modification of implanted myoblasts. Cell Transplant 1996;5:77–91.

42. Scorsin M, Hagege A, Vilquin JT, et al. Comparison of the effects of fetal cardiomyocyte and skeletal myoblast transplantation on postinfarction left ventricular function. J Thorac Cardiovasc Surg 2000;119:1169–1175.

43. Menasche P, Hagege AA, Scorsin M, et al. Myoblast transplantation for heart failure. Lancet 2001;357:279–280.

44. Reinecke H, MacDonald GH, Hauschka SD, Murry CE. Electromechanical coupling between skeletal and cardiac muscle. Implications for infarct repair. J Cell Biol 2000;149:731–740.

45. Thomson JA, Itskovitz-Eldor J, Shapiro SS, et al. Embryonic stem cell lines derived from human blastocysts. Science 1998;282:1145–1147.

46. Bianco P, Gehron Robey P. Marrow stromal stem cells. J Clin Invest 2000;105:1663–1668.

47. Kahat I, Kenyagin-Karsenti D, Druckmann M, et al. Human embryonic stem cells can differentiate into myocytes portraying cardiomycytic structural and functional properties. J Clin Invest 2001;108:407–414.

48. Wakitani S, Saito T, Caplan AI. Myogenic cells derived from rat bone marrow mesenchymal stem cells exposed to 5-azacytidine. Muscle Nerve 1995;18:1417–1426.

49. Makino S, Fukuda K, Miyoshi S, et al. Cardiomyocytes can be generated from marrow stromal cells in vitro. J Clin Invest 1999;103:697–705.

50. Klug MG, Soonpaa MH, Koh GY, Field LJ. Genetically selected cardiomyocytes from differentiating embronic stem cells form stable intracardiac grafts. J Clin Invest 1996;98:216–224.

51. Pittenger MF, Mackay AM, Beck SC, et al. Multilineage potential of adult human mesenchymal stem cells. Science 1999;284:143–147.

52. Cossu G, Mavilio F. Myogenic stem cells for the therapy of primary myopathies: wishful thinking or therapeutic perspective? J Clin Invest 2000;105:1669–1674.

53. Sussman M. Cardiovascular biology: Hearts and bones. Nature 2001;410:640–641.

54. Springer ML, Brazelton TR, Blau HM. Not the usual suspects: the unexpected sources of tissue regeneration. J Clin Invest 2001;107:1355–1356.

55. Asahara T, Murohara T, Sullivan A, et al. Isolation of putative progenitor endothelial cells for angiogenesis. Science 1997;275:964–967.

56. Takahashi T, Kalka C, Masuda H, et al. Ischemia- and cytokine-induced mobilization of bone marrow-derived endothelial progenitor cells for neovascularization. Nature Med 1999;5:434–8.

57. Shintani S, Murohara T, Ikeda H, et al. Augmentation of postnatal neovascularization with autologous bone marrow transplantation. Circulation 2001;103:897–903.

58. Kawamoto A, Gwon HC, Iwaguro H, et al. Therapeutic potential of ex vivo expanded endothelial progenitor cells for myocardial ischemia. Circulation 2001;103:634–637.

59. Kocher AA, Schuster MD, Szabolcs MJ, et al. Neovascularization of ischemic myocardium by human bone-marrow-derived angioblasts prevents cardiomyocyte apoptosis, reduces remodeling and improves cardiac function. Nature Med 2001;7:430–436.

60. Gao J, Dennis JE, Muzic RF, Lundberg M, Caplan AI. The dynamic in vivo distribution of bone marrow-derived mesenchymal stem cells after infusion. Cells Tissues Organs 2001;169:12–20.

61. Lanza RP, Cibelli JB, West MD. Prospects for the use of nuclear transfer in human transplantation. Nature Biotechnol 1999;17:1171–1174.

62. Wilmut I, Schnieke AE, McWhir J, Kind AJ, Campbell KH. Viable offspring derived from fetal and adult mammalian cells. Nature 1997;385:810–813.

63. Vacanti JP, Langer R. Tissue engineering: the design and fabrication of living replacement devices for surgical reconstruction and transplantation. Lancet 1999;354(Suppl 1):SI32–SI34.

64. Papadaki M, Bursac N, Langer R, Merok J, Vunjak-Novakovic G, Freed LE. Tissue engineering of functional cardiac muscle: molecular, structural, and electrophysiological studies. Am J Physiol (Heart Circ Physiol) 2001;280:H168–H178.

65. Leor J, Aboulafia-Etzion S, Dar A, et al. Bioengineered cardiac grafts: a new approach to repair the infarcted myocardium? Circulation 2000;102:III56–III61.

66. Akins RE, Boyce RA, Madonna ML, et al. Cardiac organogenesis in vitro: reestablishment of three-dimensional tissue architecture by dissociated neonatal rat ventricular cells. Tissue Eng 1999;5:103–118.

67. Bursac N, Papadaki M, Cohen RJ, et al. Cardiac muscle tissue engineering: toward an in vitro model for electrophysiological studies. Am J Physiol 1999;277:H433–H444.

68. Carrier RL, Papadaki M, Rupnick M, et al. Cardiac tissue engineering: cell seeding, cultivation parameters, and tissue construct characterization. Biotechnol Bioeng 1999;64:580–589.

69. Bonadio J, Smiley E, Patil P, Goldstein S. Localized, direct plasmid gene delivery in vivo: prolonged therapy results in reproducible tissue regeneration [see comments]. Nature Med 1999;5:753–759.

70. Li JM, Brooks G. Cell cycle regulatory molecules (cyclins, cyclin-dependent kinases and cyclin-dependent kinase inhibitors) and the cardiovascular system; potential targets for therapy? Eur Heart J 1999;20:406–420.

71. Williams RS. Cell cycle control in the terminally differentiated myocyte. A platform for myocardial repair? Cardiol Clin 1998;16:739–754.

72. Soonpaa MH, Field LJ. Survey of studies examining mammalian cardiomyocyte DNA synthesis. Circ Res 1998;83:15–26.

73. MacLellan WR, Schneider MD. Genetic dissection of cardiac growth control pathways. Annu Rev Physiol 2000;62:289–319.

74. Schneider MD. Myocardial infarction as a problem of growth control: cell cycle therapy for cardiac myocytes? J Cardiac Failure 1996;2:259–63.

75. Liu Y, Kitsis RN. Induction of DNA synthesis and apoptosis in cardiac myocytes by E1A oncoprotein. J Cell Biol 1996;133:325–334.

76. Kirshenbaum LA, Schneider MD. Adenovirus E1A represses cardiac gene transcription and reactivates DNA synthesis in ventricular myocytes, via alternative pocket protein- and p300-binding domains. J Biol Chem 1995;270:7791–7794.

77. Kirshenbaum LA, Abdellatif M, Chakraborty S, Schneider MD. Human E2F-1 reactivates cell cycle progression in ventricular myocytes and represses cardiac gene transcription. Dev Biol 1996;179:402–411.

78. Agah R, Kirshenbaum LA, Abdellatif M, et al. Adenoviral delivery of E2F-1 directs cell cycle reentry and p53-independent apoptosis in postmitotic adult myocardium in vivo. J Clin Invest 1997;100:2722–2728.

79. Jackson T, Allard MF, Sreenan CM, Doss LK, Bishop SP, Swain JL. Transgenic animals as a tool for studying the effect of the c-myc proto-oncogene on cardiac development. Mol Cell Biochem 1991;104:15–19.

80. Jackson T, Allard MF, Sreenan CM, Doss LK, Bishop SP, Swain JL. The c-myc proto-oncogene regulates cardiac development in transgenic mice. Mol Cell Biol 1990;10:3709–3716.

81. Soonpaa MH, Koh GY, Pajak L, et al. Cyclin D1 overexpression promotes cardiomyocyte DNA synthesis and multinucleation in transgenic mice. J Clin Invest 1997;99:2644–2654.

82. Lattanzi L, Salvatori G, Coletta M, et al. High efficiency myogenic conversion of human fibroblasts by adenoviral vector-mediated MyoD gene transfer. An alternative strategy for ex vivo gene therapy of primary myopathies. J Clin Invest 1998;101:2119–2128.

83. Murry CE, Kay MA, Bartosek T, Hauschka SD, Schwartz SM. Muscle differentiation during repair of myocardial necrosis in rats via gene transfer with MyoD. J Clin Invest 1996;98:2209–2217.

84. Tam SK, Gu W, Nadal-Ginard B. Molecular cardiomyoplasty: potential cardiac gene therapy for chronic heart failure. J Thorac Cardiovasc Surg 1995;109:918–923; discussion 923–924.

85. Quinones MJ, Leor J, Kloner RA, et al. Avoidance of immune response prolongs expression of genes delivered to the adult rat myocardium by replication-defective adenovirus. Circulation 1996;94:1394–1401.

86. Etzion S, Barbash IM, Granot Y, et al. Gene-delivery to the infarcted myocardium with ex-vivo modified cardiomyoblasts is superior to direct adenovirus-mediated gene transfer. CVR 2001, in press.

87. Houser SR, Piacentino V, III, Weisser J. Abnormalities of calcium cycling in the hypertrophied and failing heart. J Mol Cell Cardiol 2000;32:1595–1607.

88. Houser SR, Lakatta EG. Function of the cardiac myocyte in the conundrum of end-stage, dilated human heart failure. Circulation 1999;99:600–604.

89. Hajjar RJ, del Monte F, Matsui T, Rosenzweig A. Prospects for gene therapy for heart failure. Circ Res 2000;86:616–621.

90. Cooper DK, Keogh AM. The potential role of xenotransplantation in treating endstage cardiac disease: a summary of the report of the Xenotransplantation Advisory Committee of the International Society for Heart and Lung Transplantation. Curr Opin Cardiol 2001;16:105–109.

91. Lanza RP, Kuhtreiber WM. Xenotransplantation and cell therapy: progress and controversy. IBC's 4th International Conference on Xenotransplantation and Cell Therapy. Boston, MA, USA, 10–11 December 1998. Mol Med Today 1999;5:105–106.

92. Gunzburg WH, Salmons B. Xenotransplantation: is the risk of viral infection as great as we thought? Mol Med Today 2000;6:199–208.

93. Zhang M, Methot DV, Fujio Y, Walsh K, Murry CE. Cardiomyocyte grafting for cardiac repair: graft cell death and anti-death strategies. J Mol Cell Cardiol 2001;33:907–921.

94. Varda-Bloom N, Leor J, Ohad DG, et al. Cytotoxic T lymphocytes are activated following myocardial infarction and can recognize and kill healthy myocytes in vitro. J Mol Cell Cardiol 2000;32:2141–2149.

95. Vale PR, Losordo DW, Milliken CE, et al. Left ventricular electromechanical mapping to assess efficacy of ph VEGF(165) gene transfer for therapeutic angiogenesis in chronic myocardial ischemia. Circulation 2000;102:965–974.

96. Park SJ, Nguyen DQ, Bank AJ, Ormaza S, Bolman RM, III. Left ventricular assist device bridge therapy for acute myocardial infarction. Ann Thorac Surg 2000;69:1146–1151.

Index